Cardiac Arrhythmias

PRACTICAL ECG INTERPRETATION

Cardiac Arrhythmias
PRACTICAL ECG INTERPRETATION

Stelio Mangiola, M.D.

Clinical Assistant Professor of Medicine, College of Medicine and Dentistry of New Jersey, Rutgers Medical School. Director, Cardiac Care Unit, Morristown Memorial Hospital, Morristown, New Jersey.

Michael C. Ritota, M.D.

Chairman, Department of Medicine, and Director, Coronary Care Unit, Columbus Hospital, Newark, New Jersey.

J. B. Lippincott Company

Philadelphia/Toronto

Library of Congress Catalog Card Number 73-15699

ISBN 0-397-50323-7

Printed in the United States of America

1   3   5   4   2

Library of Congress Cataloging in Publication Data

Mangiola, Stelio.
    Cardiac arrhythmias.

    Bibliography: p.
    1. Arrhythmia. 2. Electrocardiography.
I. Ritota, Michael C. joint author.
II. Title. [DNLM: 1. Arrhythmia. 2. Electro-
cardiography. WG330 M277c 1973]
RC685.A65M36   616.1′28′0754   73-15699
ISBN 0-397-50323-7

Preface

This book is intended to be a practical and amply illustrated guide for the rapid identification of cardiac rhythm disturbances seen on the conventional electrocardiogram.

Emphasis is placed on the criteria for the analysis of atrial deflections, A-V conduction, and ventricular deflections. The criteria are listed in easy outline form and are illustrated by full-size tracings and diagrams. Portions of the tracings are labeled for prompt identification of the ECG waves. Lewis ladder diagrams give an immediate understanding of the site of impulse formation and of the electrophysiological mechanisms involved. Brief clinical notes provide basic information on etiology, symptomatology and treatment.

The first section of the book is devoted to the ECG interpretation of sinus rhythms and of abnormal cardiac rhythms. For each cardiac rhythm, the outline of the electrocardiographic criteria and several tracings illustrating these criteria are arranged on facing pages so that they can be seen simultaneously. A representative tracing with Lewis ladder diagram and magnified detail is shown above each outline.

Chapter 9 outlines a simplified approach to intraventricular blocks, including hemiblocks, using a minimal number of electrocardiographic leads. The chapter includes basic concepts for the approximate determination of the electrical axis in the frontal plane. Chapter 16 describes electrocardiographic criteria for the recognition of aberrant ventricular conduction mimicking ventricular extrasystoles and ventricular tachycardia. The effects on the electrocardiogram of normally functioning ventricular pacemakers and of ventricular pacemaker malfunction are analyzed in Chapter 17. The last chapter of the first section is devoted to misleading interference—artifacts—including those mimicking atrial and ventricular arrhythmias.

The second section of the book is devoted to 60 self-assessment tracings, each with a short case history, illustrating a wide range of frequently encountered arrhythmias. Each tracing is shown again on the reverse side of the page with appropriate labeling, ladder diagrams and interpretation. Here the reader can assess and further develop his skills in the identification of the rhythm abnormalities studied in the first section.

The third section consists of 91 practice strips which can be used either for classroom instruction or for further self-assessment. Brief interpretation of these strips is provided at the end of the section.

The book does not presuppose extensive knowledge of electrocardiography on the part of the reader. Theoretical considerations have been kept to a minimum. Unnecessary use of technical jargon and complex electrophysiological explanations have been omitted intentionally. We have chosen to retain old but well established and still widely used terminology such as "A-V nodal" instead of "junctional."

While the book is intended primarily for physicians, medical students and Coronary Care nurses, it may prove valuable to the rapidly growing number of nurses, physician assistants and technicians who share responsibility for the care of patients monitored in Intensive Care Units, Operating Rooms, Recovery Rooms and Emergency Rooms.

We are deeply grateful to Alvin A. Rosenberg, M.D. for his patient and thorough review of the manuscript and for his many suggestions and helpful criticism; to Warren D. Widmann, M.D. for his thoughtful review of the chapter on Artificial Pacemaker Rhythms; to Arthur J. Geller, M.D., Oscar R. Kruesi, M.D., Ralph Miller, M.D., Alvin A. Rosenberg, M.D. and I. Richard Zucker, M.D. for providing illustrative tracings; to Sal Ceraulo for his skillful drawing of figures and diagrams; to the cardiac nurses and ECG technicians on the staffs of Morristown Memorial Hospital and the Community Medical Center in Morristown, N.J.; of Dover General Hospital in Dover, N.J., of Columbus Hospital in Newark, N.J., and of the Veterans Administration Hospital in East Orange, N.J. for their interest and zeal in collecting tracings of arrhythmias for our perusal; and to Renée Gordon and Sylvia London for typing the manuscript. Finally we express our gratitude to our publishers, the J. B. Lippincott Company for cooperation and understanding and for allowing us great freedom in the layout of the book.

STELIO MANGIOLA, M.D.
MICHAEL C. RITOTA, M.D.

Contents

Cardiac Arrhythmias

PRACTICAL ECG INTERPRETATION

Chapter 1

Basic Principles

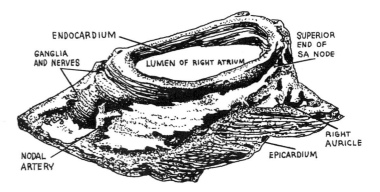

Fig. 1-2. Location and shape of the human sinus node. Reproduced from Truex.[84]

BASIC ANATOMY OF THE CONDUCTION SYSTEM

In the normal heart the cardiac impulse originates in the sinus node, spreads to the atria and reaches the atrioventricular (A-V) node. It is then transmitted to the ventricles through the His bundle, the right and left bundle branches and the Purkinje fibers. Conduction between the atria and the ventricles may also take place through accessory pathways.

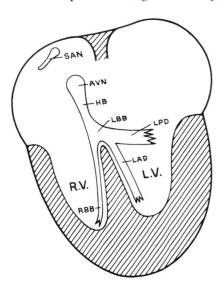

Fig. 1-1. Diagram of the sinus node and A-V conduction system of the human heart. SAN, sinus node; AVN, A-V node; HB, His bundle; LBB, left bundle branch; LPD, left posterior division; LAD, left anterior division; RBB, right bundle branch; R.V., right ventricle; L.V., left ventricle.

The sinus node

The sinus node is located in the sulcus terminalis near the junction between the superior vena cava and the right atrium, just beneath the epicardium. It has been described as a crescentic or elliptical structure measuring between 10 and 20 millimeters in length and 3 to 5 millimeters at its widest part.

The sino-atrial artery, a relatively large vessel, commonly passes through the center of the sinus node and supplies small lateral branches to the nodal tissue. The artery is one of the first branches either of the right coronary artery in about 60 percent or of the left coronary artery in about 40 percent of human hearts.

The cells of the sinus node are arranged in a fine reticular pattern within a framework of dense collagen tissue. A number of stellate cells are found in the central portion of the node and these are believed to be the source of pacemaking activity.[51]

The sinus node is richly supplied with both vagal and sympathetic nerve fibers and the former are derived mainly from the right vagus nerve.

The internodal tracts

Physiological and anatomical studies indicate that the sinus impulse spreads in the atria and to the A-V node through three pathways of specialized conducting tissue:[52]

1. *The anterior internodal tract* which divides into two parts, one going to the left atrium and known as the Bachman's bundle, the other descending to the upper margin of the A-V node.

2. *The middle internodal tract,* or Wenckebach bundle, which descends within the interatrial septum to enter the upper part of the A-V node.

3. *The posterior internodal tract,* first described by Thorel, which follows the crista terminalis, reaches the interatrial septum and enters the posterior margin of the A-V node. Thorel's tract is the longest of the three internodal tracts.

The A-V node

The A-V node is located in the right aspect of the interatrial septum just anterior to the opening of the coronary sinus and directly above the attachment of the tricuspid valve. It is a flattened structure of varying size, usually measuring 5 to 6 millimeters in length and 2 to 3 millimeters in width.

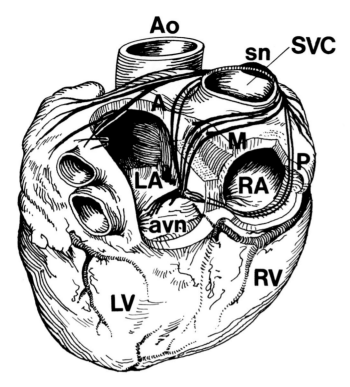

Fig. 1-3. The human heart: the internodal tracts. (After James, T. N., *in* Dreifus, L. S., and Likoff, W. (eds.): Mechanism and Therapy of Cardiac Arrhythmias. New York, Grune & Stratton, 1966) Ao, aorta; sn, sinus node; SVC, superior vena cava; RA, right atrium; RV, right ventricle; avn, atrioventricular node; LA, left atrium; A, anterior internodal tract; M, middle internodal tract; P, posterior internodal tract.

Like the sinus node, the A-V node has a central artery (ramus septi fibrosi). In 90 percent of human hearts this artery is a branch of the right coronary artery; in the remaining 10 percent it originates from the circumflex branch of the left coronary artery.

The cells of the A-V node connect freely with one another, forming a dense network. Near the distal end of the node the cells become organized in parallel fashion before entering the His bundle.

The His bundle and the bundle branches

The His bundle is an elongated structure approximately 20 millimeters long which penetrates the central fibrous body of the heart and reaches the interventricular septum where it divides into the right and the left bundle branches.

The right bundle branch, a slender group of fibers, runs along the right side of the interventricular septum and reaches the base of the anterior papillary muscle of the right ventricle where it divides into a network supplying the right ventricular myocardium.

The left bundle branch runs along the left side of the interventricular septum and divides almost immediately into an anterior (superior) division and an inferior (posterior) division. The anterior division, a relatively long and thin pathway, reaches the base of the anterior papillary muscle and supplies the anterosuperior part of the left ventricle. The posterior division, a relatively short and thick structure, passes to the base of the posterior papillary muscle and supplies the inferoposterior aspect of the left ventricle. The intraventricular conduction system is therefore composed of three conduction pathways, also called *fascicles:* the right bundle branch, the anterior division, and the posterior division of the left bundle branch.

The His bundle receives its blood supply from the artery of the A-V node. Branches of the left coronary artery supply the right bundle branch and the anterior division of the left bundle branch, whereas the posterior division has a double blood supply, from the left as well as from the right coronary artery.

Purkinje fibers

The right bundle branch and both the anterior and posterior divisions of the left bundle branch divide into a complex network of fibers, called the Purkinje fibers, which are distributed to the ventricular myocardium. The fibers are more abundant in the subendocardial layers, are longer than the common myocardial fibers and, in the human heart, are believed to lack nerve supply entirely.

Accessory pathways

Three accessory pathways have been described. They are believed to allow conduction between the atria and the ventricles in addition to or in place of the normal A-V conduction pathways. The accessory pathways are briefly described in Chapter 13.

BASIC ELECTROPHYSIOLOGY

ELECTROPHYSIOLOGICAL PROPERTIES OF THE HEART

Rhythmicity (automaticity)

The heart has the property of initiating and maintaining rhythmic activity without the help of its neurological supply. The myocardial cells which possess the property of rhythmicity are called pacemaking cells.

Under normal circumstances the pacemaking cells with the highest degree of rhythmicity and more rapid discharge rate are located in the sinus node, the primary pacemaking focus of the heart. Pacemaking cells with lesser degree of automaticity and slower inherent or natural discharge rate are present in the atria, in the A-V node and in the ventricles, forming subsidiary ectopic pacemaking foci. The more peripheral the site of the pacemaking focus the slower its rhythmicity and inherent discharge rate.

The sinus node usually controls the heart because its more rapid impulses spread to the atria, the A-V node and the ventricles abolishing the slower impulses of the ectopic pacemaking foci before they can be fired. An ectopic pacemaking focus located in the atria, the A-V node or the ventricles can take over the excitation of the heart when the sinus node fails to fire or its impulses are prevented from reaching the myocardium, or when the ectopic focus acquires a rate of discharge faster than that of the sinus node.

Some investigators have suggested that the A-V node does not possess pacemaking cells and that ectopic activity probably originates in the His bundle and not in the A-V node; A-V nodal ectopic rhythms are therefore called by some His bundle rhythms or junctional rhythms.[7,34] Since the old terminology is well established and still widely used,[5,12,16,18] we will continue to use the term A-V nodal to describe pacemaking activity that originates within or in the immediate vicinity of the A-V node.

Excitability

Both pacemaking and nonpacemaking myocardial cells have the property of responding to a natural or artificial stimulus with an abrupt change in their transmembrane potential (see below). The degree of excitability varies in different parts of the cardiac cycle but the response of a myocardial cell to a given stimulus at a particular moment is either maximal or not present at all ("all or none" law).

Conductivity

Conductivity is the property that allows the myocardial cell to propagate an impulse to a neighboring cell. An impulse of adequate strength originating in any area of the heart during its resting period creates a wave of excitation which is propagated over the whole tissue.

The conduction velocity varies in different cardiac tissues. It is maximal in the Purkinje fibers (4,000 millimeters per second) and minimal in the A-V node (200 millimeters per second). Atrial muscle and ventricular muscle have conduction velocities of 1,000 and 400 millimeters per second respectively.

Conduction between the atria and the ventricles may occur in a forward (or anterograde) fashion as well as in a retrograde fashion. Retrograde conduction is usually slower than forward conduction.

Refractoriness

During the excitation process the myocardial cell becomes completely unresponsive to any stimulus no matter how strong. This period of unresponsiveness is known as the absolute refractory period. A relative refractory period follows, during which the cell is capable of responding to a stimulus stronger than normal.

The duration of the refractory period is not constant and is influenced by the heart rate. Within limits, acceleration of the heart rate shortens the refractory

period whereas slowing has the reverse effect. The vagus nerve lengthens the refractory period of the A-V node, but shortens that of the atria. The sympathetic nerve shortens the refractory period of the entire heart.

The refractory period is longest in the A-V node, of intermediate length in the ventricular myocardium and shortest in the atrial myocardium. The right bundle branch has a refractory period longer than that of the left bundle branch.

TRANSMEMBRANE POTENTIAL

The difference in electrical potential or potential gradient between the inside and the outside of a myocardial cell can be recorded by microelectrodes. This potential is created by a flow of ions across the cell membrane, notably those of sodium and potassium, and is known as the transmembrane action potential. It can be recorded from nonpacemaking as well as from pacemaking cells.

Transmembrane action potential of a nonpacemaking cell

During the resting state a negative and steady potential gradient is present inside a nonpacemaking cell. This gradient is termed the resting potential. When an impulse propagates across the membrane, causing an excited state ("depolarization"), the inside of the cell rapidly becomes positive in relation to the extracellular fluid. A phase of recovery ("repolarization") follows and the potential again becomes negative; the repolarization phase is initially rapid, then slow, then rapid again.

By convention the phase of rapid depolarization is called phase 0. Phase 1 is the phase of early rapid repolarization, phase 2 that of slow repolarization and phase 3 is that of rapid repolarization. The resting potential is called phase 4.

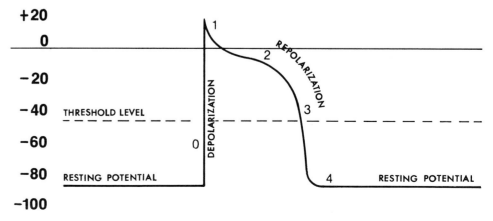

Fig. 1-4. Diagram of the transmembrane action potential of a nonpacemaking cell.

An external stimulus is capable of inducing a propagated response only when its strength is sufficient to change the transmembrane potential from its resting level to a critical level known as the threshold level or threshold potential.

Transmembrane potential of a pacemaking cell

During the resting state, or phase 4, the potential gradient inside a pacemaking cell is negative but unsteady: as soon as repolarization from the preceding excitation is completed the action potential shows a spontaneous slope which slowly reaches the threshold level. At this point rapid depolarization takes place and the action potential is transmitted through adjacent fibers.

The slow slope during the resting state is called spontaneous (diastolic) depolarization and represents the mechanism normally responsible for the rhythmic, spontaneous and automatic activity of a pacemaking cell.

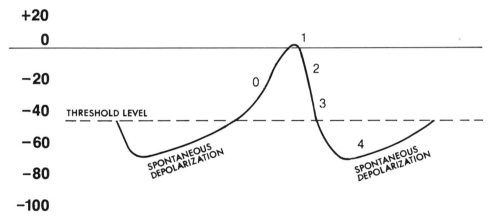

Fig. 1-5. Diagram of the transmembrane action potential of a pacemaking cell.

RATE, RHYTHM AND CONFIGURATION OF THE ECG WAVES

The electrocardiographic paper

The electrocardiogram is recorded on ruled paper which has light and heavy lines both horizontally and vertically. The light lines are 1 millimeter apart, inscribing small squares, and the heavy lines 5 millimeters apart, inscribing large squares.

The paper in the electrocardiographic machine is usually set to run at a speed of 25 millimeters per second. It therefore takes 0.04 second for the writing stylus to travel horizontally from one light line to the next, and 0.20 second to travel from one heavy line to the next. The duration (or width) of an electrocardiographic wave is therefore measured in seconds.

The distance vertically between the lines of the electrocardiographic paper is measured in millimeters. In a normally standardized machine 10 millimeters correspond to 1 millivolt. The amplitude (or voltage) of an electrocardiographic wave is therefore measured in millimeters or in millivolts.

Determination of the rate

There are various methods of determining the rate of the atrial and ventricular deflections on the electrocardiogram.

If the rhythm is regular the rate may be measured by counting the time interval (in hundredths of a second) between two consecutive deflections and dividing this number into 6,000. A quicker but less accurate calculation of the rate may be made by counting the number of large squares between two consecutive deflections and dividing this number into 300 (or the number of small squares and dividing this number into 1,500).

Another method, particularly useful when the rhythm is irregular, is that of multiplying by 20 the number of deflections inscribed in 3 seconds or by 10 the number of deflections found in 6 seconds. Most electrocardiographic paper displays marginal markers at 3-second intervals, making these calculations easier.

The rhythm of atrial and ventricular deflections

The rhythm of the atrial and ventricular deflections may be regular or irregular. The time interval between the deflections is uniform in regular rhythms and varies in irregular rhythm.

When the rhythm is irregular the time interval may vary continuously (irregularly irregular rhythm) or it may show a regular irregularity which is often repetitive. Group beating occurs when groups of beats having similar pattern and time intervals are separated by intervals of a different duration.

The configuration of atrial and ventricular deflections

Atrial and ventricular deflections may be positive or negative. When a deflection is partly positive and partly negative it is called diphasic. The duration (or width) and the amplitude (or voltage) of each deflection are variable.

In the description of the QRS complex, small letters (q, r or s) refer to small deflections (4 millimeters or less) whereas large letters (Q, R or S) indicate large deflections (5 millimeters or more).

The following rules should be remembered for the correct labeling of the QRS waves:

1. If the first wave is negative, it is a Q wave.
2. The first positive wave is an R wave.
3. The negative wave following the R wave is an S wave.
4. A positive wave following the S wave is called R′ and a negative wave following the R′ is called S′.

The term QRS complex may always be used to describe a ventricular deflection regardless of the waves that actually form it.

Ladder diagrams

Ladder diagrams (Lewis laddergrams) are frequently used to illustrate the rhythm mechanism. Black dots are often plotted to indicate the origin of the cardiac impulse and arrows are drawn to show the direction of its spreading in the atria, the A-V node and the ventricles.

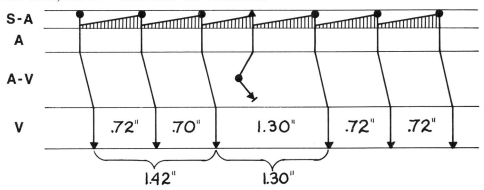

Fig. 1-6. Example of a ladder diagram. S-A, sino-atrial node; A, atria; A-V, atrioventricular node; V, ventricles. The diagram illustrates sinus rhythm with one nonconducted atrial extrasystole.

Chapter 2

Sinus Rhythms

SINUS RHYTHM

Sinus rhythm is the normal rhythm of the heart. The normal cardiac impulse originates in the sinus node and spreads to the atria, the A-V node and the ventricles, inscribing on the electrocardiogram the P wave, the P-R interval and the QRS-T complex.

The sinus P wave

The sinus P wave is positive in lead II and negative in lead aVR. In the other leads, the sinus P wave may be positive, diphasic, isoelectric, and sometimes negative. In lead V_1 it is often positive with a terminal negative component. The frontal plane axis of the sinus P wave ranges between $0°$ and $+70°$ (for the determination of the electrical axis, see Chap. 9).

The sinus P waves have a constant configuration in each lead. Their rhythm is slightly irregular, with P-P intervals varying less than 0.16 second.

The rate

The sinus rate in the adult is usually between 70 and 80 per minute. A rate between 60 and 100 per minute is arbitrarily considered to be the rate of *normal*

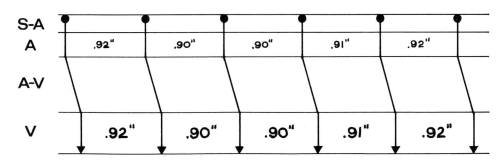

Fig. 2-1. Ladder diagram of normal sinus rhythm.

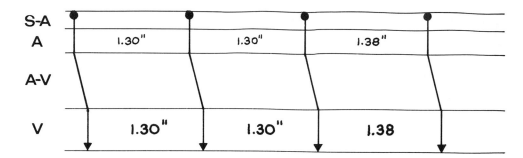

Fig. 2-2. Sinus bradycardia. Ladder diagram of the first half of Rhythm 2-1,b.

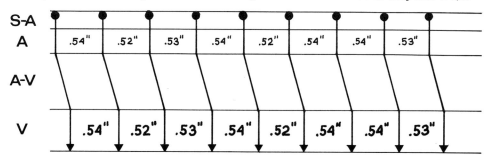

Fig. 2-3. Sinus tachycardia. Ladder diagram of the first half of Rhythm 2-1,c.

sinus rhythm. Rates above 100 per minute, usually not faster than 160 in the adult, constitute *sinus tachycardia* whereas rates below 60, usually not slower than 40 per minute, represent *sinus bradycardia.*

The P-R interval and the QRS complex

The P-R interval in normal sinus rhythm is of normal and constant duration, measuring between 0.12 and 0.20 second. When A-V dissociation or A-V block complicates sinus rhythm the P-R interval may become abnormal and vary in duration.

The QRS complex in normal sinus rhythm has normal configuration. If aberrant ventricular conduction or bundle branch block are present the QRS complex becomes wide and bizarre.

SINUS ARRHYTHMIA

Sinus arrhythmia consists of sinus rhythm occurring more irregularly, with P-P and R-R intervals varying more than 0.16 second. The rate increases for a few beats and then decreases for the next few beats. There are three types of sinus arrhythmia: respiratory, nonrespiratory and ventriculophasic.

In *respiratory sinus arrhythmia* the sinus rate increases during inspiration and decreases during expiration; during apnea the rate becomes almost regular.

In *nonrespiratory* sinus arrhythmia the changes in sinus rate bear no relationship to the phases of respiration. In *ventriculophasic sinus arrhythmia* the P-P intervals that include a QRS complex are shorter than the P-P intervals without a QRS complex; this phenomenon is often observed in A-V block (Chap. 7).

SHIFTING (OR WANDERING) PACEMAKER

The site of origin of the cardiac impulse may shift from one part to another of the sinus node or from the sinus node to the A-V node.

Shifting pacemaker within the sinus node is characterized by sinus P waves which display a gradual and temporary change in their size and shape, while the P-R interval remains relatively constant.

In *shifting pacemaker from the sinus node to (and from) the A-V node,* the P wave configuration gradually changes from positive to negative and vice versa. The P-R interval becomes shorter as the pacemaker shifts to the A-V node and again longer as the pacemaker returns to the sinus node.

Both varieties of shifting pacemaker are frequently associated with sinus arrhythmia and atrial or A-V nodal extrasystoles.

"SINUS" EXTRASYSTOLES

Extrasystoles are believed to originate in the sinus node, causing premature P waves with configuration identical to that of the normal sinus beats. Their existence is still controversial and many investigators believe that the so-called "sinus" extrasystoles are in effect atrial extrasystoles arising from a pacemaking focus located very close to the sinus node.

CLINICAL NOTES

Sinus rhythm is the normal rhythm of the heart. The rate of the sinus rhythm may be influenced by many factors, including vagal and sympathetic tone, exercise, emotions, environmental and body temperature, the metabolic status, cardiac and noncardiac diseases, and numerous drugs.

Respiratory sinus arrhythmia is frequently seen in young healthy subjects although it may also occur in diseased hearts. Nonrespiratory sinus arrhythmia is more commonly associated with heart disease, especially acute myocardial infarction. Sinus arrhythmia associated with sinus bradycardia can be a manifestation of digitalis toxicity.

Marked sinus bradycardia and sinus tachycardia may produce symptoms, especially in patients with severe cardiovascular disease; hypotension, heart failure, myocardial and cerebral ischemia may be caused or aggravated by very slow or very fast sinus rates in these patients.

The treatment of sinus bradycardia and sinus tachycardia is that of the underlying cause. Sinus bradycardia of marked degree may require the use of drugs such as atropine or isoproterenol; artificial cardiac pacing may be indicated in selected cases.

Sinus Rhythm

The normal cardiac rhythm, due to rhythmic impulses originating in the sinus node.

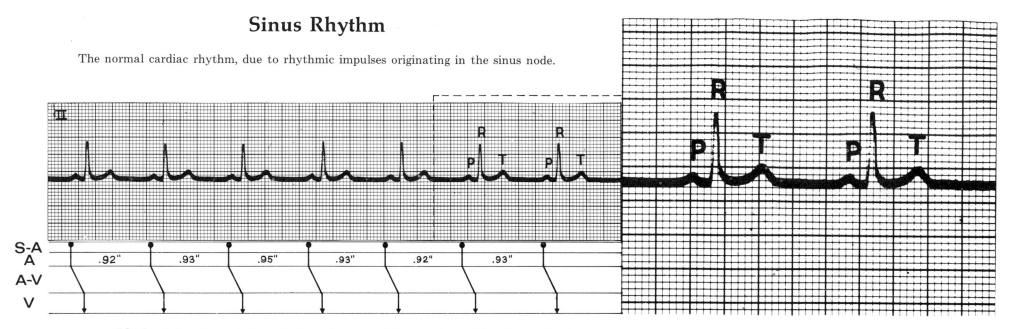

Rhythm 2-1,a. Normal sinus rhythm at a rate of 62 per minute. The P wave is of constant configuration and the rhythm slightly irregular.

ELECTROCARDIOGRAPHIC CRITERIA

A. Atrial deflections:

1. Rate:
   a. Normal sinus rhythm: between 60 and 100 per minute.
   b. Sinus bradycardia: below 60 per minute (usually not slower than 40).
   c. Sinus tachycardia: above 100 per minute (usually not faster than 160 in the adult).
2. Rhythm: slightly irregular, with P-P intervals varying less than 0.16 second.

3. Configuration:
   a. The sinus P waves are positive in lead II and negative in lead aVR.
   b. The frontal plane axis of the sinus P waves ranges between 0° and +70°.
   c. The configuration is constant in each lead.

B. A-V conduction:

1. P-R interval of normal and constant duration (0.12 to 0.20 second).
2. A-V dissociation or A-V block may cause P-R intervals of varying and abnormal duration.

C. Ventricular deflections:

1. Rate and rhythm: same as the atrial.
2. Configuration:
   a. Normal QRS complexes.
   b. Wide and bizare QRS complexes due to aberrant ventricular conduction or to bundle branch block.

Rhythm 2-1,b. Sinus bradycardia at a rate of 44 per minute. The rhythm irregularity is more obvious but the P-P intervals vary less than 0.16 second.

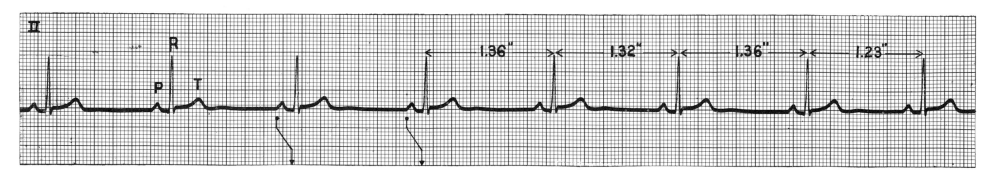

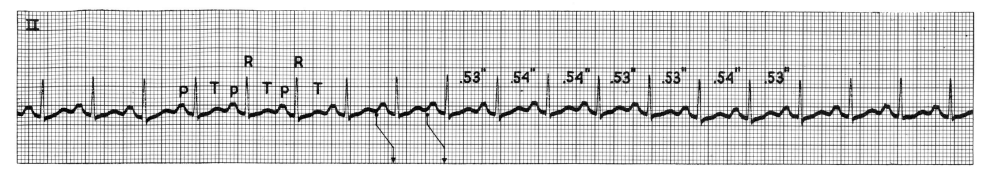

Rhythm 2-1,c. Sinus tachycardia at a rate of 110 per minute. The rhythm irregularity is only minimal (0.01 second).

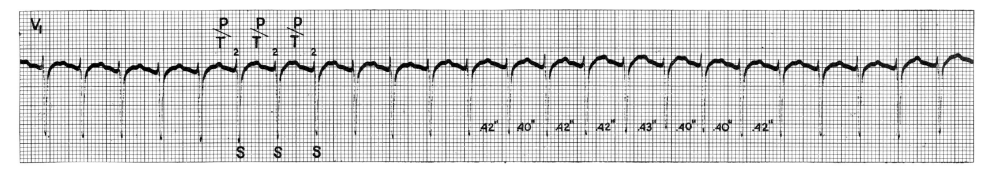

Rhythm 2-1,d. Sinus tachycardia at a rate of 145 per minute. Note the slight irregularity and the P on the T wave of the preceding beat.

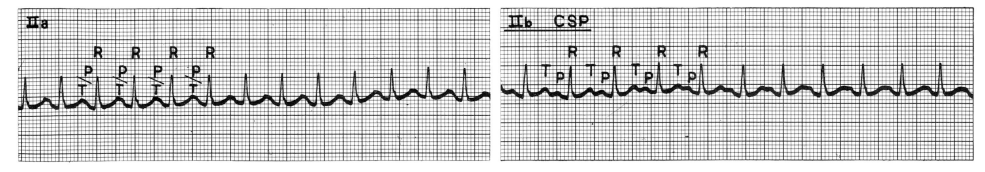

Rhythm 2-1,e. Sinus tachycardia at a rate of 152 per minute. (*Left*) IIa. The contour of each T wave is uneven because a P wave is superimposed on it ("P on T"). (*Right*) IIb. During and immediately after carotid sinus pressure (CSP) the P wave is clearly visible because of the slowing in rate induced by the vagal stimulation. As the rate speeds up the P climbs back on the T of the preceding beat.

Sinus Arrhythmia

Sinus rhythm occurring more irregularly.

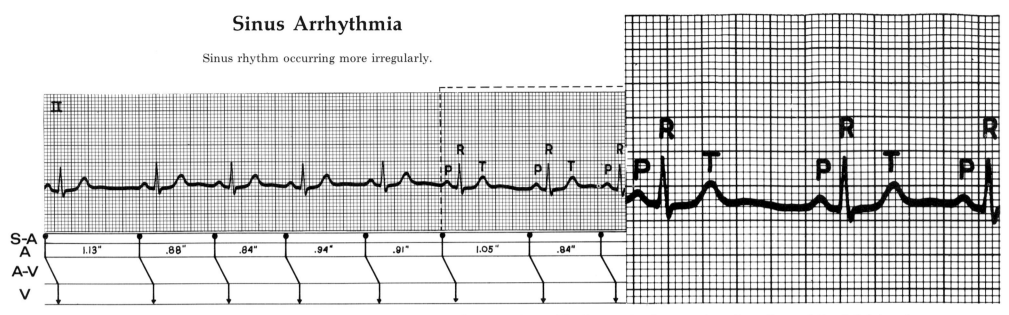

Rhythm 2-2,a. Respiratory sinus arrhythmia with average rate of 60 per minute. The P wave is of constant configuration and the P-P interval varies more than 0.16 second.

ELECTROCARDIOGRAPHIC CRITERIA

A. Sinus rhythm occurring more irregularly:

The P-P and R-R intervals vary more than 0.16 second.

B. Types:

1. Respiratory sinus arrhythmia: the rate increases during inspiration, decreases during expiration, becomes almost regular during apnea.
2. Nonrespiratory sinus arrhythmia: the changes in rate bear no relationship to the phases of respiration.
3. Ventriculophasic sinus arrhythmia: the P-P intervals that include a QRS complex are shorter than the P-P intervals without a QRS complex.

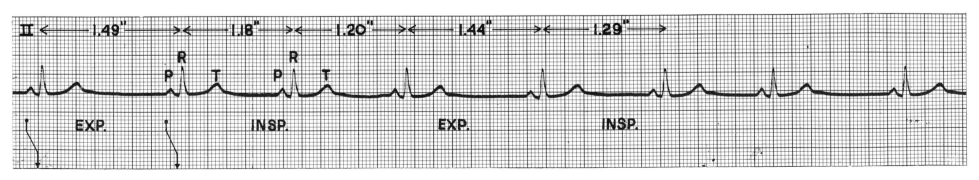

Rhythm 2-2,b. Sinus bradycardia and respiratory sinus arrhythmia with average rate of 45 per minute. The rate increases during inspiration (INSP.) and decreases during expiration (EXP.).

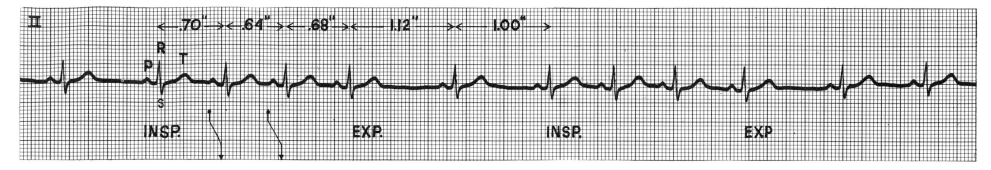

Rhythm 2-2,c. Respiratory sinus arrhythmia with average rate of 70 per minute. The rate increases during inspiration (INSP.) and decreases during expiration (EXP.).

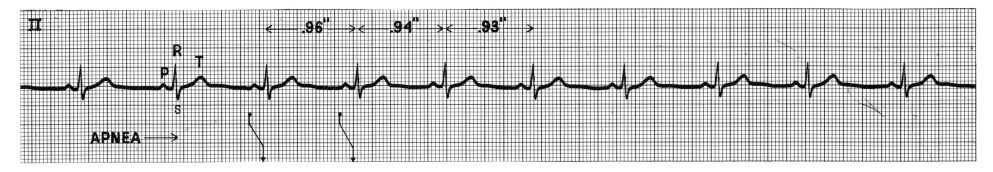

Rhythm 2-2,d. Same patient as in Rhythm 2-2,c, during apnea. The rhythm is much less irregular.

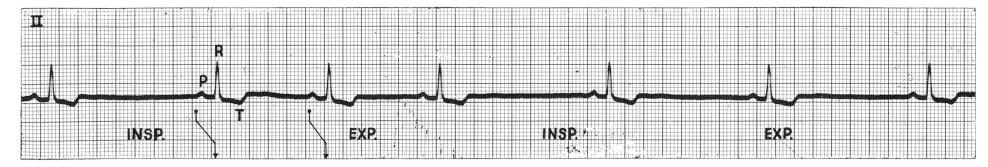

Rhythm 2-2,e. Sinus bradycardia with nonrespiratory sinus arrhythmia and average rate of 43 per minute. The changes in rate last too long and cannot be related to the phases of respiration.

Shifting (or Wandering) Pacemaker

Rhythm due to shifting in the site of origin of the cardiac impulse, within the sinus node or from the sinus to the A-V node.

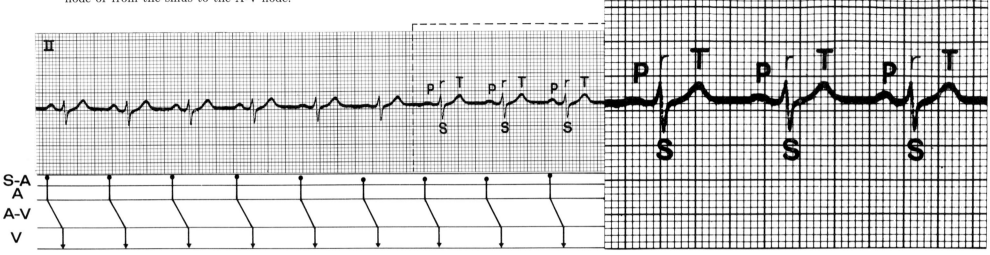

Rhythm 2-3,a. Shifting pacemaker within the sinus node.

ELECTROCARDIOGRAPHIC CRITERIA

A. Atrial deflections:

1. Shifting pacemaker within the sinus node: gradual and temporary change in configuration of the sinus P waves.
2. Shifting pacemaker to (and from) the A-V node: gradual and temporary change in configuration of the P waves which from positive become negative and vice versa.

B. A-V conduction:

1. Shifting pacemaker within the sinus node: the P-R interval remains relatively constant in duration.
2. Shifting pacemaker to (and from) the A-V node: the P'-R interval becomes gradually shorter than 0.12 second and then again of normal duration.

C. Ventricular deflections: as in sinus rhythm.

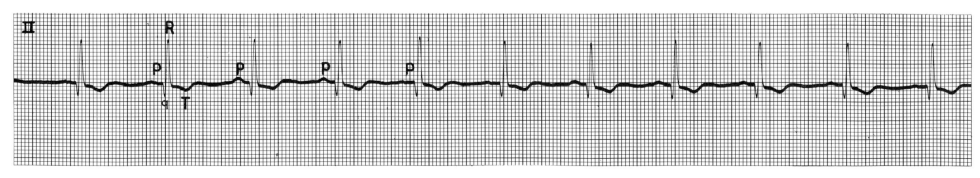

Rhythm 2-3,b. Shifting pacemaker within the sinus node. Note the gradual and temporary change in configuration of the sinus P waves.

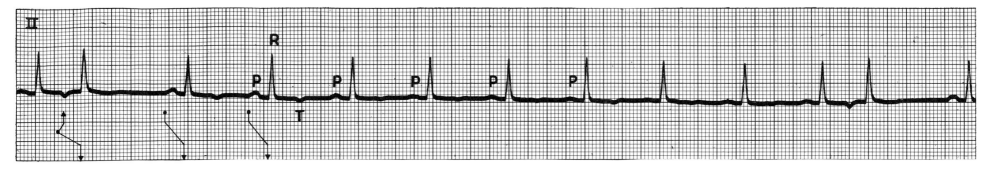

Rhythm 2-3,c. Shifting pacemaker within the sinus node following isolated A-V nodal extrasystoles.

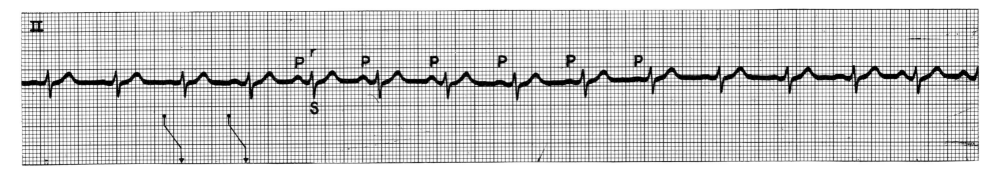

Rhythm 2-3,d. Shifting pacemaker within the sinus node.

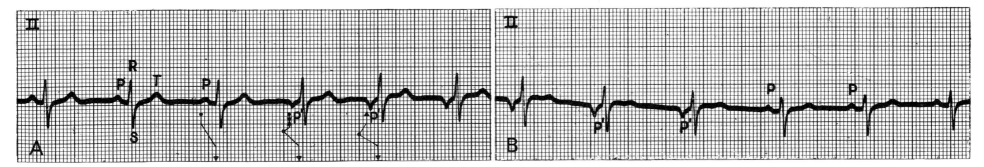

Rhythm 2-3,e. Shifting pacemaker. A, from the sinus node to the A-V node and B, from the A-V node to the sinus node.

Chapter 3

Extrasystoles and Escape Beats

Extrasystoles and escape beats are ectopic beats that originate in an ectopic pacemaking focus located in the atria, the A-V node or the ventricles. In relation to the dominant cardiac rhythm, extrasystoles are premature and escape beats are late.

EXTRASYSTOLES

Extrasystoles, also called premature beats or premature contractions, are ectopic beats that occur *prematurely* in relation to the basic cardiac rhythm. They originate in an ectopic pacemaking focus situated in the atria, the A-V node or the ventricles.

Extrasystoles may occur isolated, in pairs or in runs. Six or more consecutive extrasystoles constitute an ectopic tachycardia. When every other beat is an extrasystole the rhythm is called bigeminy; when an extrasystole occurs every third beat the rhythm is described as trigeminy; every fourth beat as quadrigeminy.

The electrocardiographic diagnosis of an extrasystole is based on the study of the atrial deflection, the A-V conduction sequence, the ventricular deflection, the coupling interval and the postextrasystolic pause. The latter two manifestations will be considered first.

The coupling interval

The time interval between the beginning of an extrasystole and the beginning of the preceding beat is known as the coupling interval. This interval is termed *constant* when its duration is constant or varies less than 0.08 second; when it varies more than 0.08 second the coupling interval is called *variable*.

The coupling interval of extrasystoles arising from a single pacemaking focus

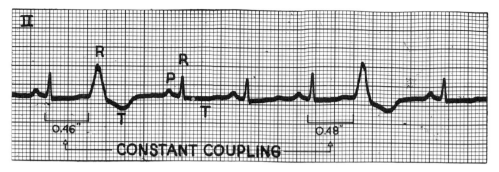

Fig. 3-1. Unifocal ventricular extrasystoles with constant coupling interval.

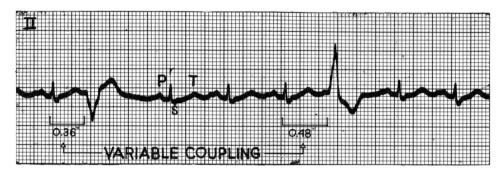

Fig. 3-2. Multifocal ventricular extrasystoles with variable coupling interval.

(unifocal extrasystoles) is constant; that of extrasystoles originating from multiple foci (multifocal extrasystoles) is variable. Extrasystoles with variable coupling interval may also be due to parasystole (see Chap. 11).

The coupling interval may be very short so that the extrasystole falls on the T wave of the preceding beat. It may also be long so that the extrasystole occurs late in diastole, usually just after the P wave of the next sinus beat but before the QRS complex of sinus origin can be inscribed; this type of extrasystole is called *end-diastolic*.

The postextrasystolic pause

Extrasystoles are usually followed by a pause which is termed noncompensatory or compensatory according to its duration.

Noncompensatory pause. The pause is *noncompensatory* when it does not completely compensate for the prematurity of the extrasystole. The ectopic impulse disturbs the regularity of the dominant rhythm and, as a result, the conducted beat following the extrasystole occurs sooner than expected.

During sinus rhythm for example, an extrasystole is followed by a noncompensatory pause when the premature impulse reaches and discharges the sinus node, resetting its cycle. One sinus impulse is aborted while it was forming;

the next one is fired after an interval usually equal to a sinus cycle. As a result, the sinus beat following the extrasystole occurs sooner than it would have, had the regularity of the sinus rhythm not been disturbed.

On the electrocardiogram the pause is said to be noncompensatory when the sum of the coupling interval and the postextrasystolic pause is less than the sum of the intervals between three consecutive sinus beats.

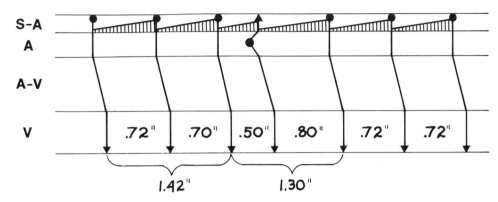

Fig. 3-3. Ladder diagram of sinus rhythm with one atrial extrasystole followed by noncompensatory pause. The extrasystolic impulse does not reach the ventricles (nonconducted APC).

Atrial and A-V nodal extrasystoles are usually followed by a noncompensatory pause. Ventricular extrasystoles may behave in the same manner when their impulses are able to travel retrogradely to the atria and discharge the sinus node (retrograde conduction).

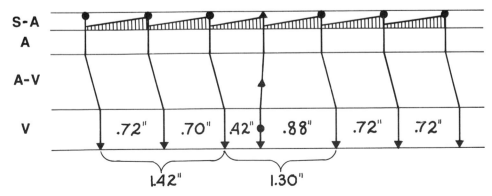

Fig. 3-4. Ladder diagram of sinus rhythm with one ventricular extrasystole. The pause is noncompensatory because the ectopic ventricular impulse is conducted retrogradely to the atria and discharges the sinus node.

Compensatory pause. The pause is *compensatory* when it completely compensates for the prematurity of an extrasystole. The regularity of the dominant rhythm is not disturbed and the conducted beat following the extrasystole occurs when expected.

During sinus rhythm, for example, an extrasystole is followed by a compensatory pause when the ectopic impulse cannot reach and discharge the sinus node; another possibility is that the impulse discharges the sinus node but temporarily inhibits its automaticity.

On the electrocardiogram the pause is said to be compensatory when the sum of the coupling interval and the postextrasystolic pause is equal to (or slightly greater than) the sum of the intervals between three consecutive sinus beats.

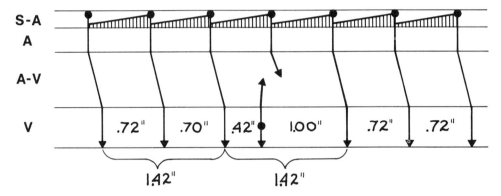

Fig. 3-5. Ladder diagram of sinus rhythm with one ventricular extrasystole followed by compensatory pause.

Ventricular extrasystoles are usually followed by a compensatory pause. Atrial and A-V nodal extrasystoles may be associated with a compensatory pause when their impulse is unable to reach and discharge the sinus node.

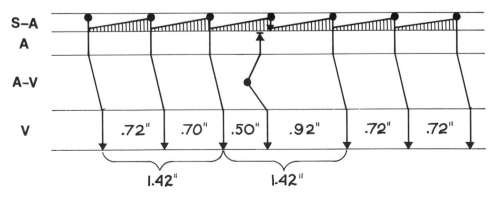

Fig. 3-6. Ladder diagram of sinus rhythm with one A-V nodal extrasystole. The postextrasystolic pause is compensatory because the ectopic A-V nodal impulse cannot reach and discharge the sinus node.

Absence of postextrasystolic pause.   When the postextrasystolic pause is absent, the extrasystole is termed *interpolated*. The ectopic impulse has little or no effect on the dominant rhythm and the extrasystole is sandwiched between two consecutive sinus beats.

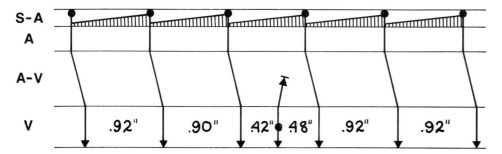

Fig. 3-7. Ladder diagram of sinus rhythm with one interpolated ventricular extrasystole.

Interpolated extrasystoles usually occur when the coupling interval is short and/or sinus bradycardia is present. The P-R interval of the sinus beat following an A-V nodal or ventricular extrasystole is often prolonged, owing to concealed retrograde conduction (Chap. 15).

Interpolated ventricular extrasystoles are not infrequent, whereas interpolated atrial and A-V nodal extrasystoles occur rarely.

ATRIAL EXTRASYSTOLE

Also known as atrial premature contraction (APC), an atrial extrasystole is the result of the premature firing of an ectopic atrial focus. Its impulse spreads through the atria, in a fashion different from that of a sinus impulse, and to the A-V node, which it may or may not traverse to reach the ventricles.

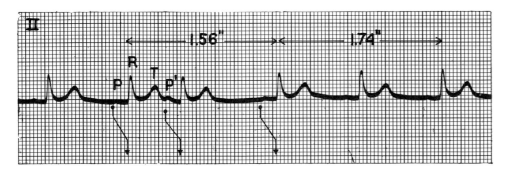

Fig. 3-8. Sinus rhythm with one atrial extrasystole. The postextrasystolic pause is noncompensatory.

The P′ wave

The P′ wave of an atrial extrasystole is premature; like the sinus P waves, it is usually positive in lead II and negative in lead aVR. Its configuration, however, is somewhat different from that of the sinus P waves in the same tracing, owing to the difference in conduction of its impulse through the atrial tissue.

The P′-R interval

The duration of the P′-R interval of an atrial extrasystole is often similar to that of a sinus beat. When very premature, however, the extrasystolic impulse may find the A-V node either (1) partially refractory, and may be conducted with a long P′-R interval, or (2) totally refractory, and may not be conducted to the ventricles at all (nonconducted atrial extrasystole).

Nonconducted atrial extrasystoles are the most frequent cause of sudden pauses interrupting the sinus rhythm and can mimic sino-atrial block, an arrhythmia of much more serious prognostic significance (Chap. 8). A nonconducted atrial extrasystole can be correctly diagnosed by noticing that a premature P′ wave deforms the T wave of the beat preceding a sudden pause during sinus rhythm.

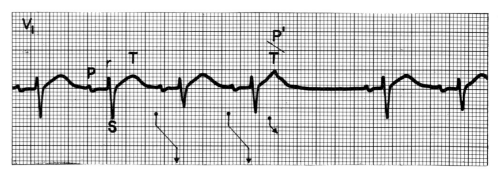

Fig. 3-9. Sinus rhythm with one nonconducted atrial extrasystole.

The QRS complex

The QRS complex of an atrial extrasystole is usually identical to that of the normal sinus beats. However, when the ectopic atrial impulse succeeds in traversing the A-V node but finds one of the bundle branches still refractory, the QRS complex becomes wide and bizarre, owing to aberrant ventricular conduction (see Chap. 16). Atrial extrasystoles with aberrant ventricular conduction mimic ventricular extrasystoles.

The coupling interval and the postextrasystolic pause

Atrial extrasystoles tend to have a constant coupling interval (the coupling interval of an atrial extrasystole is measured from the beginning of the ectopic P′ wave to the beginning of the preceding sinus P wave).

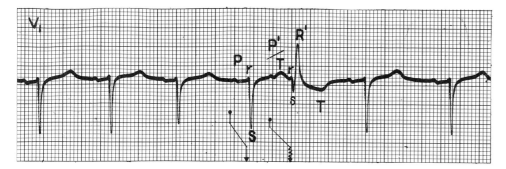

Fig. 3-10. Sinus rhythm and one atrial extrasystole with aberrant ventricular conduction, right bundle branch block type.

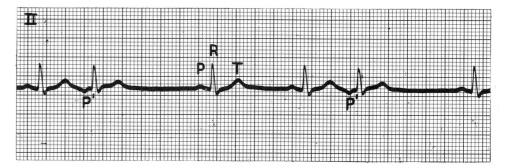

Fig. 3-11. Sinus rhythm with two A-V nodal extrasystoles.

The postextrasystolic pause of an atrial extrasystole is frequently noncompensatory: the ectopic atrial impulse discharges the sinus node prematurely and resets its cycle. When the ectopic atrial impulse cannot reach and discharge the sinus node the pause becomes compensatory. Interpolated atrial extrasystoles are very rare.

CLINICAL NOTES

Atrial extrasystoles may occur in normal individuals or may be associated with heart disease, such as rheumatic or coronary heart disease, with acute or chronic lung disease, and with hyperthyroidism. They are frequently caused by congestive heart failure and may lead to atrial tachycardia, atrial flutter, or atrial fibrillation. Frequent atrial extrasystoles may be a manifestation of digitalis toxicity.

The treatment of atrial extrasystoles is that of the underlying condition. Digitalis is the treatment of choice when they are caused by congestive heart failure. Quinidine, propranolol and procainamide are used to abolish frequent atrial extrasystoles.

A-V NODAL EXTRASYSTOLE

Also known as nodal premature contraction (NPC), an A-V nodal extrasystole is caused by the premature firing of an ectopic A-V nodal focus. Its impulse usually spreads backward to the atria as well as forward to the ventricles.

The P′ wave

In spreading backward to the atria the ectopic A-V nodal impulse creates a premature and inverted P′ wave (negative in lead II where the sinus P wave is positive and positive in lead aVR where the sinus P wave is negative). The inverted P′ wave may precede, or may be hidden within, or may follow the QRS

complex, according to the order in which the atria and the ventricles are activated.

When the P′ wave precedes the QRS complexes the A-V nodal extrasystole is called "high" nodal, on the assumption that the pacemaking focus is located high in the A-V node and therefore its impulses are able to reach the atria before they can reach the ventricles. When the P′ wave cannot be seen because it is hidden within the QRS complex and when the P′ wave follows the QRS complex, the extrasystole is called "mid" and "low" nodal respectively, on the assumption that the pacemaking focus in the A-V node is located in its mid and low portion respectively.

In fact, what determines the order of activation of atria and ventricles is not the location of the ectopic focus in the A-V node but the conduction velocity above and below the A-V nodal focus. The inverted P′ wave precedes the QRS complex ("high" nodal) when retrograde conduction of its impulse is *faster* than forward conduction, regardless of the location of the focus in the A-V node. On the other hand, the P′ wave follows the QRS complex ("low" nodal) when

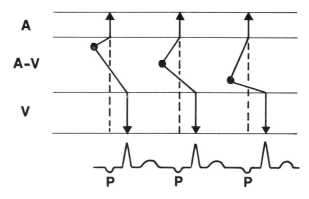

Fig. 3-12. Ladder diagram showing that "high" nodal beats can occur regardless of the location of the ectopic focus in the A-V node.

retrograde conduction of its impulse is *slower* than forward conduction, regardless of the location of the focus in the A-V node.

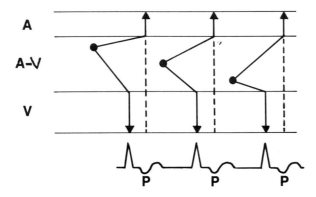

Fig. 3-13. Ladder diagram showing that "low" nodal beats can occur regardless of the ectopic focus in the A-V node.

The absence of the inverted P' wave preceding or following the QRS complex of A-V nodal origin may have one of the following causes: (1) the A-V nodal impulse reaches both the atria and the ventricles at the same time and thus the P' wave is hidden within the QRS complex ("mid" nodal), or (2) A-V dissociation or block above the A-V nodal focus prevents the A-V nodal impulse from reaching the atria which thus continue to beat undisturbed.

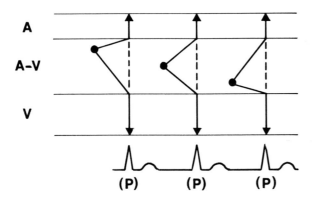

Fig. 3-14. Ladder diagram showing that "mid" nodal beats can occur regardless of the location of the ectopic focus in the A-V node.

The terms "high," "mid" and "low" nodal are well established and very useful in describing the relationship between the P wave and the QRS complex when A-V nodal extrasystoles are recorded. Although these terms are admittedly incorrect, we still continue to use them for didactic reasons. The quotation marks will serve as a reminder that these terms do not reflect the location of the ectopic focus in the A-V node.

A-V and V-A conduction

The duration of P'-R interval of a "high" nodal extrasystole is usually 0.12 second or less. In some cases it may be longer when a conduction delay below the focus slows down the conduction of the impulse to the ventricles. Nonconducted A-V nodal extrasystoles occur when the impulse is very premature and finds the conduction tissue below the focus totally refractory. They can often be diagnosed by noticing that a premature and inverted P' wave deforms the T wave of the beat preceding a sudden pause.

The R-P' interval of a "low" nodal extrasystole is usually between 0.10 and 0.20 second but may be longer, depending on the conduction velocity above and below the A-V nodal focus: a conduction delay above the focus, for example, slows down the retrograde spread of the impulse to the atria and increases the duration of the R-P' interval.

The QRS complex

The premature QRS complex of an A-V nodal extrasystole may be identical to that of the normal sinus beats. Often, however, it has a slightly different configuration which is attributed to one of the following mechanisms:
1. A-V nodal impulses can spread through the accessory pathways described by Mahaim and thus invade the ventricular myocardium in a slightly abnormal fashion.[66]
2. Impulses originating in the distal portion of the A-V node can be conducted down only part of the His bundle.[66]
3. A-V nodal extrasystoles with configuration slightly different from that of the normal sinus beats are in effect ventricular extrasystoles originating in the proximal region of the bundle branches.[71]

Aberrant ventricular conduction causes the QRS complex of an A-V nodal extrasystole to become wide and bizarre. A-V nodal extrasystole with aberrant ventricular conduction often cannot be differentiated from ventricular extrasystoles.

The coupling interval and the postextrasystolic pause

A-V nodal extrasystoles, like atrial extrasystoles, tend to have a constant coupling interval and a noncompensatory pause. When the ectopic A-V nodal impulse cannot reach and discharge the sinus node, the postextrasystolic pause becomes compensatory. Occasionally A-V nodal extrasystoles are interpolated.

CLINICAL NOTES

A-V nodal extrasystoles may occur in normal individuals or may be associated with heart disease, such as coronary heart disease, and with lung disease. They are frequently caused by congestive heart failure and may lead to A-V nodal tachycardia. Frequent A-V nodal extrasystoles may be a manifestation of digitalis toxicity.

The treatment of A-V nodal extrasystoles is that of the underlying condition. Quinidine, propranolol and procainamide are often used. In addition to discontinuance of digitalis, diphenylhydantoin may be particularly useful when the A-V nodal extrasystoles are caused by digitalis toxicity.

VENTRICULAR EXTRASYSTOLE

Also known as ventricular premature contraction (VPC), a ventricular extrasystole is caused by the premature firing of an ectopic focus located in one of the ventricles. Its impulse spreads first to the ventricle where it originates and then to the opposite ventricle, with delay.

The atrial mechanism

The atrial mechanism may be sinus rhythm or an ectopic supraventricular rhythm. During sinus rhythm, ventricular extrasystolic impulses may sometimes be conducted retrogradely to the atria and cause premature and inverted P' waves.

The QRS complex

The premature QRS complex of a ventricular extrasystole is wide and bizarre because the ectopic impulse invades first the ventricle where it originates and then spreads to the opposite ventricle, with delay. A ventricular extrasystole may originate in the left or in the right ventricle:

Left VPC. An extrasystolic impulse originating in the left ventricle invades the right ventricle with delay. Consequently, its QRS complex has a pattern that resembles *right* bundle branch block: in lead V_1 the QRS is predominantly positive and often M-shaped.

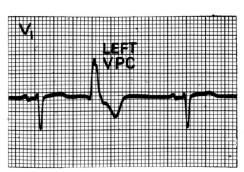 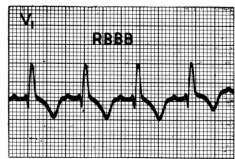

Fig. 3-15. (*Left*) Sinus rhythm with one left VPC. Its pattern resembles right bundle branch block. (*Right*) Sinus tachycardia with right bundle branch block (RBBB).

Right VPC. An extrasystolic impulse arising in the right ventricle invades the left ventricle with delay. As a result, its QRS complex has a pattern that resembles *left* bundle branch block: in lead V_1 the QRS is predominantly negative, either without an r wave or with a small r wave followed by a wide and deep S wave.

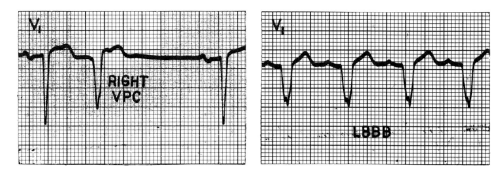

Fig. 3-16. (*Left*) Sinus rhythm with one right VPC. Its pattern resembles left bundle branch block. (*Right*) Sinus rhythm with left bundle branch block (LBBB).

A ventricular extrasystole may occasionally have a QRS pattern within normal limits. His bundle electrograms have shown that this may occur when the pacemaking focus is located in one of the intraventricular conduction fascicles and its impulse travels distally to reach the ventricle and, at the same time, centrally to reach the His bundle and the opposite bundle branch.[33,62] Another explanation for this apparent paradox is that, in the lead used, the initial or the terminal portion of the QRS complex happens to be isoelectric; if this is the case, a rhythm strip recorded in a different lead will show that the QRS is actually wide.

When two or more ventricular extrasystoles occur in the same tracing their configuration is uniform if the extrasystoles are unifocal and variable when they are multifocal.

The coupling interval

The coupling interval is constant in unifocal ventricular extrasystoles and variable when the extrasystoles are multifocal.

The coupling interval may be very short so that the ventricular extrasystole falls on the T wave of the preceding beat, in the so-called vulnerable zone. The extrasystole may then induce repetitive firing and the appearance of ventricular tachycardia or ventricular fibrillation: for this reason a VPC with its "R on T" is also called "malignant VPC."

A long coupling interval is seen when a ventricular extrasystole, although premature, occurs late in diastole. This type of extrasystole is called "end-diastolic" and is usually inscribed right after a sinus P wave, before the normal QRS complex can be inscribed. When the impulse of an end-diastolic VPC

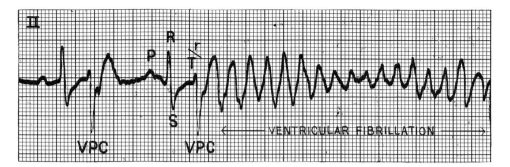

Fig. 3-17. Sinus rhythm with first-degree A-V block and two malignant VPC's falling on the T wave of the preceding sinus beat. The second VPC triggers ventricular fibrillation.

succeeds in activating only part of the ventricles while a normal sinus impulse activates the remainder, a ventricular fusion beat results. Ventricular fusion beats have a configuration intermediate between that of a ventricular extrasystole and that of a normal sinus beat (see Chap. 6).

The postextrasystolic pause

Ventricular extrasystoles are usually followed by a compensatory pause because they do not disturb the regularity of the dominant cardiac rhythm. When there is retrograde conduction to the atria, however, the ectopic ventricular impulse reaches and discharges the sinus node and the postextrasystolic pause becomes noncompensatory. Interpolated ventricular extrasystoles, sandwiched between two normal sinus beats, are not infrequently seen, especially when the coupling interval is short and sinus bradycardia is present.

The rule of bigeminy[57]

The rule states that a long ventricular cycle tends to precipitate a ventricular extrasystole. When the basic rhythm is irregular, as in sinus arrhythmia, atrial fibrillation or sino-atrial block, a ventricular extrasystole often occurs following a long R-R interval (see Rhythm 8-1,e); the long pause following the extrasystole in turn may precipitate another extrasystole and the bigeminal rhythm thus has a tendency to perpetuate itself. The precise mechanism causing the "rule of bigeminy" has not been established.

CLINICAL NOTES

Ventricular extrasystoles may be seen in normal individuals and are associated with anxiety states and the excessive use of coffee, tea and tobacco. A characteristic pattern of ventricular extrasystoles occurring in normal subjects has been recently described;[71] nearly always they arise from the anterior wall of the right

ventricle, close to its anterior papillary muscle, and therefore have a QRS complex resembling left bundle branch block (right VPC's).

Numerous forms of heart disease and a variety of drugs may cause ventricular extrasystoles. They frequently occur in coronary heart disease, especially acute myocardial infarction, and in digitalis toxicity.

The treatment of ventricular extrasystoles is that of the underlying condition. Healthy subjects usually do not require any treatment other than reassurance and moderation in the use of coffee, tea and tobacco. The following features are considered indication for aggressive treatment of ventricular extrasystoles during acute myocardial infarction:

1. Very short coupling intervals with "R on T" phenomenon (malignant VPC's).
2. Runs of two or more.
3. Varying configuration and coupling interval (multifocal VPC's).
4. VPC's occurring more frequently than five per minute.

Drugs used in the treatment of ventricular extrasystoles include lidocaine, procainamide, quinidine, propranolol, diphenylhydantoin. Digitalis should be discontinued when the arrhythmia is considered to be caused by digitalis toxicity.

ESCAPE BEATS

Escape beats are ectopic beats that occur *late* in relation to the dominant cardiac rhythm. They originate in subsidiary pacemaking foci located in the atria, the A-V node or the ventricles and represent a safety or rescuing mechanism that operates when a pause occurs in the heart rhythm. The pause may be caused by slowing, failure or block of the sinus impulses, by A-V block, by an extrasystole or by the end of a paroxysm of ectopic tachycardia.

Escape beats resemble atrial, A-V nodal or ventricular extrasystoles. The only difference is that escape beats always occur late whereas extrasystoles are always

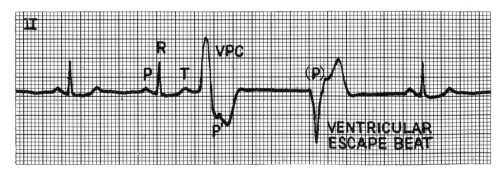

Fig. 3-18. Sinus rhythm and a ventricular extrasystole with retrograde conduction to the atria. The postextrasystolic pause is interrupted by a ventricular escape beat.

premature. Escape beats, like extrasystoles, may occur isolated, in pairs or in runs. Six or more consecutive escape beats constitute an escape rhythm.

The interval between the beginning of an escape beat and the beginning of the preceding beat is called escape interval. The escape interval is usually of constant duration.

Supraventricular escape beats may rarely display aberrant ventricular conduction. This phenomenon is discussed in Chapter 16.

CLINICAL NOTES

The clinical significance of escape beats is that of the underlying arrhythmia which causes their appearance. Treatment, when necessary, includes discontinuation of any causative drugs, the use of atropine or isoproterenol and, in symptomatic patients with an underlying arrhythmia resistant to drug treatment, artificial pacing.

Atrial Extrasystole (APC)

Ectopic beat due to the premature firing of an ectopic atrial focus.

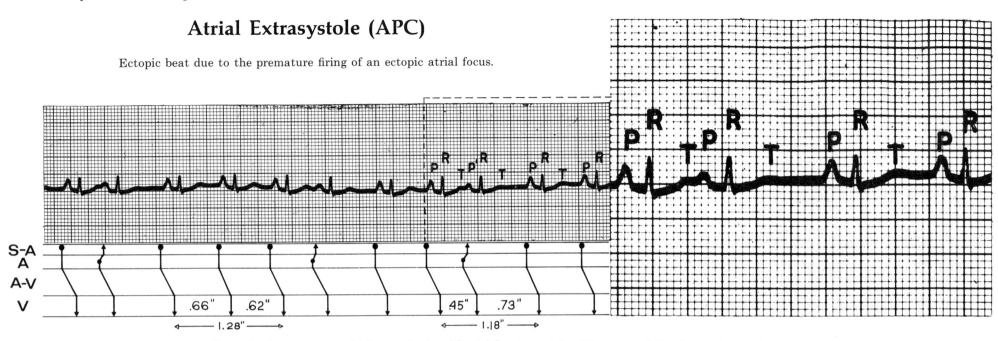

Rhythm 3-1,a. Sinus rhythm at a rate of 92 per minute with atrial extrasystoles. The pause following each APC is non-compensatory.

ELECTROCARDIOGRAPHIC CRITERIA

A. Atrial deflection:

1. Premature P' wave.
2. The P' wave is positive in lead II and inverted in lead aVR, as in sinus rhythm.
3. The configuration of the P' wave is somewhat different from that of the sinus P waves.

B. A-V conduction:

1. Conducted atrial extrasystole:

    a. The P'-R interval is similar to that of the sinus beats.

    b. Very premature P' wave with P'-R interval longer than that of the sinus beats.

2. Nonconducted atrial extrasystole: very premature P' wave not followed by QRS complex and causing a pause. Most often the nonconducted P' wave deforms the T wave of the beat preceding the pause.

C. Ventricular deflection:

1. Premature QRS complex.

    a. Identical to that of the sinus beats.

    b. Wide and bizarre: APC with aberrant ventricular conduction.

D. Coupling interval.

1. Usually constant.
2. May be variable.

E. Postextrasystole pause:

1. Usually noncompensatory.
2. Rarely compensatory.
3. Very rarely absent: interpolated APC.

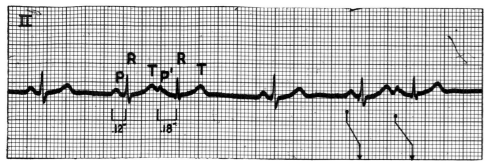

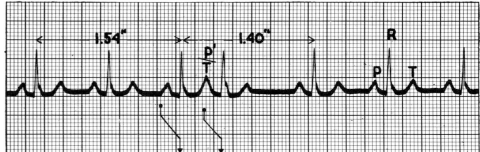

Rhythm 3-1,b. Sinus rhythm at a rate of 67 per minute with atrial extrasystoles. Note the P'-R interval of the APC (0.18 sec.) longer than the P-R interval of the sinus beats (0.12 sec.).

Rhythm 3-1,c. Sinus rhythm at a rate of 75 per minute and one atrial extrasystole with its P' on the T wave of the preceding beat. The postextrasystolic pause is noncompensatory.

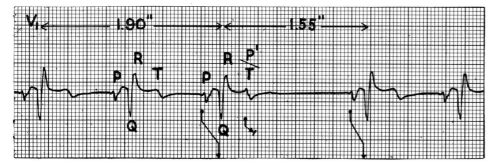

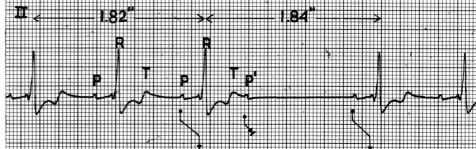

Rhythm 3-1,d. Sinus rhythm at a rate of 62 per minute with one nonconducted atrial extrasystole. Note the premature P' wave deforming the T wave of the beat preceding the sudden pause. The pause is noncompensatory.

Rhythm 3-1,e. Sinus rhythm at a rate of 66 per minute with one nonconducted atrial extrasystole. The pause is here compensatory.

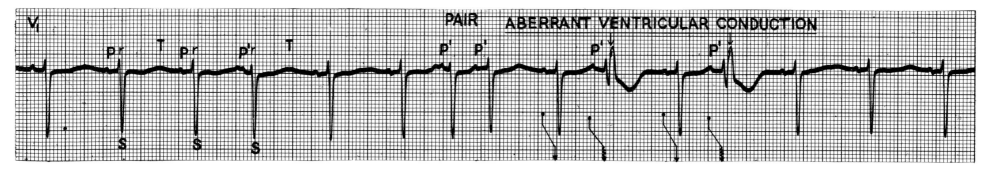

Rhythm 3-1,f. Sinus rhythm at a rate of 77 per minute and atrial extrasystoles without and with aberrant ventricular conduction (right bundle branch block type). Both APC's with aberrant conduction could be mistaken for ventricular extrasystoles if the premature P' wave preceding each beat is missed. Note the pair of APC's in the middle of the strip.

A-V Nodal Extrasystole (NPC)

Ectopic beat due to the premature firing of an ectopic A-V nodal focus.

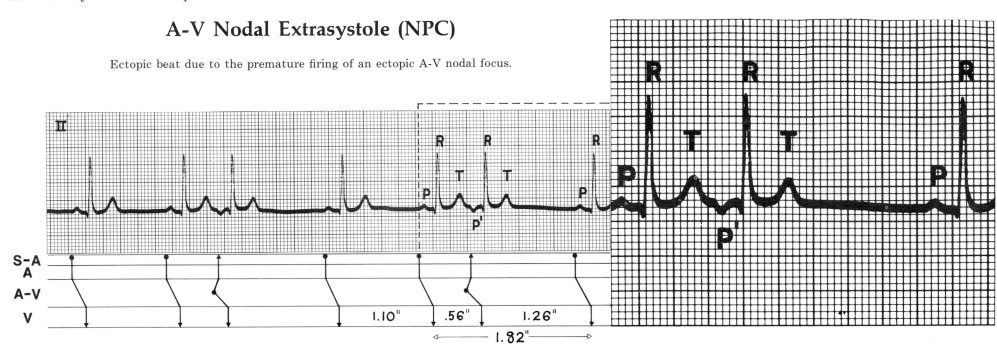

Rhythm 3-2,a. Sinus bradycardia at a rate of 55 per minute with "high" nodal extrasystoles.

ELECTROCARDIOGRAPHIC CRITERIA

A. Atrial deflection:

1. Premature P′ wave, negative in lead II:
   a. Preceding the QRS complex: "high" nodal
   b. Following the QRS complex: "low" nodal
2. Absent P′ wave:
   a. P′ wave hidden within the QRS complex: "mid" nodal.
   b. The atria cannot be reached by the A-V nodal impulse and continue to beat undisturbed.

B. A-V and V-A conduction:

1. P′-R interval: usually 0.12 second or less.
2. R-P′ interval: usually between 0.10 and 0.20 second.

C. Ventricular deflection:

1. Premature QRS complex:
   a. Identical to that of the sinus beats.
   b. Slightly different in configuration but normal in duration.
   c. Wide and bizarre: NPC with aberrant ventricular conduction.

D. Coupling interval:

1. Usually constant.
2. May be variable.

E. Postextrasystolic pause:

1. Usually noncompensatory.
2. Rarely compensatory.
3. Occasionally absent: interpolated NPC.

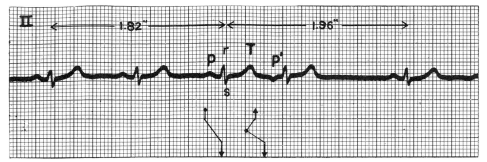

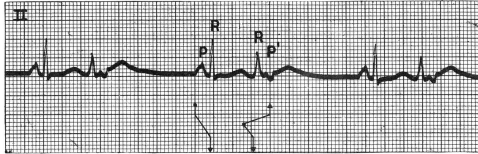

Rhythm 3-2,b. Sinus rhythm at a rate of 67 per minute with a "high" nodal extrasystole. The pause is compensatory.

Rhythm 3-2,c. Sinus rhythm with "low" nodal extrasystoles in bigeminy. The average ventricular rate is 68 per minute.

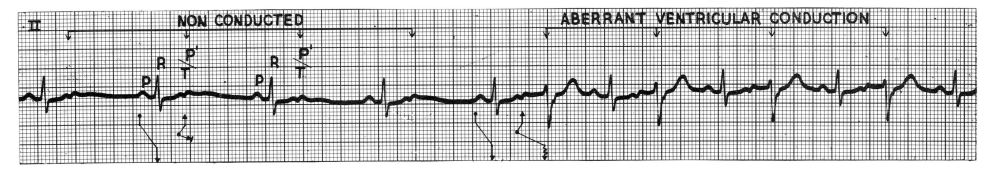

Rhythm 3-2,d. In the first half of the strip nonconducted A-V nodal bigeminy is present with a ventricular rate of 50 per minute (nonconducted atrial or A-V nodal bigeminy may be responsible for very slow ventricular rates simulating marked sinus bradycardia); the NPC impulses deform the T waves of the first four beats and are unable to reach the ventricles. In the second half of the strip the NPC impulses are still in bigeminy but they manage to spread to the ventricular myocardium which they activate in an abnormal fashion (aberrant ventricular conduction).

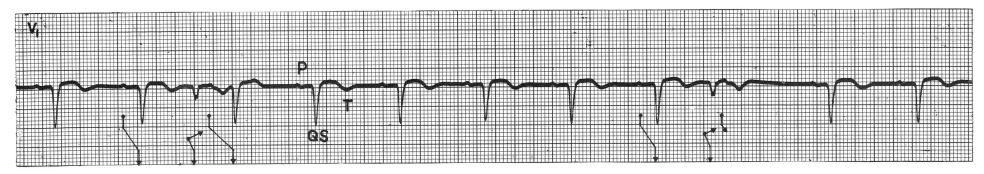

Rhythm 3-2,e. Sinus rhythm at a rate of 67 per minute with two A-V nodal extrasystoles. The first NPC squeezes in between two consecutive sinus impulses and is therefore interpolated. The second is followed by a compensatory pause. Note that the sinus beat which follows the interpolated NPC finds the A-V junction not completely recovered and is conducted to the ventricles with delay (P-R interval 0.26 second).

Ventricular Extrasystole (VPC)

Ectopic beat due to the premature firing of an ectopic focus located in one of the ventricles.

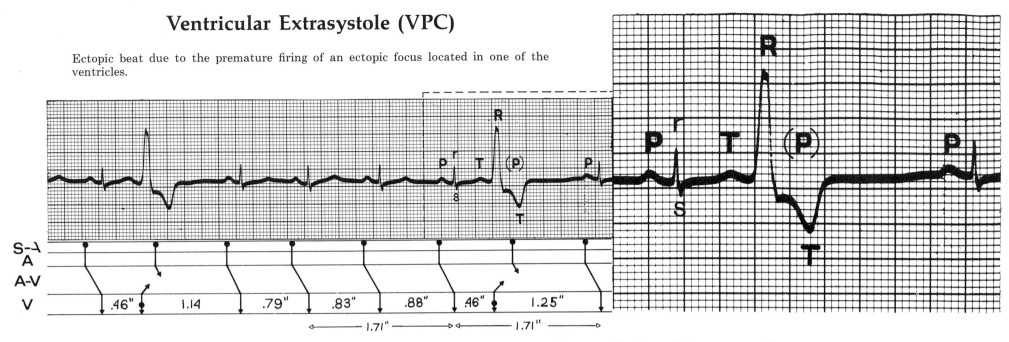

Rhythm 3-3,a. Sinus rhythm at a rate of 75 per minute with two unifocal ventricular extrasystoles.

ELECTROCARDIOGRAPHIC CRITERIA

A. Atrial deflections:

1. Rate, rhythm and configuration depend on the atrial mechanism (sinus or ectopic).
2. During sinus rhythm a premature and inverted P' wave may follow the QRS complex of the extrasystole: VPC with retrograde conduction.

B. Ventricular deflection:

1. Premature, wide and bizarre QRS complex:
   a. Left VPC: QRS pattern resembling right bundle branch block (predominantly positive and often M-shaped in lead V_1).
   b. Right VPC: QRS pattern resembling left bundle branch block (predominantly negative in lead V_1).
2. When two or more VPC's occur in the same tracing:
   a. Uniform configuration: unifocal VPC's.
   b. Variable configuration: multifocal VPC's.

C. Coupling interval:

1. Constant: unifocal VPC's

2. Variable:
   a. Multifocal VPC's.
   b. Ventricular parasystole.
3. Very short: malignant VPC.
4. Long: end-diastolic VPC.

D. Postextrasystole pause:

1. Usually compensatory.
2. Rarely noncompensatory.
3. Occasionally absent: interpolated VPC.

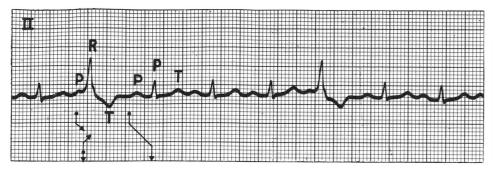

Rhythm 3-3,b. Sinus rhythm at a rate of 98 per minute with two end-diastolic ventricular extrasystoles.

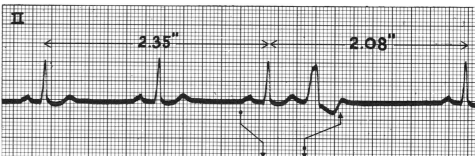

Rhythm 3-3,c. Sinus bradycardia at a rate of 50 per minute and one VPC with retrograde conduction to the atria. The postextrasystolic pause is noncompensatory.

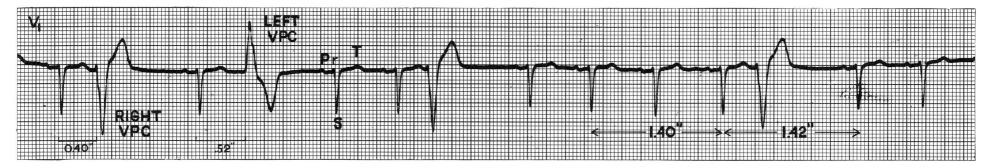

Rhythm 3-3,d. Sinus rhythm at a rate of 95 per minute with multifocal right and left ventricular extrasystoles. The coupling interval is variable and the pause following each extrasystole is compensatory.

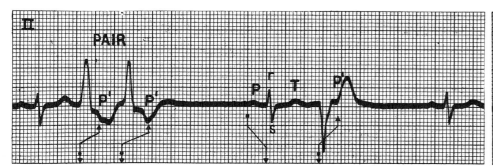

Rhythm 3-3,e. Sinus rhythm with multifocal ventricular extrasystoles, isolated or in pairs, each with retrograde conduction to the atria.

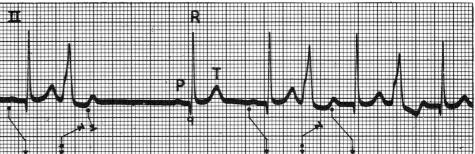

Rhythm 3-3,f. Sinus rhythm at a rate of 74 per minute with unifocal ventricular extrasystoles. The first one is followed by a compensatory pause. The other two are interpolated.

Escape Beats

Ectopic beats due to the "late" firing of an ectopic atrial, A-V nodal or ventricular focus.

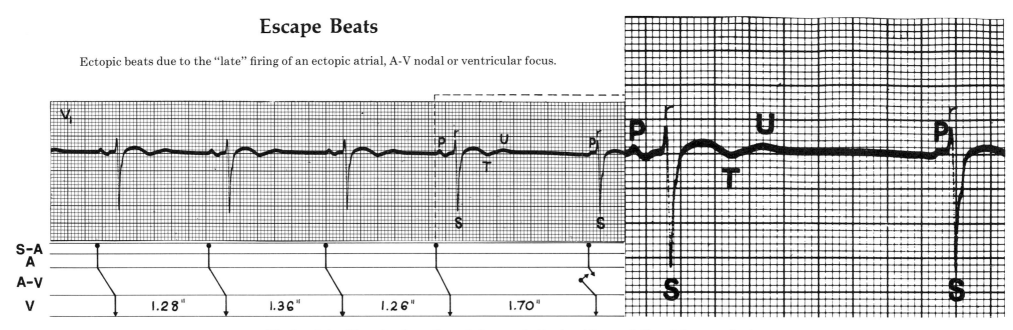

Rhythm 3-4,a. Sinus bradycardia and sinus arrhythmia with one A-V nodal escape beat.

ELECTROCARDIOGRAPHIC CRITERIA

A. Always occur "late".

B. May occur whenever there is a cardiac pause caused by:

1. Slowing or failure of the sinus impulses.

2. Sino-atrial block.
3. A-V block.
4. An extrasystole.
5. The end of a paroxysm of ectopic tachycardia.

C. Origin:

1. Atrial.

2. A-V nodal.
3. Ventricular.

D. Atrial and Ventricular deflections: see Extrasystoles

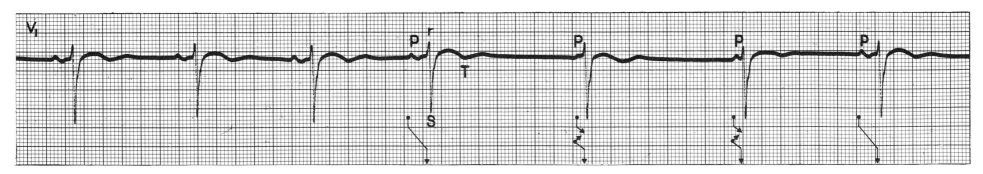

Rhythm 3-4,b. Same patient as in 3-4,a. Two consecutive A-V nodal escape beats can be seen.

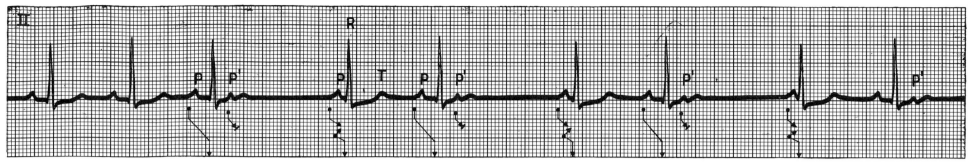

Rhythm 3-4,c. Sinus rhythm at a rate of 70 per minute with nonconducted atrial extrasystoles, each followed by an A-V nodal escape beat.

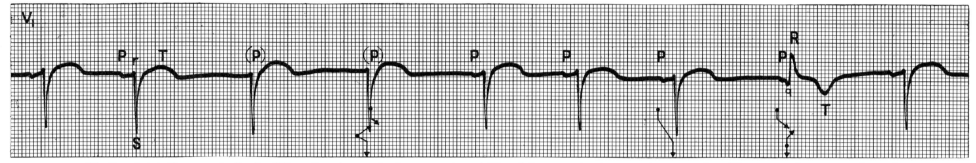

Rhythm 3-4,d. Sinus arrhythmia. When the sinus rate decreases, two A-V nodal escape beats occur in succession. The escape beat near the end of the strip is probably of ventricular origin.

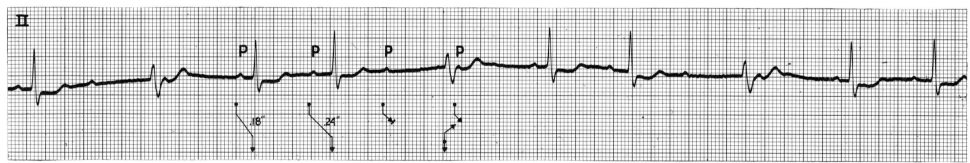

Rhythm 3-4,e. Sinus rhythm with second degree A-V block type I (Wenckebach). The pause following each blocked P wave is terminated by a ventricular escape beat.

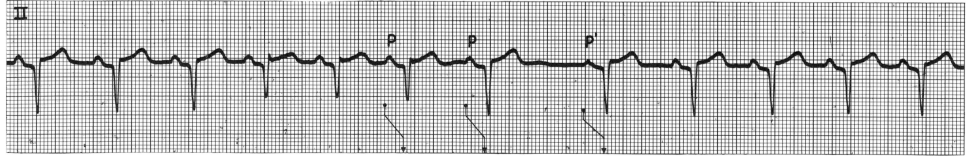

Rhythm 3-4,f. Sinus arrhythmia with average rate 70 per minute. A long pause is terminated by an atrial escape beat. Note the different configuration of the escape P′ wave.

Chapter 4

Atrial Ectopic Rhythms

Atrial ectopic rhythms, also called atrial tachyarrhythmias, are caused by the repetitive and rapid firing of one or more foci located anywhere in the atria other than in the sinus node. They consist of six or more consecutive atrial ectopic beats which temporarily seize control of the heart and render the slower sinus impulses ineffectual.

Classification of atrial ectopic rhythms

Atrial ectopic rhythms include atrial tachycardia, chaotic atrial rhythm, atrial flutter, and atrial fibrillation.

The most important of the factors that determine the occurrence of one atrial ectopic rhythm instead of another appears to be the discharge rate of the ectopic focus or foci. For convenience and for didactic reasons arbitrary rates have been set in the classification of the various atrial ectopic rhythms. These rates may provide a useful guide although it should be remembered that there is overlapping and that exceptions not infrequently occur.

Atrial Rates

Atrial tachycardia	140 to 220 per minute
Chaotic atrial rhythm	100 to 200 per minute
Atrial flutter	220 to 350 per minute
Atrial fibrillation	350 to 650 per minute

In addition to the atrial rate, the rhythm and the configuration of the atrial deflections are important factors for the differentiation of one atrial ectopic rhythm from the other. When an atrial tachyarrhythmia cannot be clearly categorized the term supraventricular tachycardia may be used.

Basic mechanism

The ectopic impulses spread through the atria, creating atrial deflections with a configuration different from that of the sinus P waves, and arrive at the A-V node which they try to traverse in order to reach the ventricles. When the atrial rate is slower than 180 to 200 per minute, every atrial ectopic impulse may be conducted to the ventricles (1:1 conduction). Physiological refractoriness in the A-V node is responsible for 2:1 conduction of atrial impulses, especially when their rate is faster than 180 to 200 per minute. Pathological increase of the A-V nodal refractory period and drug effect, particularly digitalis, cause higher degrees of block and variable A-V block.

In spreading down to the ventricles the ectopic atrial impulses (1) may follow the normal conduction sequence, giving rise to normal QRS complexes, or (2) may reach the bifurcation of the His bundle at a time when only one bundle branch can conduct while the other has not yet recovered from its refractory period; this results in the intermittent appearance of wide and bizarre QRS complexes (aberrant ventricular conduction). Permanent failure of conduction in one of the bundle branches (bundle branch block) causes all QRS complexes to become wide and bizarre; the atrial arrhythmia may then mimic ventricular tachycardia. Another cause of wide and bizarre QRS complexes in atrial ectopic rhythms is the Wolff-Parkinson-White syndrome.

ATRIAL TACHYCARDIA

This arrhythmia is also called paroxysmal atrial tachycardia (PAT) and results from the repetitive and rapid firing of an ectopic atrial focus at a rate usually between 140 and 220 beats per minute. The ectopic impulses spread through the atria in a fashion different from that of the sinus impulses, creating P' waves which replace the sinus P waves.

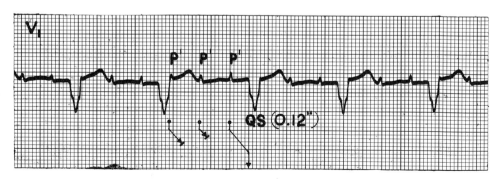

Fig. 4-1. Atrial tachycardia with 3:1 A-V block and bundle branch block.

Atrial deflections

The P' waves of atrial tachycardia have a rate usually between 140 and 220 per minute; during quinidine therapy the rate may be slower.

The P' wave rhythm is regular or slightly irregular. In short paroxysms of atrial tachycardia the rhythm may be more irregular.

The P′ waves are usually positive in lead II and negative in lead aVR, as in sinus rhythm. Their configuration, however, is somewhat different from that of the sinus P waves recorded in the same lead before or after the paroxysm of tachycardia. The baseline between the P′ waves is isoelectric.

A-V conduction

In untreated atrial tachycardia with atrial rate slower than 180 to 200 per minute all ectopic impulses may be conducted to the ventricles (1:1 conduction). Physiological refractoriness in the A-V node is responsible for 2:1 conduction of the atrial impulses, especially when their rate is faster than 180 to 200 per minute.

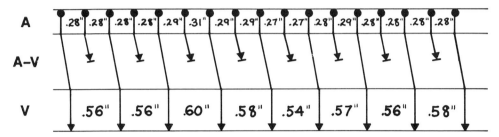

Fig. 4-2. Atrial tachycardia with 2:1 conduction. Ladder diagram of Rhythm 4-1,c.

Pathological increase of the A-V nodal refractory period and drug effect, especially digitalis, cause higher degrees of block and variable A-V block.

If 1:1 conduction continues to occur in spite of atrial rate faster than 180 to 200 per minute the presence of Wolff-Parkinson-White syndrome should be suspected; the circus movement present in this syndrome, in fact, frequently has a rate exceeding 200 per minute.

The P′-R interval may be short, normal or prolonged, depending on the conduction velocity in the A-V node. If the conduction is constant the P′-R interval is of constant duration. P′-R intervals of variable duration may be

associated (a) with regular ventricular response caused by A-V dissociation or complete A-V block, or (b) with regularly irregular ventricular response (group beating) caused by variable second degree A-V block.

The P′ wave immediately preceding the QRS complex may not be the one conducted to the ventricles, in which case it is called "skipped" P′ wave: an earlier P′ wave is responsible for the QRS complex and, in spreading to the ventricles, it "skips" one or more P′ waves inscribed in the P′-R interval.

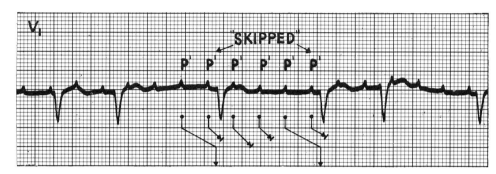

Fig. 4-3. Atrial tachycardia with variable A-V block. Note "skipped" P′ waves.

Ventricular deflections

The ventricular rate in untreated atrial tachycardia usually ranges between 140 and 180 per minute. A preexisting A-V conduction defect or drug treatment may induce 3:1, 4:1 (or greater) A-V block and cause slower ventricular rates.

The ventricular rhythm is regular or slightly irregular when the A-V conduction ratio is constant and when there is complete A-V block, and regularly irregular in the presence of variable A-V block.

In atrial tachycardia the QRS configuration may be entirely normal or may vary slightly because of superimposed P′ waves. Aberrant ventricular conduction is responsible for the intermittent occurrence of wide and bizarre QRS complexes, whereas in bundle branch block, the QRS configuration is consistently wide and

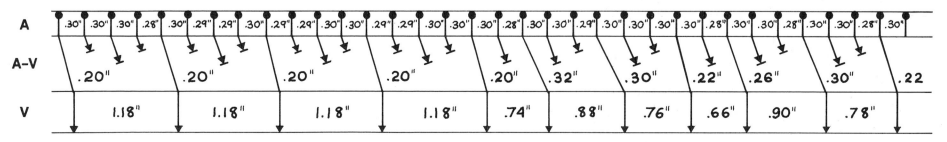

Fig. 4-4. Atrial tachycardia with 4:1 A-V block, then variable A-V block. Ladder diagram of Rhythm 4-1,d.

bizarre. Another cause for abnormal QRS complexes in atrial tachycardia is the Wolff-Parkinson-White syndrome.

CLINICAL NOTES

Atrial tachycardia is usually paroxysmal, with abrupt onset and termination and, therefore, is usually called paroxysmal atrial tachycardia (PAT). It may occur in apparently healthy individuals or in the presence of heart disease, especially rheumatic and coronary heart disease, and is often associated with the Wolff-Parkinson-White syndrome. Digitalis toxicity is the most frequent cause of atrial tachycardia with block. Less common causes include hyperthyroidism, acute or chronic lung disease and hypertension.

Healthy individuals tolerate paroxysmal atrial tachycardia fairly well when the ventricular rate is slower than 180 to 200 per minute. Patients with heart disease may develop angina, congestive heart failure or episodes of cerebral ischemia, owing to the reduction in cardiac output, even when the ventricular rate is not too rapid.

Atrial tachycardia is usually a transient arrhythmia and may sometimes be terminated by vagal stimulating maneuvers such as carotid sinus pressure. In the presence of heart disease drug treatment is often necessary and includes the use of digitalis. This drug, on the other hand, should be discontinued if atrial tachycardia with block appears during digitalis therapy. Other drugs used include propranolol, phenylephrine hydrochloride, quinidine, procainamide. Electrical cardioversion may be indicated.

CHAOTIC ATRIAL RHYTHM

This interesting arrhythmia is also called multifocal atrial tachycardia and is caused by the repetitive and rapid firing of two or more ectopic atrial foci at a rate usually between 100 and 200 per minute, though sometimes slower.

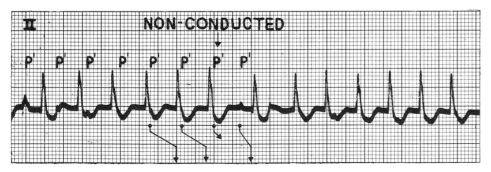

Fig. 4-5. Chaotic atrial rhythm (multifocal atrial tachycardia).

As in atrial tachycardia, the ectopic impulses spread through the atria in a fashion different from that of the sinus impulses, creating ectopic P' waves which replace the sinus P waves.

Atrial deflections

The P' waves of chaotic atrial rhythm have a rate usually between 100 and 200 per minute. In contrast to atrial tachycardia, the atrial rhythm is grossly irregular and the P' waves are of varying configuration. As in atrial tachycardia the baseline between the P' waves is isoelectric.

A-V conduction

The duration of the P'-R interval frequently changes from one beat to the next. Nonconducted P' waves may occur.

Ventricular deflections

The ventricular rate in untreated chaotic atrial rhythm usually ranges between 100 and 150 per minute. In most cases it is somewhat slower than the atrial rate, owing to the nonconducted P' waves. The ventricular rhythm is grossly irregular, owing to both the varying P'-R interval and the nonconducted P' waves, and the arrhythmia may simulate atrial fibrillation. The QRS configuration is usually normal but intermittent aberrant ventricular conduction is not uncommon. When bundle branch block is present all QRS complexes are wide and bizarre.

CLINICAL NOTES

Chaotic atrial rhythm almost always occurs in the presence of serious lung or heart disease. The most common cause is chronic cor pulmonale. Coronary heart disease with congestive heart failure and digitalis toxicity are also common causes. Many patients with chaotic atrial rhythm have diabetes mellitus.[42]

The treatment of chaotic atrial rhythm is primarily that of the underlying condition. Digitalis may be of value when congestive heart failure is present; however, if chaotic atrial rhythm appears during treatment with digitalis and toxicity is suspected, the drug should be discontinued and administration of potassium chloride, diphenylhydantoin or propranolol considered. Other drugs used to treat this arrhythmia include quinidine and procainamide. Attention to blood gases, adequate ventilation and serum electrolytes is of great importance inasmuch as the commonest cause is chronic cor pulmonale. Electrical cardioversion may be indicated when other measures have failed and the patient is not on digitalis.

ATRIAL FLUTTER

Atrial flutter results from the repetitive and rapid firing of an ectopic atrial focus (theory of unifocal impulse formation) at a rate usually between 220 and 350 per minute. Another theory postulates the presence of a circus movement in a ring of atrial tissue situated between the two venae cavae.

The ectopic impulses spread through the atria in a fashion different from that of the sinus impulses, creating "saw-tooth" flutter (F) waves which replace the sinus P waves.

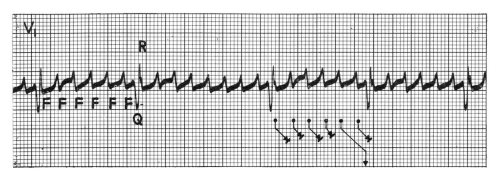

Fig. 4-6. Atrial flutter with variable A-V block.

Atrial deflections

The atrial flutter waves, or F waves, have a rate usually between 220 and 350 per minute. The rate may become slower than 220 per minute during quinidine therapy and faster than 350 per minute when digitalis is used.

The rhythm of the F waves is regular in untreated atrial flutter and slightly irregular following the use of drugs such as quinidine or digitalis. In short paroxysms of atrial flutter the F wave rhythm may become clearly irregular.

The F waves have a characteristic "saw-tooth" or "picket-fence" configuration, at least in some leads. They are identical in size and shape and in lead II no isoelectric baseline can be seen between them. In lead V_1 the flutter waves may resemble the P′ waves of atrial tachycardia; when this happens, the faster atrial rate may still allow the correct diagnosis of atrial flutter.

In atrial flutter with 2:1 conduction every other F wave may be hidden in the QRS complex and the rhythm then resembles sinus tachycardia, or atrial or A-V nodal tachycardia. Carotid sinus pressure in these cases may temporarily increase the degree of block and unmask the hidden F waves.

A-V conduction

In untreated atrial flutter every other F wave is not conducted to the ventricles because of the physiological refractory period of the A-V node (2:1 conduction). In very rare cases 1:1 conduction may occur in spite of the very rapid atrial

rate and the Wolff-Parkinson-White syndrome is almost invariably associated. Higher degrees of block and variable A-V block are seen when digitalis is used or when an A-V conduction defect was preexistent. Even-numbered A-V con-

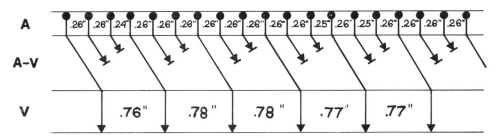

Fig. 4-7. Atrial flutter with 3:1 A-V block. Ladder diagram of Rhythm 4-3,c.

duction ratios, especially 4:1, are much more frequent than odd-numbered ratios.

The interval between the QRS complex and the preceding F wave (F-R interval) is of constant duration when the conduction ratio is constant. F-R intervals of variable duration may be associated (a) with regular ventricular response caused by A-V dissociation or complete A-V block, or (b) with regularly irregular ventricular response (group beating) caused by variable second degree A-V block.

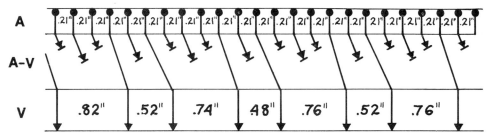

Fig. 4-8. Atrial flutter with variable 4:1 and 2:1 A-V block. Ladder diagram of Rhythm 4-3,e.

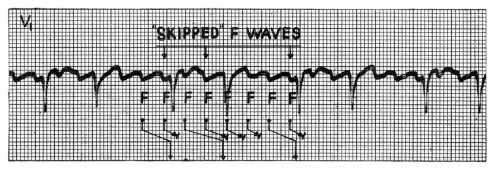

Fig. 4-9. Atrial flutter with variable 2:1 and 4:1 A-V block. Note group beating and "skipped" F waves.

The true F-R interval in most cases is believed to be between 0.25 and 0.45 second in duration. The F wave immediately preceding the QRS complex is usually not the one that is conducted to the ventricles and it is known as "skipped" F wave: an earlier F wave, in spreading to the ventricles, "skips" one or more F waves inscribed in the F-R interval.

Ventricular deflections

The ventricular rate is usually 150 to 160 per minute, since, in untreated atrial flutter, the atrial rate is often 300 to 320 per minute and there is 2:1 conduction. In rare cases of 1:1 conduction the QRS rate may be extremely rapid. Slower ventricular rates occur with 3:1, 4:1 or higher degrees of A-V block.

The ventricular rhythm is regular or slightly irregular when there is a constant A-V conduction ratio or complete A-V block, and regularly irregular (group beating) when there is variable second degree A-V block.

The QRS configuration is usually normal but rapid ventricular rates may be associated with intermittent aberrant ventricular conduction. The ST segment, the T waves and the QRS complexes may be deformed by the F waves. In the presence of bundle branch block or of the Wolff-Parkinson-White syndrome the wide and bizarre QRS complexes mimic ventricular tachycardia.

CLINICAL NOTES

Atrial flutter may be paroxysmal and occur in apparently healthy individuals. Often, however, it is chronic and occurs in the presence of heart disease such as rheumatic, coronary, hypertensive and congenital heart disease. Less common causes include hyperthyroidism and acute or chronic cor pulmonale.

Atrial flutter with fast ventricular rate may cause acute or chronic congestive heart failure, especially in elderly patients with severe forms of heart disease. Symptoms of myocardial and cerebral ischemia also frequently occur in such patients.

Atrial flutter is preferably treated with digitalis when the ventricular rate is rapid or if heart failure is present. The drug slows down the ventricular rate by increasing the refractory period of the A-V node and may, at the same time, increase the atrial rate, transforming the atrial flutter into atrial fibrillation. At times, withdrawal of digitalis causes conversion to normal sinus rhythm. In the rare case in which atrial flutter is caused by digitalis toxicity the drug, of course, should be discontinued.

Atrial flutter can usually be converted to normal sinus rhythm by low-energy DC precordial shock; the procedure can be performed more safely if the patient has not taken any digitalis for the previous 24 to 48 hours. Appropriate doses of quinidine can also induce conversion to normal sinus rhythm.

Following the conversion, quinidine and/or propranolol may be effective in preventing recurrences.

ATRIAL FIBRILLATION

Atrial fibrillation is caused by the repetitive and rapid firing of multiple ectopic atrial foci (theory of multifocal impulse formation) at a rate between 350 and 650 per minute. Other theories postulate the presence of a circus movement in a ring of atrial tissue situated between the two venae cavae (theory of unifocal impulse formation), or that atrial fibrillation originates in the sinus node or in a single ectopic atrial focus and is associated with multiple re-entry mechanisms in the atrial tissue (theory of multiple re-entry).

The atrial fibrillation impulses spread to the atria, creating very rapid and irregular waves which replace the sinus P waves.

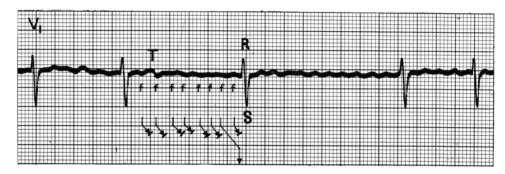

Fig. 4-10. Atrial fibrillation.

Atrial deflections

The normal sinus P waves are replaced by fibrillatory waves, called f waves in contrast to the F waves of atrial flutter. Their rate, often impossible to count with accuracy, varies between 350 and 650 per minute and their rhythm is clearly irregular.

The configuration of the f waves is typically variable: their size and shape continuously change. They are usually best seen in leads V$_1$ and II.

In "coarse" atrial fibrillation the f waves are prominent and, when they show some regularity resembling atrial flutter, the arrhythmia is called by some "flutter-fibrillation" or "impure flutter."

In "fine" atrial fibrillation the f waves are very small and may not be visible at all in some or most leads. When the f waves are not seen, the diagnosis of atrial fibrillation can still be made on the basis of the irregularly irregular ventricular rhythm with absent P waves.

A-V conduction

The physiological refractory period of the A-V node allows only a limited number of fibrillatory waves to be conducted to the ventricles. Many impulses penetrate the A-V node only partially, modifying its refractory period and thus influencing the conduction of subsequent impulses (concealed conduction). A prolonged refractory period in the A-V node, owing to disease or drug effect, especially digitalis, allows even fewer fibrillatory waves to reach the ventricles, causing slower ventricular response.

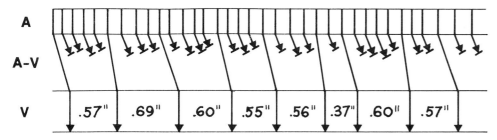

Fig. 4-11. Atrial fibrillation. Ladder diagram of Rhythm 4-4,b.

Ventricular deflections

In untreated atrial fibrillation the average ventricular rate usually ranges between 120 and 200 per minute. A ventricular response faster than 200 per minute is unusual and may be associated with the Wolff-Parkinson-White syndrome. Following treatment with digitalis or propranolol the refractory period of the A-V node lengthens and the ventricular rate becomes slower.

The ventricular rhythm is typically irregularly irregular. The irregularity is less noticeable with fast ventricular rates and more obvious with slow ventricular rates.

When the ventricular rhythm becomes regular in atrial fibrillation, high grade or complete A-V block has occurred and a focus located below the block (A-V nodal or ventricular) has taken over the control of the ventricles.

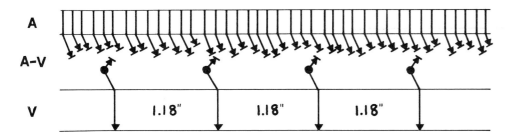

Fig. 4-12. Atrial fibrillation with high grade or complete A-V block and A-V nodal escape rhythm. Ladder diagram of Rhythm 4-4,g.

When A-V nodal impulses originating below the area of high grade or complete A-V block are conducted down to the ventricles with second degree A-V block

type I (Wenckebach), the ventricular rhythm in atrial fibrillation becomes regularly irregular, causing group beating.

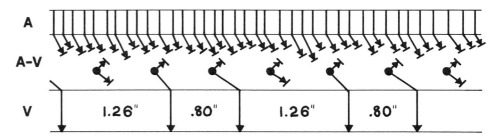

Fig. 4-13. Atrial fibrillation with high grade or complete A-V block and nonparoxysmal A-V nodal tachycardia. The conducted A-V nodal impulses reach the ventricles with second degree A-V block type I (Wenckebach). This is the ladder diagram of Rhythm 4-4,f.

The QRS complexes may be normal in configuration but their amplitude may vary, owing to superimposed f waves or to respiratory changes. Occasional wide and bizarre QRS complexes due to intermittent aberrant ventricular conduction are not infrequently seen, especially with fast ventricular rates. Bundle branch block causes all QRS complexes to be wide and bizarre and the rhythm may then mimic ventricular tachycardia. Another cause for wide and bizarre QRS complexes in atrial fibrillation is the Wolff-Parkinson-White syndrome.

CLINICAL NOTES

Atrial fibrillation may be paroxysmal and may occur in apparently healthy individuals. Most often, however, it persists for long periods of time and is associated with heart disease such as rheumatic, coronary, or hypertensive heart disease, particularly in the presence of congestive heart failure. Less common causes include cardiomyopathy, hyperthyroidism, acute or chronic cor pulmonale, pericarditis and, very seldom, digitalis toxicity. The use of digitalis in atrial tachycardia or atrial flutter may change the rhythm into atrial fibrillation.

Atrial fibrillation is more likely to cause symptoms when the average ventricular rate is rapid and heart disease is present, especially when complicated by congestive heart failure. Angina and symptoms of cerebral ischemia may be caused or aggravated by atrial fibrillation with rapid ventricular response.

Atrial fibrillation is most often treated with digitalis; the drug decreases the ventricular rate and sometimes causes conversion to normal sinus rhythm. Propranolol may be useful in slowing the ventricular rate when therapeutic doses of digitalis are ineffective. Electrical cardioversion with DC precordial shock is performed in selected cases after withholding digitalis for 24 to 48 hours. Following conversion to sinus rhythm quinidine may be effective in preventing recurrences.

Atrial Tachycardia (PAT)

Ectopic rhythm due to the repetitive and rapid firing of an ectopic
atrial focus at a rate usually between 140 and 220 per minute.

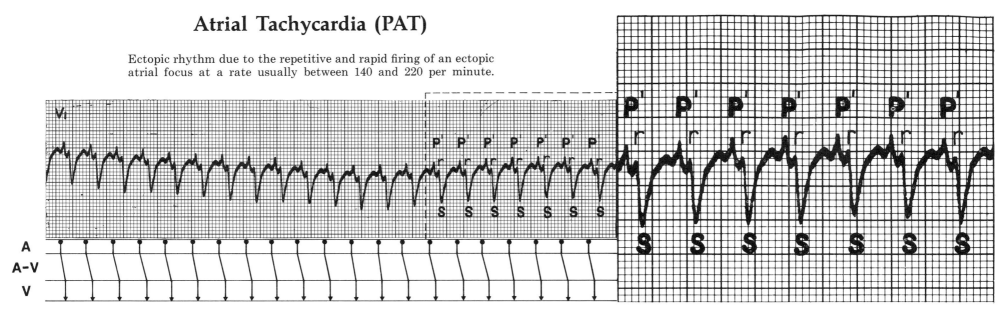

Rhythm 4-1,a. Atrial tachycardia with rate 190 per minute and 1:1 conduction.

ELECTROCARDIOGRAPHIC CRITERIA

A. Atrial deflections:

1. Rate: usually between 140 and 220 per minute.
   During quinidine therapy the atrial rate may
   be slower.
2. Rhythm: regular or slightly irregular. In short
   paroxysms of atrial tachycardia the atrial
   rhythm may be more irregular.
3. Configuration:
   a. P′ waves usually positive in lead II and neg-
      ative in lead aVR, as in sinus rhythm. Their
      configuration, however, is somewhat differ-
      ent from that of the sinus P waves.
   b. Isoelectric baseline between P′ waves.
   c. "Skipped" P′ waves may occur.

B. A-V conduction:

1. P′-R interval of constant duration (short, normal or prolonged): constant A-V conduction
   ratio.
2. P′-R interval of variable duration:
   a. With regular ventricular response: A-V dis-
      sociation or complete A-V block.
   b. With regularly irregular ventricular re-
      sponse (group beating): variable second de-
      gree A-V block.

C. Ventricular deflections:

1. Rate (usually between 140 and 180 per minute):
   a. Same as the atrial rate: 1:1 conduction.
   b. One half the atrial rate: 2:1 conduction.

   c. 1/3, 1/4, (etc.) the atrial rate: 3:1, 4:1 (etc.)
      A-V block.
2. Rhythm:
   a. Regular: constant A-V conduction ratio or
      complete A-V block.
   b. Regularly irregular (group beating): varia-
      ble second degree A-V block.
3. Configuration:
   a. Normal.
   b. Wide and bizarre: intermittent aberrant
      ventricular conduction, bundle branch block
      or Wolff-Parkinson-White syndrome.

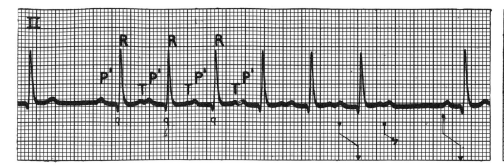

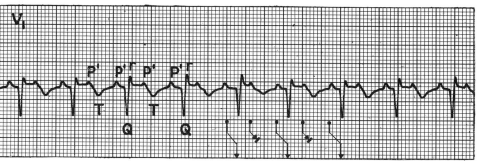

Rhythm 4-1,b. Sinus rhythm and short paroxysms of atrial tachycardia with 1:1 conduction and rate of about 120 per minute. Note the configuration of the P′ waves slightly different from that of the sinus P waves and the slightly irregular rhythm.

Rhythm 4-1,c. Atrial tachycardia with 2:1 conduction. The atrial rate is 210 per minute and the ventricular rate 105 per minute. The ventricular rhythm is slightly irregular.

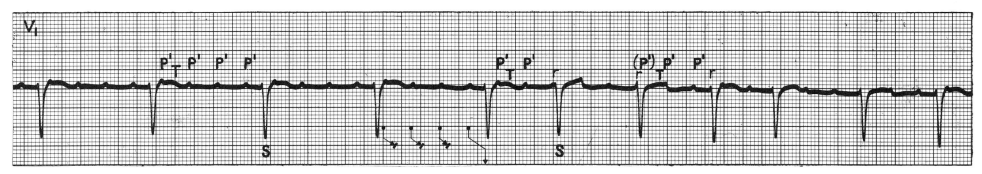

Rhythm 4-1,d. Atrial tachycardia with 4:1 A-V block in the first half of the strip and variable A-V block in the other half. The atrial rate is 200 per minute; the ventricular rate is 50 per minute at first, then it averages 75 per minute.

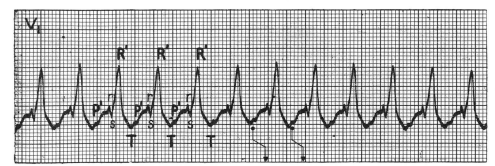

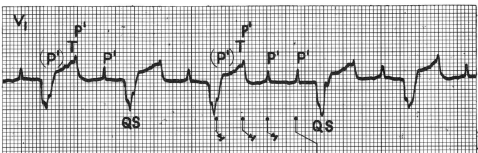

Rhythm 4-1,e. Atrial tachycardia with 1:1 conduction and bundle branch block, mimicking ventricular tachycardia. The rate is 140 per minute.

Rhythm 4-1,f. Atrial tachycardia with variable (3:1 and 4:1) second degree A-V block and bundle branch block. The atrial rate is 200 per minute and the average ventricular rate 60 per minute.

Chaotic Atrial Rhythm (Multifocal Atrial Tachycardia)

Ectopic rhythm due to the repetitive and rapid firing of two or more ectopic atrial foci at a rate usually between 100 and 200 per minute.

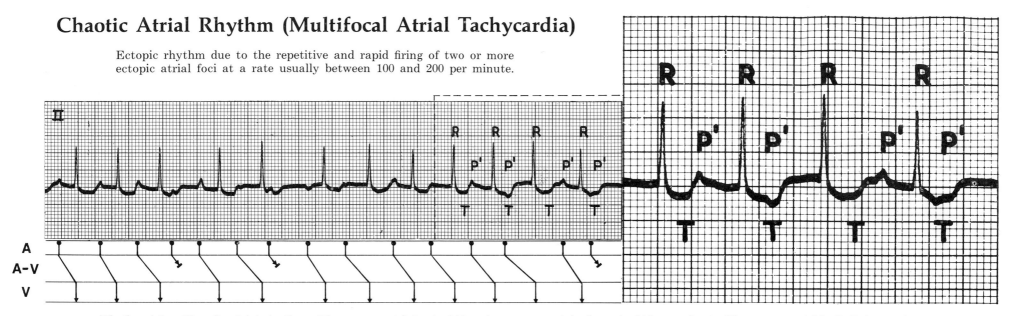

Rhythm 4-2,a. Chaotic atrial rhythm with average atrial rate 140 and average ventricular rate 110 per minute. There are variable P′-R intervals and non-conducted P′ waves.

ELECTROCARDIOGRAPHIC CRITERIA

A. Atrial deflections:

1. Rate: between 100 and 200 per minute, occasionally slower.
2. Rhythm: grossly irregular.
3. Configuration:
   a. P′ waves of varying shape and contour.
   b. Isoelectric baseline between P′ waves.

B. A-V conduction:

1. P′-R interval of varying duration.
2. Nonconducted P′ waves may occur.

C. Ventricular deflections:

1. Rate: usually 100 to 150 per minute in untreated cases.
2. Rhythm: grossly irregular (may mimic atrial fibrillation).
3. Configuration:
   a. Normal.
   b. Wide and bizarre: intermittent aberrant ventricular conduction or bundle branch block.

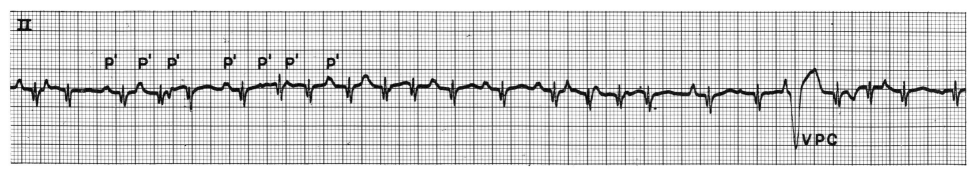

Rhythm 4-2,b. Chaotic atrial rhythm with average ventricular rate 130 per minute. Note the irregular atrial rhythm, the P′ waves of varying configuration, and the varying P′-R intervals. The wide and bizarre QRS complex near the end of the strip probably represents a VPC.

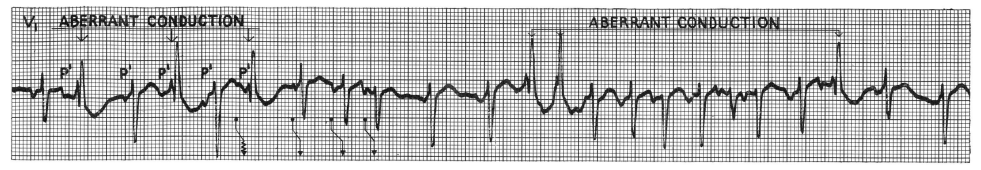

Rhythm 4-2,c. Chaotic atrial rhythm with frequent aberrant ventricular conduction simulating VPC's isolated or in pairs. The average ventricular rate is 135 per minute and the tracing mimics atrial fibrillation.

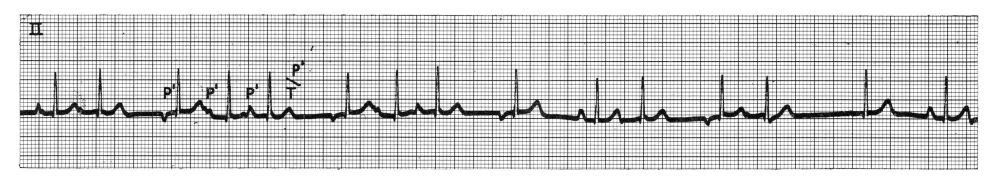

Rhythm 4-2,d. Chaotic atrial rhythm with average ventricular rate 90 per minute. Note the P' waves of varying configuration, the P'-R intervals of varying duration and the irregular rhythm.

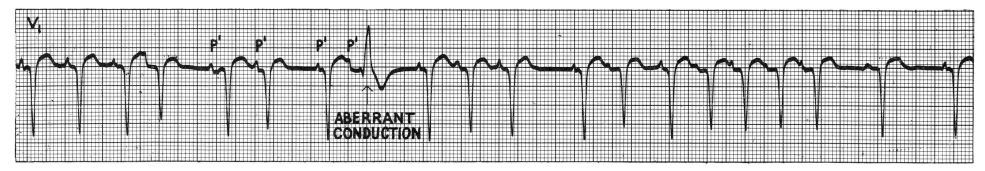

Rhythm 4-2,e. Chaotic atrial rhythm with one aberrantly conducted beat mimicking a VPC. The average ventricular rate is 115 per minute.

Atrial Flutter

Ectopic rhythm due to the repetitive and rapid firing of an ectopic atrial focus (theory of unifocal impulse formation) at a rate usually between 220 and 350 per minute.

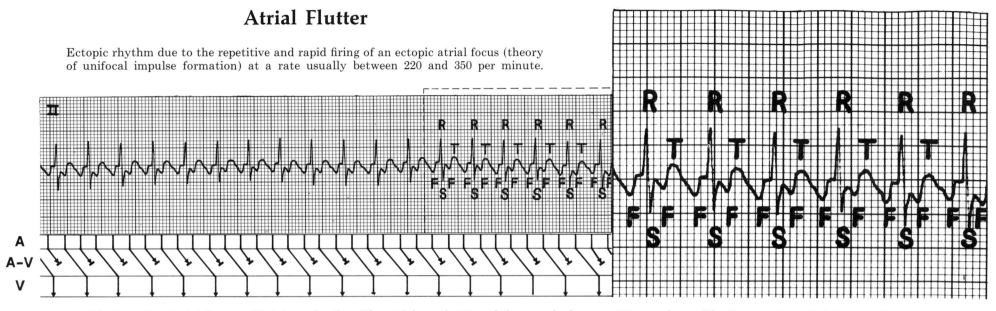

Rhythm 4-3,a. Atrial flutter with 2:1 conduction. The atrial rate is 320 and the ventricular rate 160 per minute. The F waves immediately preceding the QRS complexes are not the ones conducted to the ventricles ("skipped" F waves).

ELECTROCARDIOGRAPHIC CRITERIA

A. Atrial deflections:

1. Rate: between 220 and 350 per minute. During quinidine therapy the atrial rate may become slower than 220 per minute.
2. Rhythm: regular or slightly irregular.
3. Configuration:
   a. "Saw-tooth" F waves, identical in size and shape.
   b. No isoelectric baseline between F waves in lead II.
   c. "Skipped" F waves may occur.

B. A-V conduction:

1. F-R interval of constant duration: constant A-V conduction ratio.
2. F-R interval of variable duration:
   a. With regular ventricular response: A-V dissociation or complete A-V block.
   b. With regularly irregular ventricular response (group beating): variable second degree A-V block.

C. Ventricular deflections:

1. Rate (usually 150 to 160 per minute in untreated atrial flutter):
   a. Same as the atrial rate: 1:1 conduction.
   b. One half the atrial rate: 2:1 conduction.
   c. $\frac{1}{3}$, $\frac{1}{4}$, etc. the atrial rate: 3:1, 4:1, etc. A-V block.
2. Rhythm:
   a. Regular or slightly irregular: constant A-V conduction ratio or complete A-V block.
   b. Regularly irregular (group beating): variable second degree A-V block.
3. Configuration (the F waves may deform ST-T and QRS):
   a. Normal.
   b. Wide and bizarre: intermittent aberrant ventricular conduction, bundle branch block or Wolff-Parkinson-White syndrome.

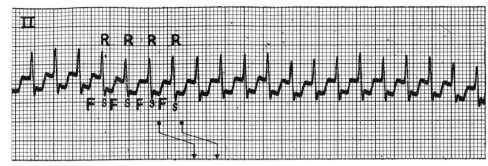

Rhythm 4-3,b. Atrial flutter at a rate of 250 per minute with 1:1 conduction. Each ectopic atrial impulse is conducted to the ventricles.

Rhythm 4-3,c. Atrial flutter with 3:1 A-V block. The atrial rate is 228 and the ventricular rate 76 per minute.

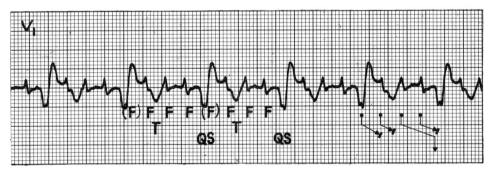

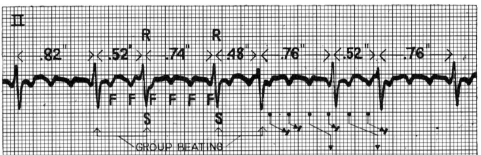

Rhythm 4-3,d. Atrial flutter with 4:1 A-V block. A flutter wave is hidden within each QRS complex and the one immediately preceding the QRS is a "skipped" F wave. The atrial rate is 280 and the ventricular rate 70 per minute.

Rhythm 4-3,e. Atrial flutter with variable 2:1 and 4:1 second degree A-V block. Note the "skipped" F waves and the group beating. The average ventricular rate is 88 per minute.

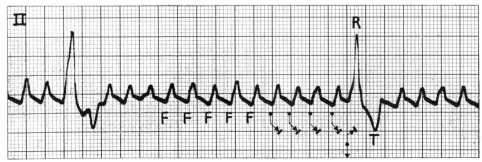

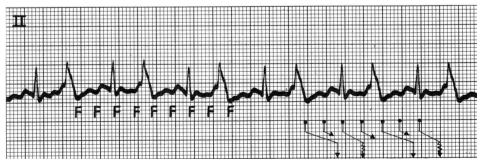

Rhythm 4-3,f. Atrial flutter with complete A-V block. The ventricular rate is only 20 per minute. Flutter waves deform the QRS complex, the ST segment and the T wave.

Rhythm 4-3,g. Atrial flutter with 2:1 conduction and intermittent aberrant ventricular conduction mimicking VPC's in bigeminy. The atrial rate is 300 and the ventricular rate 150 per minute.

Atrial Fibrillation

Ectopic rhythm due to the repetitive and rapid firing of multiple ectopic atrial foci (theory of multifocal impulse formation) at a rate between 350 and 650 per minute.

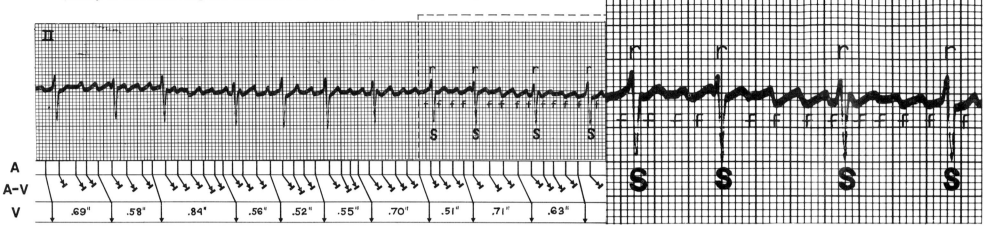

Rhythm 4-4,a. "Coarse" atrial fibrillation with average ventricular rate 90 per minute. The rhythm of the f waves is irregular and their configuration is typically variable: their size and shape continuously change.

ELECTROCARDIOGRAPHIC CRITERIA

A. Atrial deflections:

1. Rate: usually between 350 and 650 per minute.
2. Rhythm: irregular.
3. Varying configuration and amplitude:
   a. Usually best seen in leads V_1 and II.
   b. Prominent f waves ("coarse" atrial fibrillation). When these prominent waves show some regularity resembling atrial flutter, the arrhythmia is called by some "flutter-fibrillation" or "impure flutter."
   c. Small f waves which in some leads may not be visible at all ("fine" atrial fibrillation).

B. Ventricular deflections:

1. Rate: usually averages 120 to 200 per minute in untreated atrial fibrillation.
2. Rhythm:
   a. Irregularly irregular. The faster the ventricular rate, the less obvious the irregularity.
   b. Regular: high grade or complete A-V block. A focus located below the block (A-V nodal or ventricular) controls the ventricles.
   c. Regularly irregular (group beating): high grade or complete A-V block. A-V nodal impulses originating below the block are conducted to the ventricles with variable second degree A-V block.
3. Configuration (the f waves may deform ST-T and QRS):
   a. Normal, sometimes of varying amplitude.
   b. Wide and bizarre: intermittent aberrant ventricular conduction, bundle branch block or Wolff-Parkinson-White syndrome.

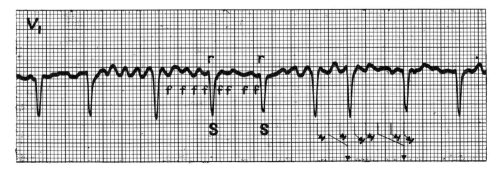

Rhythm 4-4,b. "Coarse" atrial fibrillation with average ventricular rate 100 per minute.

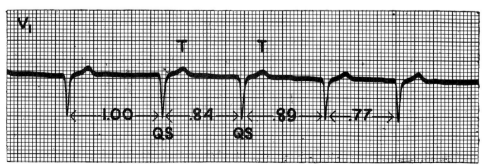

Rhythm 4-4,c. "Fine" atrial fibrillation with average ventricular rate 70 per minute. The f waves are almost not visible at all. The correct diagnosis can still be made on the basis of the irregularly irregular ventricular rhythm with absent P waves.

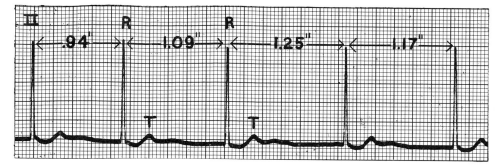

Rhythm 4-4,d. "Fine" atrial fibrillation with slow ventricular rate averaging 52 per minute.

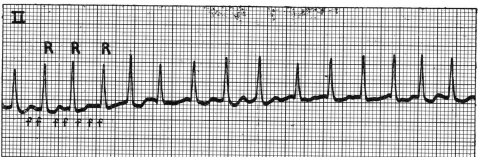

Rhythm 4-4,e. Atrial fibrillation with fast ventricular rate averaging 170 per minute. The irregularity is much less obvious. Note the f waves deforming the ST segment and T wave.

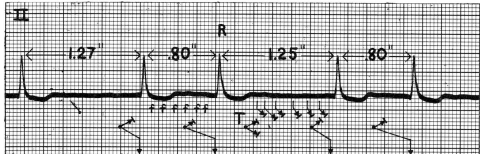

Rhythm 4-4,f. "Fine" atrial fibrillation with high grade or complete A-V block. A-V nodal impulses arising below the block are conducted to the ventricles with second degree A-V block type I and cause group beating.

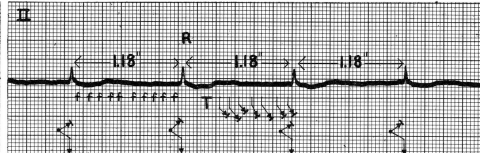

Rhythm 4-4,g. "Fine" atrial fibrillation with high grade or complete A-V block and A-V nodal escape rhythm. Note the regular ventricular rhythm at a rate of 52 per minute.

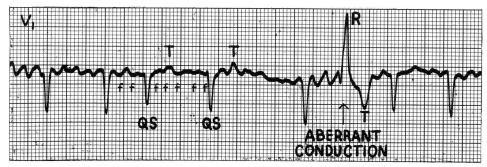

Rhythm 4-4,h. "Coarse" atrial fibrillation. One beat shows aberrant ventricular conduction mimicking a VPC.

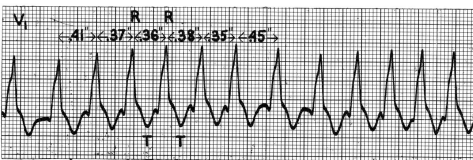

Rhythm 4-4,i. Atrial fibrillation with bundle branch block mimicking ventricular tachycardia. The correct interpretation can be made by noticing the irregularly irregular ventricular rhythm.

Chapter 5

A-V Nodal Ectopic Rhythms

Idionodal escape rhythm	40 to 60 per minute
Nonparoxysmal A-V nodal tachycardia	60 to 160 per minute
Paroxysmal A-V nodal tachycardia	160 to 220 per minute

A-V nodal ectopic rhythms result from the repetitive firing of an ectopic focus located within or in the immediate vicinity of the A-V node. They consist of six or more consecutive A-V nodal ectopic beats which temporarily seize control of the ventricles and, if the impulses can be conducted retrogradely, of the atria as well.

Some investigators have suggested that the A-V node does not have pacemaking cells and that ectopic activity probably originates in the His bundle and not in the A-V node. A-V nodal ectopic rhythms are therefore called by some His bundle rhythms or junctional rhythms.[7,34] Since the old terminology is well established and still widely used,[5,12,16,18] we shall continue to use the term A-V nodal to describe pacemaking activity that originates within or in the immediate vicinity of the A-V node.

Classification of A-V nodal ectopic rhythms

A-V nodal pacemaking foci have an inherent or natural firing rate of 40 to 60 per minute. Under normal circumstances the faster sinus or ectopic atrial impulses continuously discharge the slower A-V nodal impulses before they can be fired. When the sinus or ectopic atrial foci fail to fire or when their impulses fail to reach the A-V node, an A-V nodal focus can manifest its activity and temporarily control the ventricles, the atria, or both. The resulting "passive" rhythm is called *idionodal escape rhythm.*

An A-V nodal focus may also acquire enhanced automaticity and produce impulses at a rate faster than 60 per minute but usually not exceeding 220 per minute. Under these circumstances the A-V node can temporarily seize control of the heart with an "active" rhythm called *A-V nodal tachycardia.* A-V nodal tachycardia is divided in two categories, according to the discharge rate of the A-V nodal focus: nonparoxysmal, and paroxysmal. In nonparoxysmal A-V nodal tachycardia the rate is 60 to 160 per minute, whereas in the paroxysmal form the rate is 160 to 220 per minute.

The inverted P' waves*

The ectopic A-V nodal impulses, whatever their rate, may spread forward to the ventricles and backward to the atria. In spreading backward to the atria they create inverted P' waves (negative in lead II where the sinus P waves are positive, and positive in lead aVR where the sinus P waves are negative) which precede, are hidden within, or follow the QRS complexes, according to the order in which the atria and the ventricles are activated.

When the P' waves precede the QRS complexes the A-V nodal ectopic rhythm is called "high" nodal, on the assumption that the pacemaking focus is located high in the A-V node and therefore its impulses are able to reach the atria before they can reach the ventricles. When the P' waves cannot be seen because they are hidden within the QRS complexes and when the P' waves follow the QRS complexes, the rhythm is called "mid" and "low" nodal respectively, on the assumption that the pacemaking focus in the A-V node is located in the mid portion and in the low portion respectively.

In fact, what determines the order of activation of atria and ventricles is not the location of the ectopic focus in the A-V node but the conduction velocity above and below the A-V nodal focus. The inverted P' waves precede the QRS complexes ("high" nodal) when retrograde conduction of its impulses is *faster* than forward conduction and follow the QRS complexes ("low" nodal) when retrograde conduction is *slower* than forward conduction, regardless of the location of the focus in the A-V node. The absence of inverted P' waves preceding or following the QRS complexes of A-V nodal origin may have one of the following causes: (1) the A-V nodal impulses reach both the atria and the ventricles at the same time and thus the P' waves are hidden within the QRS complexes ("mid" nodal), or (2) the presence of A-V dissociation or block above the A-V nodal focus prevents the A-V nodal impulses from reaching the atria which thus continue to beat undisturbed. Diagrams illustrating the potential relationship between retrograde and forward conduction in A-V nodal ectopic beats are shown in Chapter 3.

The terms "high," "mid" and "low" nodal are well established and very useful in describing the relationship between the P wave and the QRS complex when A-V nodal tachycardia is recorded, and we shall continue to use them for didactic reasons. The quotation marks will serve as a reminder that these terms do not reflect the location of the ectopic focus in the A-V node.

*The text of this section is nearly identical to that on the same subject in Chapter 3. It is being repeated here for the convenience of the reader.

IDIONODAL ESCAPE RHYTHM

This rhythm is the result of the repetitive firing of an ectopic A-V nodal focus at a rate of 40 to 60 per minute. This passive rhythm consists of a succession of six or more A-V nodal escape beats. The ectopic impulses may spread backward to the atria, creating inverted P′ waves which replace the sinus P waves, and forward to the ventricles.

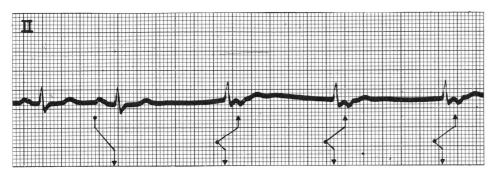

Fig. 5-1. Normal sinus rhythm followed by "low" idionodal escape rhythm.

Atrial deflections

When visible, the retrograde P′ waves of idionodal escape rhythm have a rate between 40 and 60 per minute and a regular or slightly irregular rhythm. They are inverted as compared to the sinus P waves, being negative in lead II and positive in lead aVR; in lead V_1 they are completely positive without the terminal negative component often present in sinus rhythm. The inverted P′ waves precede, are hidden within, or follow the QRS complexes of nodal origin ("high," "mid" or "low" idionodal escape rhythm).

During idionodal escape rhythm the atria may be under the control of sinus impulses or of ectopic atrial impulses (atrial tachycardia, flutter and fibrillation) which cannot reach the A-V node because of A-V dissociation or because of block above the A-V nodal focus.

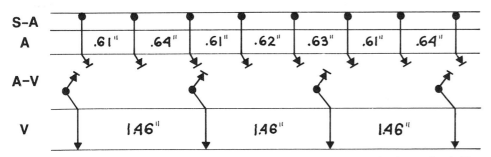

Fig. 5-2. Idionodal escape rhythm during sinus rhythm and block above the A-V nodal focus. Ladder diagram of the first half of Rhythm 5-1,*c*.

A-V or V-A conduction

In "high" idionodal escape rhythm the duration of the P′-R interval usually does not exceed 0.12 second. When there is conduction delay below the focus, however, the P′-R interval may become of normal duration or prolonged (as compared to the length of the P-R interval of normal sinus rhythm).

In "low" idionodal escape rhythm the R-P′ interval is usually 0.10 to 0.20 second in duration. When there is conduction delay above the A-V nodal focus the R-P′ interval becomes longer and may exceed 0.20 second.

Ventricular deflections

The ventricular rate is 40 to 60 per minute and the rhythm usually regular or slightly irregular. At the onset of an idionodal escape rhythm the rate may gradually increase for the first few beats; this is called the Treppe phenomenon and is due to a "warming up" process of the dormant A-V nodal focus.

The QRS configuration may be entirely normal or slightly different from that of the normal sinus beats. Bundle branch block causes wide and bizarre QRS complexes.

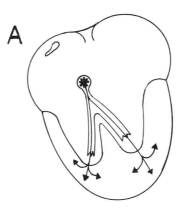 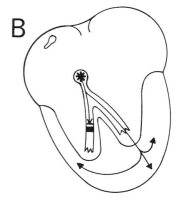

Fig. 5-3. Diagrams illustrating the spreading of an ectopic A-V nodal impulse to the ventricles. (*Left*) Normal conduction to the ventricles. (*Right*) Abnormal conduction to the ventricles because of block of the impulse in the right bundle branch.

CLINICAL NOTES

Any of the causes of sinus bradycardia, sinus arrest, sino-atrial block and A-V block may produce idionodal escape rhythm. They include coronary and rheumatic heart disease, myocarditis, many other cardiac and noncardiac diseases, and drugs such as digitalis, reserpine and guanethidine.

The reduction in cardiac output associated with the slow ventricular rate may induce angina and cause or aggravate congestive heart failure. The treatment is directed toward the underlying cause and may require discontinuance of the causative drug, the use of atropine sulfate, isoproterenol or artificial pacing.

A-V NODAL TACHYCARDIA

A-V nodal tachycardia, also called accelerated A-V nodal rhythm, is caused by the repetitive firing of an ectopic A-V nodal focus at a rate faster than its inherent or natural rate of 40 to 60 per minute. This "active" rhythm consists of a succession of six or more A-V nodal extrasystoles.

According to the discharge rate of the ectopic A-V nodal focus, A-V nodal tachycardia is divided in two forms: *nonparoxysmal* and *paroxysmal*.

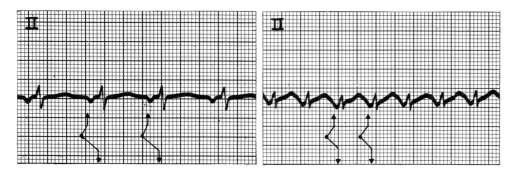

Fig. 5-4. Nonparoxysmal (rate 95 per minute) and paroxysmal (rate 170 per minute) "high" nodal tachycardia.

Atrial deflections

When visible, the retrograde P' waves of A-V nodal tachycardia have a rate between 60 and 160 per minute (nonparoxysmal form) or between 160 and 220 per minute (paroxysmal form). The rhythm of the P' waves is regular or slightly irregular.

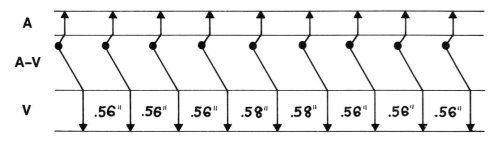

Fig. 5-5. Nonparoxysmal "high" nodal tachycardia. Ladder diagram of Rhythm 5-2,b.

The P' waves are inverted as compared to the sinus P waves, being negative in lead II and positive in lead aVR; in lead V₁ they are completely positive without the terminal negative component often present in sinus P waves. The inverted P' waves precede, are hidden within, or follow the QRS complexes of nodal origin ("high," "mid," or "low" A-V nodal tachycardia).

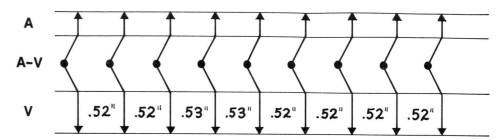

Fig. 5-6. Nonparoxysmal "mid" nodal tachycardia. Ladder diagram of Rhythm 5-2,d.

During A-V nodal tachycardia the atria may be under the control of sinus impulses or of ectopic atrial impulses (atrial tachycardia, flutter and fibrillation) which cannot reach the A-V node because of A-V dissociation or because of block above the A-V nodal focus.

A-V and V-A conduction

In untreated A-V nodal tachycardia with rate of the ectopic focus slower than 180 to 200 per minute, all A-V nodal impulses may be conducted to the ventricles (1:1 conduction). Physiological refractoriness below the A-V nodal focus is responsible for 2:1 conduction of the ectopic impulses, especially when the rate is faster than 180 to 200 per minute. If 1:1 conduction continues to occur in spite of A-V nodal rate faster than 180 to 200 per minute, the presence of Wolff-Parkinson-White syndrome should be suspected. Pathological increase of the refractory period and drug effect, especially digitalis, cause higher degrees of block and variable A-V block.

In "high" A-V nodal tachycardia the P'-R interval usually does not exceed 0.12 second in duration. When there is conduction delay below the focus, however, the P'-R interval becomes of normal length or prolonged (as compared with the length of the P-R interval of normal sinus rhythm).

The P'-R interval is of constant duration when the conduction velocity above and below the A-V nodal focus is constant. Variable duration of the P'-R interval may result from (a) variable speed of retrograde and forward conduction, or (b) the presence of two A-V nodal foci, one above and the other below an area of block (double A-V nodal rhythm, producing A-V dissociation).

In "low" A-V nodal tachycardia the duration of the R-P′ interval is often 0.10 to 0.20 second. When there is conduction delay above the focus the R-P′ interval becomes longer and may exceed 0.20 second.

Ventricular deflections

The ventricular rate is the same as the atrial when all A-V nodal impulses are conducted to the ventricles (1:1 conduction). When the A-V nodal rate exceeds 180 to 200 per minute the ventricular rate usually becomes half that of the atria (2:1 conduction). Slower ventricular rates occur with 3:1, 4:1 or higher degrees of A-V block.

The ventricular rhythm is regular or slightly irregular when the A-V conduction ratio is constant. Variable second degree A-V block below the A-V nodal focus produces regularly irregular ventricular rhythm and may cause group beating.

The QRS configuration may be entirely normal or slightly different from that of the normal sinus beats. The intermittent occurrence of wide and bizarre QRS complexes may result from aberrant ventricular conduction. Bundle branch block causes all the QRS complexes to become wide and bizarre. Another cause for wide and bizarre QRS configuration in A-V nodal tachycardia is the Wolff-Parkinson-White syndrome.

CLINICAL NOTES

Nonparoxysmal A-V nodal tachycardia almost always occurs in the presence of cardiac disease, especially rheumatic and coronary heart disease, or it is caused by digitalis toxicity. Less common causes include cardiomyopathies, hypertensive heart disease, infections and intracardiac surgery.[69] Often of gradual onset and termination, its rate can be temporarily slowed by carotid sinus pressure, as in sinus rhythm.

The paroxysmal form frequently occurs in healthy individuals but may also complicate heart disease. It is of sudden onset and termination and carotid sinus pressure either terminates the tachycardia abruptly or has no effect at all.

A-V nodal tachycardia causes no symptoms when the ventricular rate is relatively slow. Fast ventricular rates may induce or aggravate heart failure and symptoms of myocardial and cerebral ischemia, especially in elderly patients with advanced heart disease.

Nonparoxysmal A-V nodal tachycardia is often difficult to treat. If caused by digitalis toxicity the drug should be discontinued. Atropine may accelerate the sinus rhythm and overdrive the A-V nodal focus. Suppressive drugs such as quinidine, lidocaine, procainamide and propranolol and, in selected cases, the use of DC cardioversion may prove effective in restoring normal sinus rhythm.

Paroxysmal A-V nodal tachycardia is often of brief duration and does not require any treatment. Carotid sinus pressure may terminate the arrhythmia. In persistent cases, digitalization or DC precordial shock are often beneficial.

Idionodal Escape Rhythm

Ectopic rhythm due to the repetitive firing of an
A-V nodal focus at a rate of 40 to 60 per minute.

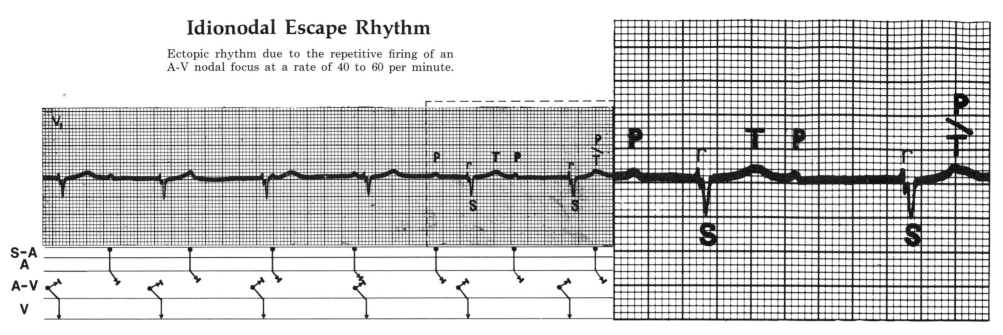

Rhythm 5-1,a. Idionodal escape rhythm at a rate of 50 per minute. The atria are under the control of the sinus node. The sinus impulses cannot
reach the A-V node and the A-V nodal impulses cannot spread retrogradely to the atria, because of block above the A-V nodal focus.

ELECTROCARDIOGRAPHIC CRITERIA

A. Atrial deflections:

1. Rate: between 40 and 60 per minute.
2. Rhythm: regular or slightly irregular.
3. Configuration:
   a. Inverted P′ waves which precede, are hidden within, or follow the QRS complexes of nodal origin ("high," "mid," or "low" idionodal escape rhythm).
   b. The atria may be under the control of sinus impulses or of ectopic atrial impulses which cannot reach the A-V node because of A-V dissociation or because of block above the A-V nodal focus.

B. A-V and V-A conduction:

1. "High" idionodal escape rhythm:
   a. P′-R interval 0.12 second or shorter.
   b. P′-R interval longer than 0.12 second when there is conduction delay below the A-V nodal focus.
2. "Low" idionodal escape rhythm:
   a. R-P′ interval 0.10 to 0.20 second.
   b. R-P′ interval longer than 0.20 second when there is conduction delay above the A-V nodal focus.

C. Ventricular deflections:

1. Rate: 40 to 60 per minute.
2. Rhythm: regular or slightly irregular.
3. Configuration:
   a. Normal or slightly aberrant.
   b. Wide and bizarre: bundle branch block.

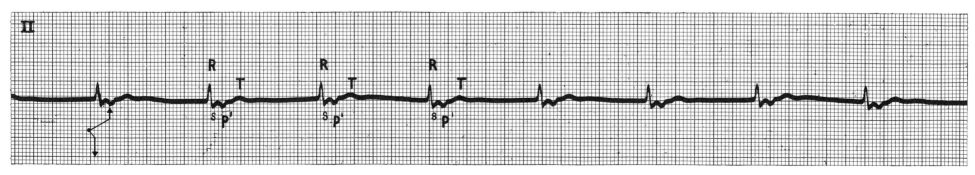

Rhythm 5-1,b. "Low" idionodal escape rhythm at a rate of 52 per minute.

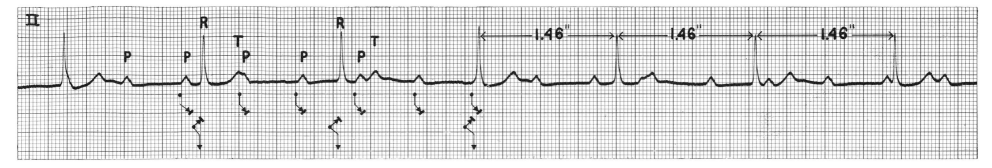

Rhythm 5-1,c. Idionodal escape rhythm at a rate of 41 per minute. Sinus rhythm controls the atria and there is block above the A-V nodal focus.

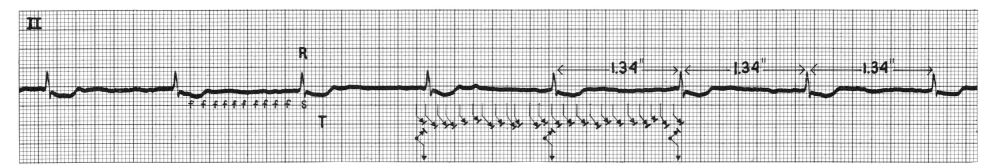

Rhythm 5-1,d. Atrial fibrillation and idionodal escape rhythm at a rate of 44 per minute. The atrial fibrillation impulses cannot reach the A-V node and the ventricles because of block above the A-V nodal focus.

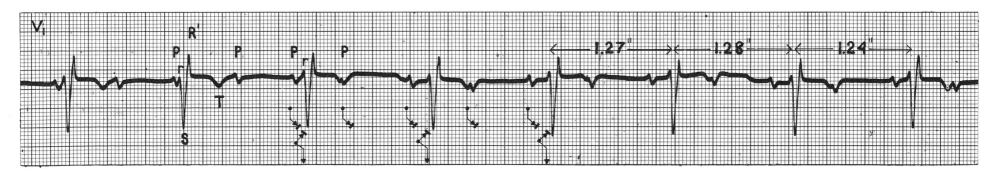

Rhythm 5-1,e. Idionodal escape rhythm at a rate of about 47 per minute. The ventricular rhythm is slightly irregular and the QRS complexes are wide and bizarre because of bundle branch block. The sinus node controls the atria and its impulses cannot reach the A-V node and the ventricles because of block above the A-V nodal focus.

A-V Nodal Tachycardia

Ectopic rhythm due to the repetitive firing of an A-V nodal focus at a rate of 60 to 160 per minute (nonparoxysmal form) or 160 to 220 per minute (paroxysmal form).

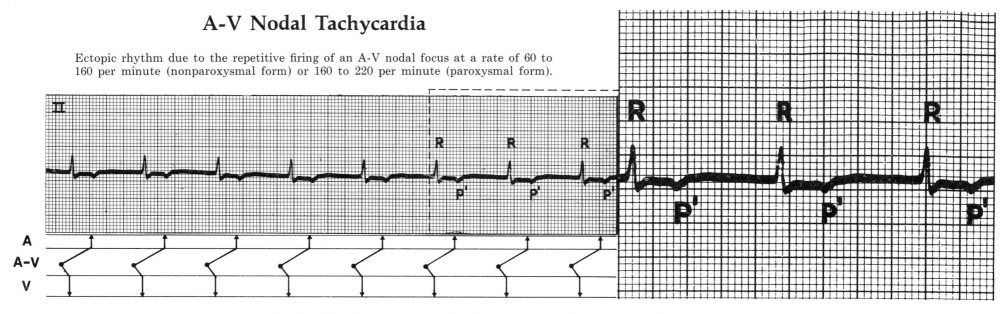

Rhythm 5-2,a. Non-paroxysmal "low" nodal tachycardia at a rate of 70 per minute.

ELECTROCARDIOGRAPHIC CRITERIA

A. Atrial deflections:

1. Rate:
   a. Nonparoxysmal A-V nodal tachycardia: between 60 and 160 per minute.
   b. Paroxysmal A-V nodal tachycardia: between 160 and 220 per minute.
2. Rhythm regular or slightly irregular.
3. Configuration:
   a. Inverted P' waves which precede, are hidden within or follow the QRS complexes of nodal origin ("high," "mid," or "low" A-V nodal tachycardia).
   b. The atria may be under the control of sinus impulses or of ectopic atrial impulses which cannot reach the A-V node and the ventricles because of A-V dissociation or because of block above the A-V nodal focus.

B. A-V and V-A conduction:

1. "High" A-V nodal tachycardia:
   a. P'-R interval 0.12 second or shorter; longer than 0.12 second when there is conduction delay below the A-V nodal focus.
   b. P'-R interval of constant length: constant conduction velocity above and below the A-V nodal focus.
   c. P'-R interval of variable length:
      1. Variable speed of retrograde and forward conduction
      2. Double A-V nodal rhythm (two A-V nodal foci, one above and the other below an area of block).
2. "Low" A-V nodal tachycardia:
   a. R-P' interval 0.10 to 0.20 second.
   b. R-P' interval longer than 0.20 second when there is conduction delay above the A-V nodal focus.

C. Ventricular deflections:

1. Rate:
   a. Same as the atrial: 1:1 conduction.
   b. One half the atrial: 2:1 conduction.
   c. $\frac{1}{3}$, $\frac{1}{4}$, etc. the atrial: 3:1, 4:1, etc. A-V block.
2. Rhythm:
   a. Regular or slightly irregular.
   b. Regularly irregular (group beating).
3. Configuration:
   a. Normal or slightly aberrant.
   b. Wide and bizarre: intermittent aberrant ventricular conduction, bundle branch block or Wolff-Parkinson-White syndrome.

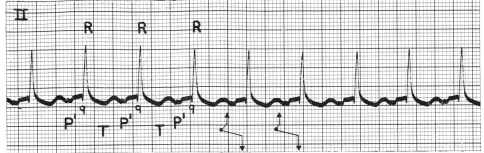

Rhythm 5-2,b. Nonparoxysmal "high" nodal tachycardia at a rate of 102 per minute.

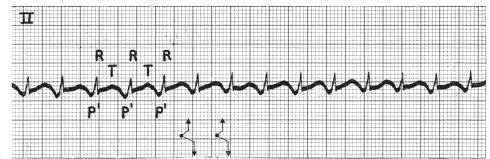

Rhythm 5-2,c. Paroxysmal "high" nodal tachycardia at a rate of 170 per minute and 1:1 conduction.

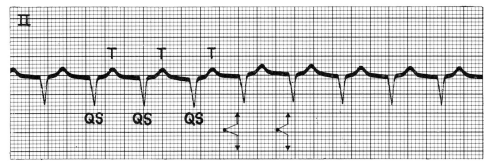

Rhythm 5-2,d. Nonparoxysmal "mid" nodal tachycardia. The rate is 115 per minute.

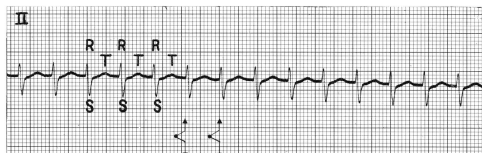

Rhythm 5-2,e. Paroxysmal "mid" nodal tachycardia. The rate is 170 per minute.

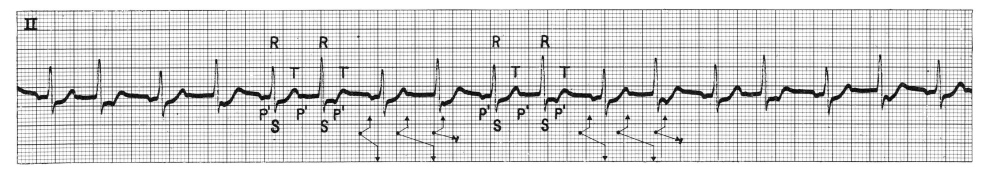

Rhythm 5-2,f. Nonparoxysmal A-V nodal tachycardia with 3:2 second degree A-V block (Wenckebach) below the nodal focus. The atrial rate is 155 per minute and the average ventricular rate 104 per minute.

Chapter 6

A-V Dissociation

A-V dissociation is a dual rhythm during which the atria and the ventricles beat independently of each other under the control of separate pacemaking foci. The sinus node or an atrial focus controlling the atria and an A-V nodal or ventricular focus controlling the ventricles can coexist without continuously discharging each other because either (1) their rates are nearly identical, or (2) their rates are different but incomplete block (forward or retrograde) prevents the impulses of the faster focus from reaching and discharging the slower one.

When there is complete interruption of conduction between the atria and the ventricles, the atria and the ventricles also beat independently but the mechanism is fundamentally different; in order to avoid confusion, this arrhythmia should be called complete A-V block and not A-V dissociation.

A-V dissociation has also been called "interference dissociation" and "dissociation with interference" but the term interference has been used by different authors in completely different senses and, in order to avoid confusion, this term will not be used in this book.

Mechanism of production

The mechanism producing A-V dissociation is either a disturbance in impulse formation or a disturbance in impulse conduction. Sometimes both mechanisms operate in the same patient.

Disturbance in impulse formation. In sinus bradycardia, marked sinus arrhythmia or inhibition of the sinus node by a retroconducted ectopic impulse, slowing of the sinus rate may allow an A-V nodal or a ventricular focus to escape and take control of the ventricles, causing dissociation. A-V dissociation also occurs when an A-V nodal or ventricular focus acquires enhanced automaticity and seizes control of the ventricles while the sinus node or an ectopic atrial focus continues to activate the atria.

Disturbance in impulse conduction. In second degree A-V block, slowing of the ventricular rate may allow an A-V nodal focus (located below the area of block) or a ventricular focus to activate the ventricles independently of the atria and cause A-V dissociation.

When the rate of the pacemaking focus controlling the atria is nearly identical to the rate of the focus controlling the ventricles, the two foci can coexist because their impulses spread to the respective heart chambers almost simultaneously. When their rate is different, on the other hand, incomplete block (forward or retrograde) must be present between the two foci in order for A-V dissociation to occur.

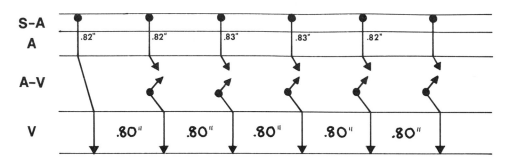

Fig. 6-1. A-V dissociation between sinus rhythm and non-paroxysmal A-V nodal tachycardia. The rate of the sinus node and that of the A-V node are nearly identical. Ladder diagram of the first half of Rhythm 6-1,b.

A faster sinus or ectopic atrial focus can coexist with a slower A-V nodal or ventricular focus when second degree A-V block prevents some of the more rapid atrial impulses from reaching the A-V node and the ventricles. Similarly, a faster A-V nodal or ventricular focus can coexist with a slower sinus or ectopic atrial focus if retrograde block prevents the more rapid A-V nodal or ventricular impulses from reaching the atria. Differential refractoriness within the A-V node is another mechanism which can prevent faster A-V nodal or ventricular impulses from reaching the atria and the sinus node; this phenomenon is discussed and illustrated in Chapter 10.

In A-V dissociation the two rhythms, one controlling the atria and the other the ventricles, may be completely independent of each other. Impulses from the atria, on the other hand, may occasionally succeed in reaching the A-V node and the ventricles, causing so-called ventricular captures and ventricular fusion beats. Conversely, impulses from the A-V node or the ventricles may occasionally reach the atria and cause so-called atrial captures and atrial fusion beats.

Ventricular captures and fusion beats

While A-V dissociation is present, impulses from the focus controlling the atria (sinus or ectopic) may occasionally be conducted to the ventricles and "capture" them. This occurs whenever a sinus or ectopic supraventricular impulse arrives at an opportune time, once the A-V nodal and ventricular pathways have recovered from their activation by the preceding impulse.

If both the ventricles are completely activated by the capturing impulse, a ventricular capture occurs. When, on the other hand, the capturing impulse

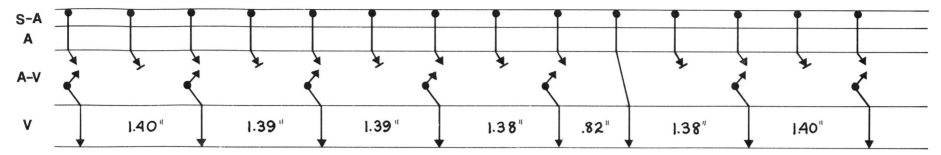

Fig. 6-2. Sinus rhythm with 2:1 A-V block. A-V dissociation is present between every other sinus impulse and an idionodal escape rhythm. One sinus impulse reaches the ventricles (ventricular capture). Ladder diagram of Rhythm 6-1d.

succeeds in activating only part of the ventricles, while an ectopic ventricular impulse activates the remainder, then a ventricular fusion beat (incomplete capture) occurs.

It should be remembered that captures and fusion beats are named after the cardiac chambers that are captured and not after the capturing impulse. For example, a sinus impulse in reaching the ventricles during A-V dissociation produces a ventricular capture and not a sinus capture. Similarly, an A-V nodal impulse conducted retrogradely to the atria produces an atrial capture and not an A-V nodal capture.

A *ventricular capture* appears as a premature beat during A-V dissociation, always related to a preceding P wave when the atrial mechanism is sinus rhythm. Its QRS complex is usually normal in configuration. The pause following an isolated ventricular capture has the same duration as the interval between two consecutive QRS complexes of the dominant ventricular rhythm (noncompensatory pause).

A *ventricular fusion beat* also appears as a premature beat during A-V dissociation, always related to a preceding P wave when the atrial mechanism is sinus rhythm. Its QRS complex has a configuration intermediate between that of a ventricular capture and that of an ectopic ventricular beat, and can be recognized with certainty only when a ventricular capture is present in the same tracing: the intermediate contour of the fusion beat can then be easily spotted. Varying degrees of ventricular fusion may occur and the QRS complex of the fusion beat resembles the ventricular capture more when most of the ventricles are invaded by the capturing impulse, whereas it resembles the ectopic ventricular beat more when most of the ventricles are invaded by the ectopic ventricular impulse. The pause following an isolated ventricular fusion beat has the same duration as the interval between two consecutive QRS complexes of the dominant ventricular rhythm (noncompensatory pause).

Atrial captures and fusion beats

While A-V dissociation is present, impulses from the focus controlling the ventricles (A-V nodal or ventricular) may occasionally be conducted retrogradely

to the atria and "capture" them. This occurs whenever an A-V nodal or ventricular impulse arrives at an opportune time once the atria have recovered from their activation by the preceding impulse. When the atrial rhythm is flutter or fibrillation it is impossible for atrial captures to occur, because the atria are continuously rendered refractory by the rapid atrial flutter or fibrillation impulses.

If the atria are both completely activated by the capturing impulse, an atrial capture occurs. When, on the other hand, the capturing impulse activates only part of the atria while the sinus or atrial tachycardia impulse activates the remainder, then an atrial fusion beat (incomplete capture) occurs.

An *atrial capture* appears as a premature and inverted P′ wave which follows a QRS complex during A-V dissociation. An *atrial fusion beat* appears as a premature and deformed P′ wave which has a configuration intermediate between that of an atrial capture and that of a sinus P wave. Varying degrees of atrial fusion may occur and the fusion P′ wave resembles the atrial capture more when most of the atria are invaded by the capturing impulse, whereas it resembles the sinus P wave more when most of the atria are invaded by the sinus impulse.

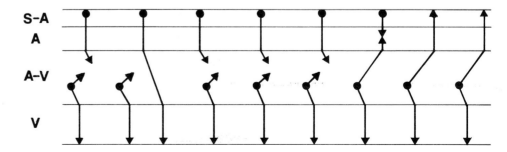

Fig. 6-3. Diagram of A-V dissociation between sinus rhythm and nonparoxysmal A-V nodal tachycardia. The 3rd ventricular arrow represents a ventricular capture by the sinus impulse. The last three atrial arrows represent an atrial fusion beat followed by two atrial captures.

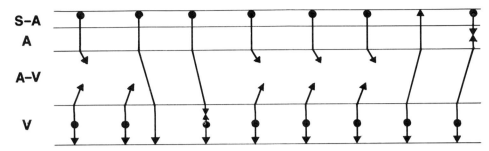

Fig. 6-4. Diagram of A-V dissociation between sinus rhythm and nonparoxysmal ventricular tachycardia. The 3rd ventricular arrow represents a ventricular capture by the sinus impulse, the 4th, a ventricular fusion beat. The last two atrial arrows represent an atrial capture followed by an atrial fusion beat.

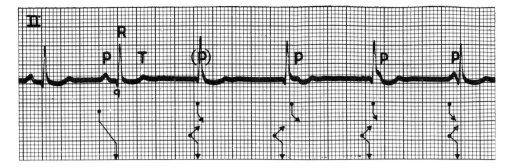

Fig. 6-5. A-V dissociation between the sinus node and the A-V node (sinus arrhythmia and non-paroxysmal A-V nodal tachycardia). The first two beats are ventricular captures by sinus impulses.

Types of A-V dissociation

A-V dissociation may occur:

1. Between the *sinus node* (or ectopic atrial foci) and the *A-V node*: the atrial mechanism is sinus rhythm, atrial tachycardia, flutter or fibrillation, while the A-V node controls the ventricles. This form of A-V dissociation may be seen with idionodal escape rhythm or A-V nodal tachycardia.

2. Between the *sinus node* (or ectopic supraventricular foci) and a *ventricular focus*: the atrial mechanism is sinus rhythm, atrial tachycardia, atrial flutter, atrial fibrillation or A-V nodal rhythm, while a ventricular focus controls the ventricles. This form of A-V dissociation may be seen in ventricular tachycardia.

3. Between the *sinus node* (or ectopic supraventricular foci) and an *artificial ventricular pacemaker*.

4. Between *two A-V nodal foci*, one situated above and the other below an area of block (double A-V nodal rhythm).

The most frequent form of A-V dissociation occurs between the sinus node and the A-V node.

A-V DISSOCIATION BETWEEN THE SINUS AND THE A-V NODE

The atria are under the control of the sinus node and the ventricles under the control of the A-V node. The two foci can coexist either because their rates are nearly identical or because there is incomplete block between them. When their rates are nearly identical the dissociation is called *isorhythmic*.

The sinus impulses spread through the atria, creating normal P waves, but cannot reach the ventricles because the A-V nodal impulses reach them first and render them refractory. The A-V nodal impulses, on their part, spread to the ventricles but cannot reach the atria rendered refractory by the sinus impulses. The two rhythms are independent and, as a result, the P waves bear no constant relationship to the QRS complexes as in normal sinus rhythm.

Atrial deflections

The atrial rate is that of sinus bradycardia (below 60 per minute), normal sinus rhythm (60 to 100 per minute), or sinus tachycardia (above 100 per minute). The sinus P waves have a slightly irregular rhythm and a constant configuration. Sinus arrhythmia causes a more irregular P wave rhythm.

When there is retrograde conduction to the atria, an inverted premature P′ wave follows a QRS complex of A-V nodal origin (atrial capture). Atrial fusion beats appear as deformed premature P′ waves with a configuration intermediate between that of an atrial capture and that of a sinus P wave.

A-V conduction

The sinus P waves bear no constant relationship to the QRS complexes of A-V nodal origin: the P waves "travel" toward, inside, and away from them. As a result, the apparent "P-R interval" continuously changes in duration.

Sinus P waves occasionally may be conducted to the ventricles with a normal or prolonged P-R interval (ventricular captures).

When A-V dissociation is superimposed on second degree A-V block, the *conductible* P waves (every other P wave in 2:1 A-V block, every third in 3:1 A-V block, etc.) are the ones that "travel" toward, inside, and away from the QRS complexes.

Ventricular deflections

The ventricular rate is between 40 and 220 per minute, depending on the rate of the A-V nodal focus.

The ventricular rhythm is regular or slightly irregular. Isolated ventricular captures appear as premature QRS complexes preceded by a P wave and followed by a pause that has the same duration as the interval between two consecutive QRS complexes of A-V nodal origin (noncompensatory pause).

The configuration of the QRS complexes is normal or slightly aberrant. Ventricular captures may display a normal QRS complex or a wide and bizarre QRS complex because of intermittent aberrant ventricular conduction. When bundle branch block is present, all QRS complexes, including the ventricular captures, have a wide and bizarre configuration.

CLINICAL NOTES

The clinical significance of A-V dissociation is that of the underlying disturbance in impulse formation or conduction. Digitalis toxicity is a very frequent etiologic factor.

The treatment should be directed toward the underlying cause and the basic rhythm disorder. When digitalis toxicity is present the drug should be discontinued. Atropine sulfate may be helpful in accelerating the sinus rate and overriding the A-V nodal focus.

A-V Dissociation Between Sinus Node and A-V Node

Dual rhythm generated by two independent pacemaking foci: the sinus node activating the atria and the A-V node activating the ventricles. The two foci can coexist because their rates are nearly identical or because there is incomplete block between them.

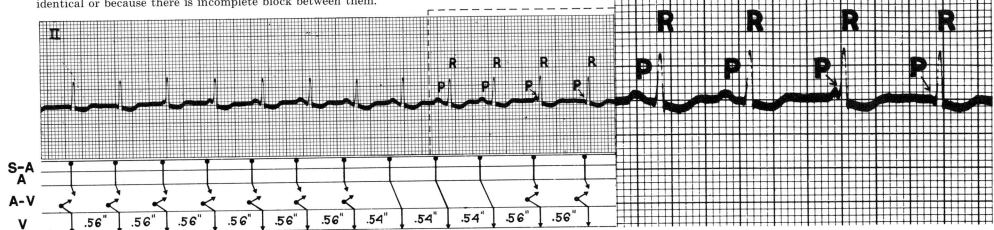

Rhythm 6-1,a. A-V dissociation between sinus and A-V node. The two foci have a nearly identical rate of about 110 per minute. The P wave "travels" away from, and toward the QRS complex. Three ventricular captures are present.

ELECTROCARDIOGRAPHIC CRITERIA

A. Atrial deflections:

1. Rate, rhythm and configuration of sinus P waves.
2. When there is retrograde conduction to the atria a premature, inverted or deformed P′ wave follows the QRS complex (atrial capture or atrial fusion beat).

B. A-V conduction:

1. The sinus P waves bear no constant relationship to the QRS complexes: the P waves "travel" toward, inside and away from them. The apparent "P-R interval" continuously changes in duration.
2. When second degree A-V block is present the conductible P waves (every other one in 2:1 A-V block, every third one in 3:1 A-V block, etc.) are the ones that "travel" toward, inside, and away from the QRS complexes.
3. Sinus P waves may be conducted to the ventricles with a normal or prolonged P-R interval (ventricular captures).

C. Ventricular deflections:

1. Rate: between 40 and 220 per minute, depending on the rate of the A-V nodal focus.
2. Rhythm:
   a. Regular or slightly irregular.
   b. Ventricular capture: premature QRS complex preceded by a P wave and followed by a noncompensatory pause.
3. Configuration:
   a. Normal or slightly aberrant.
   b. Wide and bizarre: intermittent aberrant ventricular conduction or bundle branch block.

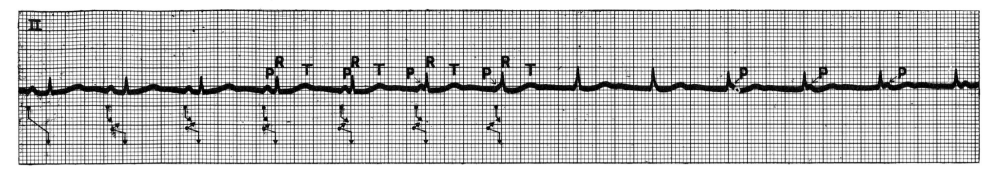

Rhythm 6-1,b. A-V dissociation between the sinus and the A-V node. The first QRS is of sinus origin then the P wave "travels" toward, inside and beyond the QRS complexes of A-V nodal origin.

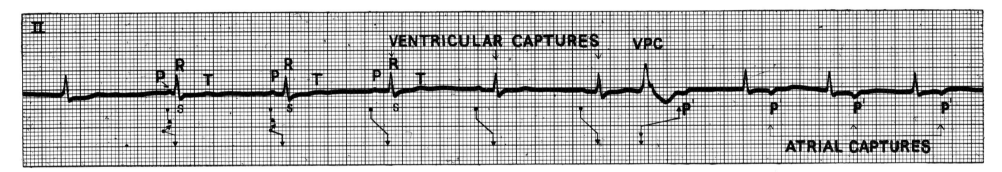

Rhythm 6-1,c. A-V dissociation between the sinus and the A-V node. The fourth, fifth, and sixth QRS complexes are ventricular captures by sinus impulses. After a VPC followed by retrograde conduction to the atria, three QRS complexes of A-V nodal origin occur, each followed by an atrial capture.

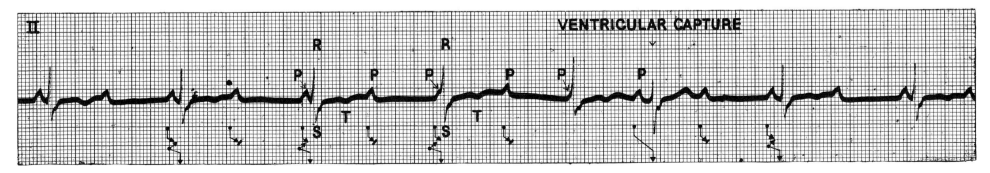

Rhythm 6-1,d. A-V dissociation between sinus and A-V node, superimposed on 2:1 second degree A-V block. The conductible P waves (every other one) "travel" toward and away from the QRS. The premature QRS complex is a ventricular capture by the sinus impulse.

Chapter 7

Atrioventricular (A-V) Block

Conduction of sinus or ectopic supraventricular impulses to the ventricles may be delayed or blocked because of prolongation of the refractory period in the A-V node or in both the bundle branches. The resulting arrhythmia is called atrioventricular (A-V) block.

Delay or failure of conduction may also occur as a normal event whenever a sinus or ectopic supraventricular impulse reaches the A-V node or the bundle branches too early, before they have recovered from their normal refractory period. In this case the use of the term block, which implies a pathological event, should be avoided. An atrial premature beat, for example, which falls on the T wave of the previous beat and is not conducted to the ventricles is more correctly called nonconducted atrial extrasystole rather than blocked atrial extrasystole. For the same reason, atrial flutter with 2:1 conduction is a better term than atrial flutter with 2:1 A-V block.

Classification of A-V block and mechanism of A-V conduction

A-V block is divided in two categories: incomplete and complete. Incomplete A-V block is subdivided into first degree, second degree (which includes type I and type II) and high grade. Complete A-V block is also called third degree.

In *first degree* A-V block all sinus or ectopic supraventricular impulses are conducted to the ventricles but conduction occurs with delay. This results in a prolonged P-R interval.

In *second degree* A-V block some sinus or ectopic supraventricular impulses are blocked while others are conducted to the ventricles with or without delay. Type I is characterized by progressive prolongation of the P-R interval before a blocked P wave, whereas in type II the P-R interval of the conducted beats is of constant duration. The two types of second degree A-V block are called by some "Mobitz type I" and "Mobitz type II." Type I is also referred to as "the Wenckebach phenomenon" or "Wenckebach A-V block," and type II as "Mobitz type A-V block." We will call the two categories type I (Wenckebach) and type II (Mobitz) or simply type I and type II.

In *high grade* A-V block two or more consecutive impulses are blocked causing long ventricular pauses.

Complete A-V block occurs when all sinus or ectopic supraventricular impulses fail to reach the ventricles. A rescuing A-V nodal or ventricular focus usually takes over the control of the ventricles.

FIRST DEGREE A-V BLOCK

First degree A-V block is due to prolongation of the relative refractory period in the A-V node or in both bundle branches. This causes a delay in the conduction of the sinus or ectopic supraventricular impulses to the ventricles and results in a prolonged P-R interval.

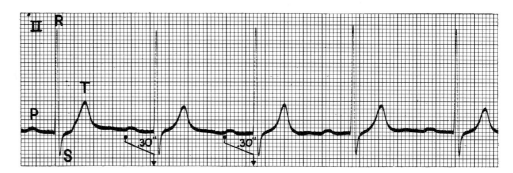

Fig. 7-1. First degree A-V block. The P-R interval measures 0.30 second.

Atrial deflections

The rate, rhythm and configuration of the atrial deflections depend upon the atrial mechanism which may be sinus or ectopic. When the P-R interval is very long or the rate is rapid, the P wave may become superimposed on the preceding T wave ("P on T").

A-V conduction

The P-R interval is longer than 0.21 second. Its duration may reach 0.60 second or even 0.80 second.

The P-R duration is usually constant although it may vary slightly with changes in heart rate, as in sinus arrhythmia.

Ventricular deflections

The ventricular rate and rhythm are the same as the atrial. The QRS configuration may be normal or, if bundle branch block is present, wide and bizarre.

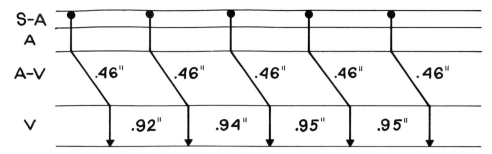

Fig. 7-2. First degree A-V block. Ladder diagram of the first half of Rhythm 7-1d.

First degree A-V block associated with bundle branch block may be caused by incomplete bilateral bundle branch block: the conduction delay responsible for the prolonged P-R interval may be occurring in the other bundle branch rather than in the A-V node.

CLINICAL NOTES

First degree A-V block may occur in apparently normal individuals.[55] More frequently, however, it is associated with heart disease, especially acute myocardial infarction and rheumatic fever. Excessive doses of digitalis, propranolol, quinidine, procainamide, and electrolyte imbalance such as hyperkalemia may also cause first degree A-V block.

The treatment of first degree A-V block is that of the underlying condition. When the conduction disturbance is of acute onset the patient should be monitored for possible increase in the degree of block.

SECOND DEGREE A-V BLOCK
TYPE I (WENCKEBACH)

Type I (Wenckebach) second degree A-V block is due to prolongation of both the absolute and the relative refractory periods of the A-V node. The conduction of the sinus or ectopic supraventricular impulses to the ventricles becomes progressively more difficult, causing progressively longer P-R intervals until a P wave is blocked and a ventricular pause occurs. The pause enables the A-V node to recover and the following P wave is again conducted, starting a new sequence. The greatest increment in prolongation of the P-R interval occurs between the first and the second P-R after the pause; the increments then become progressively smaller. For this reason, while the P-R intervals become progressively longer, the R-R intervals become progressively shorter before the pause.

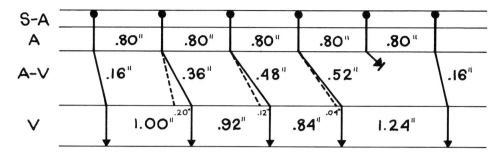

Fig. 7-3. Ladder diagram of type I (Wenckebach) second degree A-V block during sinus rhythm. The P-R interval progressively lengthens until a blocked P wave occurs. Following the blocked P wave the P-R interval returns to its original duration of 0.16 second. Note the progressive shortening of the R-R interval before the pause, due to the progressively smaller increments (small numbers) in the prolongation of the P-R interval.

Atrial deflections

The rate, rhythm and configuration of the atrial deflections depend upon the atrial mechanism which may be sinus or ectopic. The atrial wave immediately preceding the QRS complex may not be the one conducted to the ventricles in which case it is called "skipped" P, P' or F wave.

A-V conduction

The P-R interval grows progressively *longer* until a P wave is blocked and a ventricular pause occurs. The P-R interval following the pause is the shortest of the sequence and may be normal or abnormal in duration. The greatest increment in duration of the P-R interval occurs between the first and the second P-R after the pause.

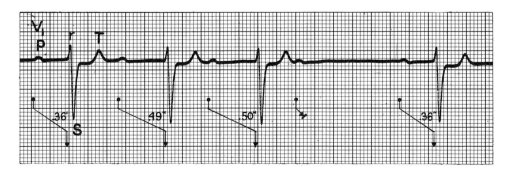

Fig. 7-4. Sinus rhythm with second degree A-V block type I. The P-R interval following the pause is the shortest of the sequence but is abnormal in duration.

The conduction ratio, or number of P waves to number of conducted QRS complexes in each so-called Wenckebach sequence, may be 2:1, 3:2, 4:3, 5:4 or greater, and may vary in the same tracing.

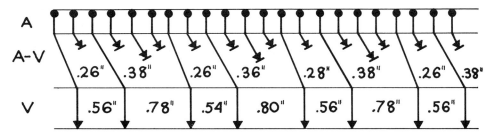

Fig. 7-5. Atrial flutter with second degree A-V block type I. The conduction ratio alternates between 2:1 and 4:1. Ladder diagram of Rhythm 7-2,f.

Second degree A-V block with 2:1 conduction ratio may be either type I (Wenckebach) or type II (Mobitz). When long and repeated rhythm strips fail to slow at least one Wenckebach sequence with a 3:2 or greater conduction ratio, the 2:1 block is considered type II.

Ventricular deflections

The ventricular rate is always slower than the atrial rate because of the blocked atrial waves.

The ventricular rhythm is regularly irregular with groups of QRS complexes separated by pauses (group beating). The R-R interval in each group becomes progressively *shorter* until the pause occurs; the pause measures less than twice the preceding R-R interval. In "atypical" Wenckebach sequences the R-R interval may fail to become shorter as expected or may suddenly lengthen.

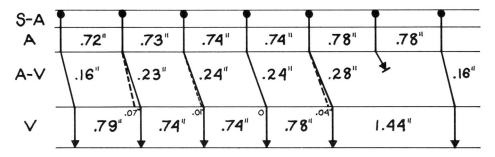

Fig. 7-6. Sinus rhythm with "atypical" Wenckebach sequence. Ladder diagram of Rhythm 7-2,c. The R-R interval does not become progressively shorter before the pause because the increments in prolongation of the P-R interval (small numbers) do not become progressively shorter as in the typical sequence illustrated in Figure 7-3.

An A-V nodal or ventricular escape beat may terminate the pause.

The QRS configuration may be normal or, in the presence of bundle branch block, wide and bizarre. When second degree A-V block type I is associated with bundle branch block, incomplete bilateral bundle branch block may be present.

CLINICAL NOTES

Type I second degree A-V block is a common and usually transient arrhythmia, often associated with acute inferior infarction, rheumatic fever, digitalis, quinidine and procainamide toxicity, and with electrolyte imbalance. The conduction disturbance rarely progresses to complete A-V block. Patients with second degree A-V block and wide QRS complexes (bundle branch block) have a less favorable prognosis than patients with narrow QRS complexes.[38]

Treatment is seldom necessary, although atropine sulfate or prophylactic artificial pacing may be required in some cases.

SECOND DEGREE A-V BLOCK TYPE II (MOBITZ)

Type II (Mobitz) second degree A-V block results from prolongation of the absolute refractory period of the A-V node or of both bundle branches, with little or no change in the duration of the relative refractory period. Conduction to the ventricles of sinus or ectopic supraventricular impulses either occurs with P-R intervals of constant duration or it does not occur at all. Long ventricular

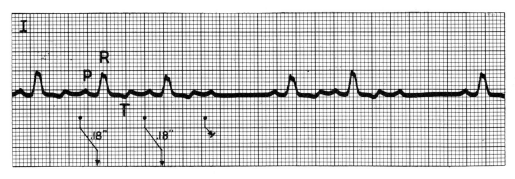

Fig. 7-7. Sinus rhythm with second degree A-V block type II. There is sudden failure of conduction not preceded by gradual lengthening of the P-R interval. The QRS complexes are wide because of associated bundle branch block.

pauses may allow idionodal or idioventricular rhythms to escape; the arrhythmia may then mimic complete A-V block. In such cases, the occurrence of ventricular captures on long rhythm strips proves that the A-V block is not complete and that A-V dissociation is responsible for the temporarily independent atrial and ventricular activity.

Atrial deflections

The rate, rhythm and configuration of the atrial deflections depend on the atrial mechanism, which may be sinus or ectopic.

The atrial wave immediately preceding the QRS complex may not be the one conducted to the ventricles, in which case it is called "skipped" P, P′ or F wave.

The P-P interval that includes a QRS complex may be shorter than the P-P interval without a QRS complex (ventriculophasic sinus arrhythmia).

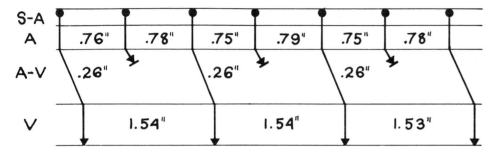

Fig. 7-8. Sinus rhythm with 2:1 second degree A-V block. Ladder diagram of Rhythm 7-3,c.

A-V conduction

One or more (not consecutive) P waves are blocked. The P-R interval of the conducted beats may be normal or prolonged but its duration, unlike that in type I, is constant.

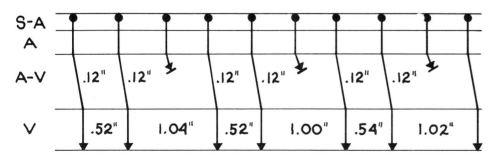

Fig. 7-9. Sinus tachycardia with 3:2 second degree A-V block type II (Mobitz). Ladder diagram of the first half of Rhythm 7-3,e.

The first P-R interval after a pause may be slightly shorter than the others. This is due to an improvement in A-V conduction following the block of a P wave.

The conduction ratio, or number of P waves to number of QRS complexes, may be 2:1, 3:2, 4:3, etc. and may vary in the same tracing. A conduction ratio of 2:1 may be due to either type II (Mobitz) or to type I (Wenckebach) second degree A-V block; if repeated and long rhythm strips fail to show at least one Wenckebach sequence, the 2:1 block is considered to be type II.

Ventricular deflections

The ventricular rate is slower than the atrial rate because of the blocked atrial waves.

The ventricular rhythm is regular when the A-V conduction ratio is constant. A variable A-V conduction ratio and the occurrence of runs of idionodal or idioventricular escape rhythm with ventricular captures cause regularly irregular ventricular rhythm.

The QRS configuration is normal. If bundle branch block is present the QRS complexes are wide and bizarre. When second degree A-V block type II is associated with bundle branch block, incomplete bilateral bundle branch block is likely to be present.

CLINICAL NOTES

Type II second degree A-V block is frequently associated with coronary heart disease and may complicate the acute phase of an anterior wall infarction. It is much less common than type I second degree block and its clinical significance is more serious: complete A-V block may suddenly ensue and cause ventricular standstill. Patients with second degree A-V block and wide QRS complexes (bundle branch block) have a less favorable prognosis than patients with the same conduction disturbance and narrow QRS complexes.[38]

The arrhythmia is often symptomatic, and congestive heart failure, angina, mental confusion, or azotemia may be induced or aggravated by the slow ventricular rates associated with this type of block.

The treatment of second degree A-V block type II should be aggressive and may require insertion of a temporary transvenous pacemaker followed by permanent pacing if the conduction defect persists. Atropine sulfate and isoproterenol I.V. drip may be used as an initial therapeutic trial or as a temporary measure, while awaiting pacemaker insertion.

HIGH GRADE A-V BLOCK

This type of advanced A-V block may be considered to fall between second degree and complete block. It is due to marked prolongation of the absolute refractory period of the A-V node or of both the bundle branches, with little or no change in the duration of the relative refractory period.

Two or more consecutive impulses are blocked. The resulting long ventricular pauses often allow idionodal or idioventricular rhythms to escape and the arrhythmia may then mimic complete A-V block: the occurrence on long rhythm strips of ventricular captures proves that the A-V block is not complete and that A-V dissociation is responsible for the temporarily independent atrial and ventricular activity.

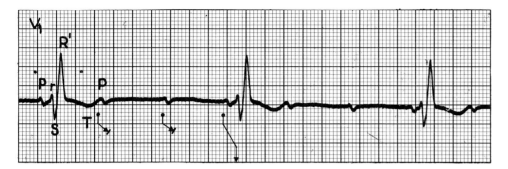

Fig. 7-10. Sinus rhythm with high grade (3:1) A-V block and bundle branch block.

Atrial deflections

The rate, rhythm and configuration of the atrial deflections depend on the atrial mechanism, which may be sinus or ectopic.

The atrial wave immediately preceding the QRS complex may not be the one conducted to the ventricles in which case it is called "skipped" P, P′ or F wave.

The P-P interval that includes a QRS complex may be shorter than the P-P interval without a QRS complex (ventriculophasic sinus arrhythmia).

A-V conduction

Two or more consecutive impulses are blocked. The conduction ratio may be 3:1, 4:1, etc. and may vary in the same tracing.

When the atria are fibrillating, the presence of high grade A-V block is suggested by long ventricular pauses and by the appearance of idionodal or idioventricular escape beats or rhythm.

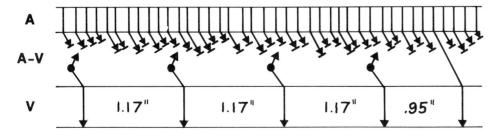

Fig. 7-11. Atrial fibrillation with high grade A-V block and A-V nodal escape rhythm. The last beat is a ventricular capture. Ladder diagram from Rhythm 7-4,*d.*

The P-R interval is of constant duration when the A-V conduction ratio is constant and may be normal or prolonged. When the conduction ratio is variable

the duration of the P-R interval may be influenced by the time interval between the preceding QRS complex and the conducted P wave (R-P interval): the longer the preceding R-P interval the shorter the P-R duration and vice versa—the shorter the preceding R-P interval the longer the P-R duration.

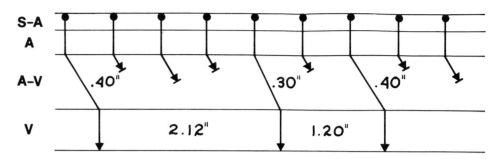

Fig. 7-12. Sinus tachycardia with high grade A-V block. The P-R interval following a long pause is shorter than that of the other conducted beats. Ladder diagram of the first half of Rhythm 7-4,b.

Ventricular deflections

The ventricular rate is slower than the atrial rate because of the blocked atrial waves.

The ventricular rhythm is regular when the A-V conduction ratio is constant. A variable conduction ratio and the occurrence of idionodal or idioventricular escape rhythm with ventricular captures produces a regularly irregular ventricular rhythm.

The QRS configuration may be normal. If bundle branch block is present the QRS complexes become wide and bizarre. When high grade A-V block is associated with bundle branch block, incomplete bilateral bundle branch block is likely to be present.

CLINICAL NOTES

High grade A-V block is always associated with heart disease. Its clinical significance and treatment are similar to those of complete A-V block.

COMPLETE A-V BLOCK

Complete or third degree A-V block results from complete interruption of conduction, temporary or permanent, in the A-V node or in both the bundle branches. All sinus or ectopic supraventricular impulses are blocked and a rescuing focus, located below the area of block, takes over the control of the ventricles. The atria and the ventricles thus beat independently of each other.

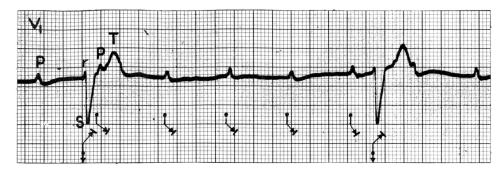

Fig. 7-13. Sinus rhythm with complete A-V block. The ventricles are under the control of a rescuing ventricular focus.

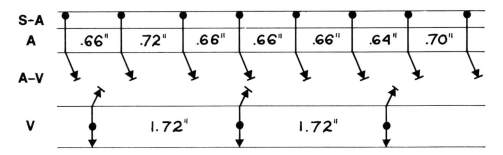

Fig. 7-14. Sinus rhythm with complete A-V block and idioventricular escape rhythm. The ventricular rate is 35 per minute. Ladder diagram of the first half of Rhythm 7-5,*c*.

As emphasized in Chapter 6, the atria and the ventricles may also beat independently because of A-V dissociation. A-V dissociation may mimic complete A-V block, particularly when it is superimposed on second degree or high grade A-V block and the ventricular rhythm is slow. A diagnosis of complete A-V block should be made only when long rhythm strips fail to show the occurrence of ventricular captures; if even one supraventricular impulse is conducted to the ventricles the A-V block should be called incomplete (second degree or high grade) and not complete.

Atrial deflections

The rate, rhythm and configuration of the atrial deflections depend on the atrial mechanism which may be sinus or ectopic.

The P-P interval includes a QRS complex may be shorter than the P-P interval without a QRS complex (ventriculophasic sinus arrhythmia).

A-V conduction

There is no conduction between the atria and the ventricles in a forward direction. The atrial deflections bear no constant relationship to the QRS complexes and the "P-R interval" continuously changes in duration.

Rarely, retrograde conduction to the atria of an idionodal or idioventricular impulse occurs in complete A-V block (unidirectional block), causing an inverted P' wave which immediately follows the QRS complex.

Ventricular deflections

The ventricular rate depends on the ventricular mechanism: idioventricular escape rhythm has a rate below 40 per minute, whereas in idionodal escape rhythm the rate is between 40 and 60 per minute. The ventricular rhythm is regular or slightly irregular.

If the QRS configuration is normal the rescuing focus is located in the A-V node, below the area of block. When the QRS complexes are wide and bizarre the rescuing focus is located either (1) in one of the ventricles or (2) in the A-V

node, but the presence of bundle branch block causes abnormal conduction of the A-V nodal impulses to the ventricles.

Certain features are believed to help differentiate an idioventricular rhythm from an idionodal rhythm with bundle branch block[18]: (1) The ventricular rate is usually slower in idioventricular rhythm because the rescuing focus is situated more distally in the conduction pathways. (2) The QRS configuration of idionodal beats with bundle branch block is typical of right or left bundle branch block, whereas idioventricular beats are wider and more bizarre, only resembling right or left bundle branch block. (3) In idionodal rhythm the rate and configuration of the QRS complex tend to be stable; when changes in configuration occur, they are usually not associated with changes in rate. Conversely, in idioventricular rhythm there is a tendency to some variability of both rate and configuration of the QRS complexes; this variability may be due either to multifocal ventricular impulses or to unifocal impulses with changes in discharge rate and direction of myocardial propagation.

CLINICAL NOTES

Complete A-V block may complicate coronary heart disease, hypertensive cardiovascular disease and congenital heart disease such as ventricular septal defect, ostium primum atrial septal defect, and complete or corrected transposition of the great vessels. Digitalis toxicity may also cause complete A-V block. Among less frequent causes are intracardiac surgery, Lenegre's disease (a degenerative sclerotic process limited to the conduction system) and intracardiac tumors.

Complete A-V block is usually treated with artificial pacing especially in symptomatic patients, since drugs needed to control heart failure and other associated arrhythmias may then be used with impunity. Isoproterenol I.V. drip may be tried as a temporary measure. When complete A-V block is caused by digitalis toxicity, discontinuation of the drug may be effective in restoring normal conduction.

First Degree A-V Block

A-V conduction delay causing prolongation of the P-R interval.

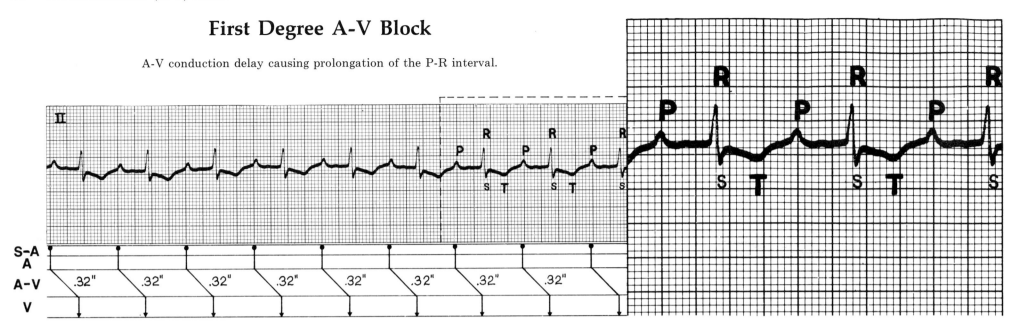

Rhythm 7-1,a. Sinus rhythm at a rate of 75 per minute with first degree A-V block. The P-R interval measures 0.32 second.

ELECTROCARDIOGRAPHIC CRITERIA

A. Atrial deflections:

1. Rate, rhythm and configuration depend on the atrial mechanism (sinus or ectopic).
2. When the P-R interval is very long or the rate is rapid, the P wave may become superimposed on the preceding T wave ("P on T").

B. A-V conduction:

1. Prolonged P-R interval: 0.21 second or longer.
2. P-R duration:
   a. Usually constant.
   b. May vary with changes in heart rate as in sinus arrhythmia.

C. Ventricular deflections:

1. Rate and rhythm: same as the atrial.
2. Configuration:
   a. Normal.
   b. Wide and bizarre: bundle branch block (incomplete bilateral bundle branch block may be present).

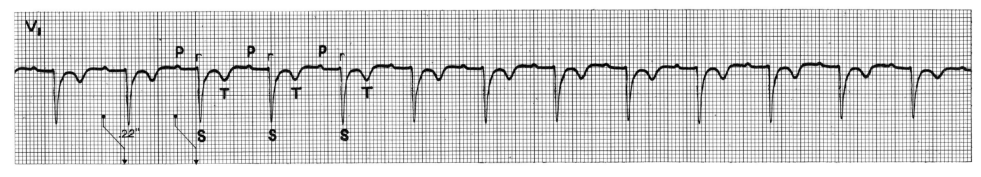

Rhythm 7-1,b. Sinus rhythm at a rate of 80 per minute and first degree A-V block. The P-R interval measures 0.22 second.

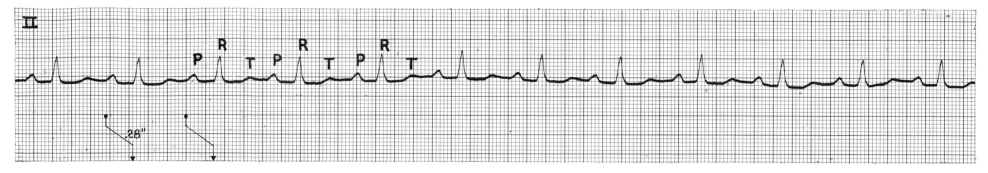

Rhythm 7-1,c. Sinus rhythm at a rate of 70 per minute. There is first degree A-V block and the P-R interval measures 0.28 second.

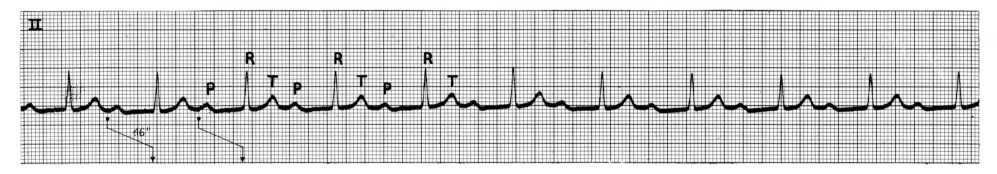

Rhythm 7-1,d. Sinus rhythm at a rate of 66 per minute and first degree A-V block with P-R interval measuring 0.46 second.

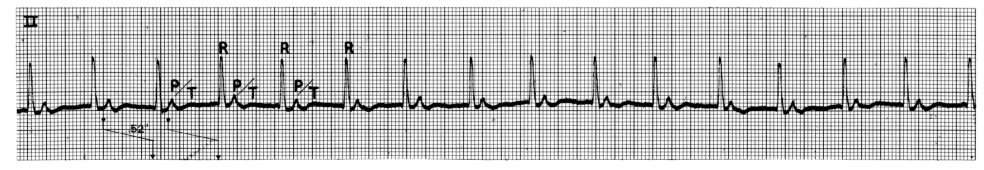

Rhythm 7-1,e. Sinus rhythm at a rate of 90 per minute with first degree A-V block. The P-R interval measures 0.52 second and the P wave is superimposed on the preceding T wave ("P on T").

Second Degree A-V Block Type I (Wenckebach)

A-V conduction disturbance causing progressively longer P-R interval until a P wave is blocked and a ventricular pause occurs.

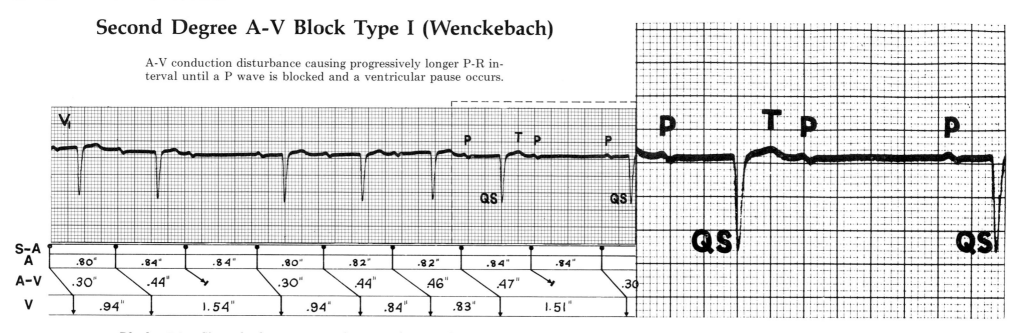

Rhythm 7-2,a. Sinus rhythm at a rate of 72 per minute and second degree A-V block type I. The average ventricular rate is 57 per minute.

ELECTROCARDIOGRAPHIC CRITERIA

A. Atrial deflections:

1. Rate, rhythm and configuration depend on the atrial mechanism (sinus or ectopic).
2. "Skipped" P, P' or F waves may occur.

B. A-V conduction:

1. The P-R interval grows progressively *longer* until a P wave is blocked and a ventricular pause occurs.
2. The P-R interval following the pause is the shortest of the sequence and may be normal or abnormal in duration.
3. The greatest increment in duration of the P-R interval occurs between the first and the second P-R after the pause; the increments then become progressively smaller.
4. Conduction ratio:
   a. May be 2:1, 3:2, 4:3, 5:4, etc. and may vary in the same tracing.
   b. A conduction ratio of 2:1 may result from type I (Wenckebach) or type II (Mobitz) second degree A-V block.

C. Ventricular deflections:

1. Rate: slower than the atrial because of the blocked atrial waves.
2. Rhythm: regularly irregular (group beating):
   a. The R-R intervals become progressively *shorter* until the pause occurs; the pause measures less than twice the preceding R-R interval.
   b. In "atypical" Wenckebach the R-R interval may fail to become shorter as expected or may suddenly lengthen.
   c. An A-V nodal or ventricular escape may terminate the pause.
3. Configuration:
   a. Normal.
   b. Wide and bizarre: bundle branch block (incomplete bilateral bundle branch block may be present).

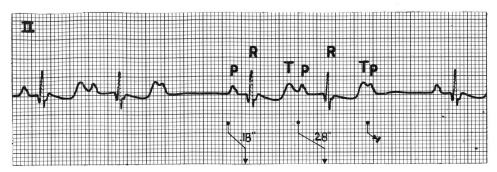

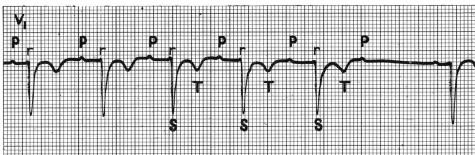

Rhythm 7-2,b. Sinus rhythm at a rate of 82 per minute and second degree A-V block type I with 3:2 Wenckebach sequences. The average ventricular rate is 55 per minute.

Rhythm 7-2,c. Sinus rhythm at a rate of 82 per minute and second degree A-V block type I. The Wenckebach sequence is here 6:5.

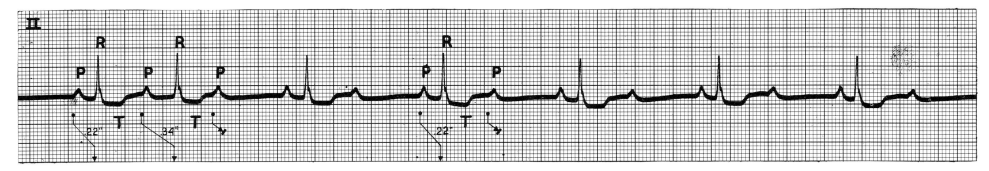

Rhythm 7-2,d. Sinus rhythm at a rate of 81 per minute and second degree A-V block type I. The 3:2 sequence at the beginning of the strip reveals that the block is type I and not type II. The P-R interval of the conducted beat after each pause is prolonged (0.22 second).

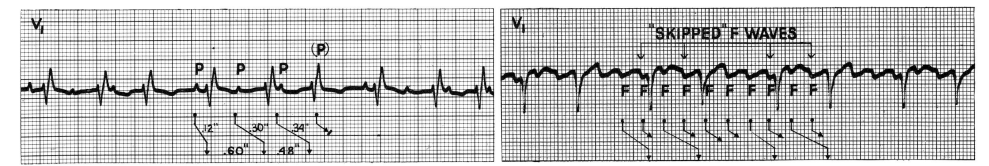

Rhythm 7-2,e. Atrial tachycardia with type I second degree A-V block and bundle branch block. The atrial rate is 140 per minute and the average ventricular rate 100 per minute. The conduction disturbance may be due to incomplete bilateral bundle branch block.

Rhythm 7-2,f. Atrial flutter with second degree A-V block and 2:1 alternating with 4:1 Wenckebach sequences. Note the "skipped" F waves and the group beating. The atrial rate is 300 per minute and the average ventricular rate 90 per minute.

Second Degree A-V Block Type II (Mobitz)

A-V conduction disturbance causing the intermittent block of an impulse. The P-R interval of the conducted beats is of constant duration.

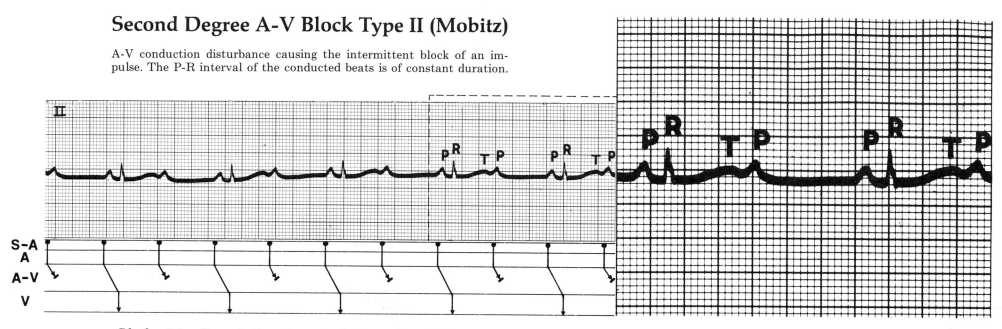

Rhythm 7-3,a. Sinus rhythm at a rate of 92 per minute with 2:1 second degree A-V block type II. The ventricular rate is 46 per minute.

ELECTROCARDIOGRAPHIC CRITERIA

A. Atrial deflections:

1. Rate, rhythm and configuration depend on the atrial mechanism (sinus or ectopic).
2. "Skipped" P, P′ or F waves may occur.
3. The P-P interval that includes a QRS complex may be shorter than the P-P interval without a QRS complex (ventriculophasic sinus arrhythmia).

B. A-V conduction:

1. One or more (not consecutive) P waves are blocked.

2. P-R duration of the conducted beats:
   a. Usually constant (normal or prolonged).
   b. The P-R interval of the beat following a long pause may be slightly shorter than the others.
3. Conduction ratio:
   a. May be 2:1, 3:2, 4:3, etc. and may vary in the same tracing.
   b. A conduction ratio of 2:1 may result from either type I or type II second degree A-V block.

C. Ventricular deflections:

1. Rate: slower than the atrial because of the blocked P waves.
2. Rhythm:
   a. Regular: constant A-V conduction ratio.
   b. Regularly irregular: variable conduction ratio or runs of escape rhythm with ventricular captures.
3. Configuration:
   a. Normal
   b. Wide and bizarre: bundle branch block (incomplete bilateral bundle branch block is likely to be present).

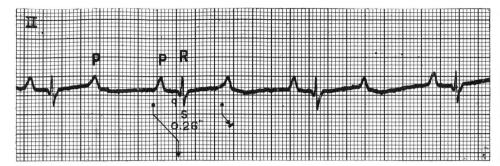

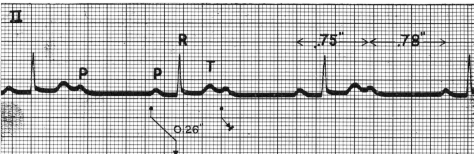

Rhythm 7-3,b. Sinus rhythm at a rate of 84 per minute and 2:1 second degree A-V block type II. The P-R interval of the conducted beats is prolonged (0.26 second) and the ventricular rate is 42 per minute.

Rhythm 7-3,c. Sinus rhythm at a rate of 80 per minute and 2:1 second degree A-V block type II. There is ventriculophasic sinus arrhythmia and the P-R of the conducted beats is prolonged (0.26 second). The ventricular rate is 40 per minute.

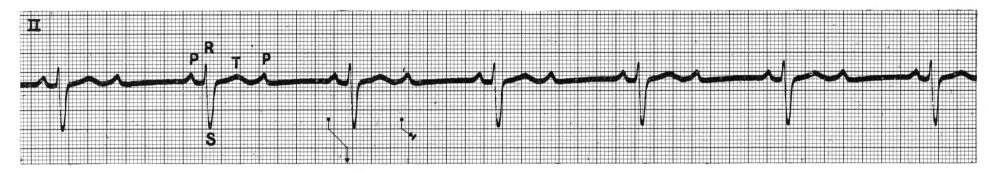

Rhythm 7-3,d. Sinus rhythm at a rate of 80 per minute with 2:1 second degree A-V block type II and bundle branch block. The conduction disturbance is probably due to incomplete bilateral bundle branch block. The ventricular rate is 40 per minute.

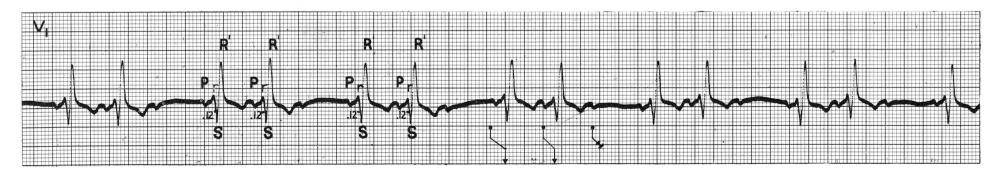

Rhythm 7-3,e. Sinus tachycardia at a rate of 120 per minute with 3:2 second degree A-V block type II and bundle branch block. The average ventricular rate is 75 per minute. This is not a type I block because the P-R interval of the conducted beats is of constant duration. The conduction disturbance is probably due to incomplete bilateral bundle branch block.

High Grade A-V Block

A-V conduction disturbance causing the intermittent block of two or more consecutive impulses.

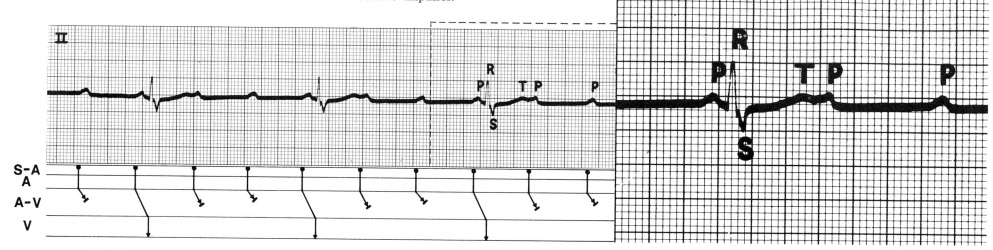

Rhythm 7-4,a. Sinus rhythm at a rate of 85 per minute with high grade 3:1 A-V block and bundle branch block. The conduction defect is probably due to incomplete bilateral bundle branch block.

ELECTROCARDIOGRAPHIC CRITERIA

A. Atrial deflections:

1. Rate, rhythm and configuration depend on the atrial mechanism (sinus or ectopic).
2. "Skipped" P, P′ or F waves may occur.
3. The P-P interval that includes a QRS complex may be shorter than the P-P interval without a QRS complex (ventriculophasic sinus arrhythmia).

B. A-V conduction:

1. Two or more consecutive impulses are blocked.
2. Conduction ratio:

   a. May be 3:1, 4:1, etc.
   b. In atrial fibrillation: long ventricular pauses and appearance of escape beats or escape rhythm.
3. P-R duration of the conducted beats:

   a. Normal or prolonged.
   b. Constant when the conduction ratio is constant.
   c. May vary when the conduction ratio is variable (inversely proportional to the preceding R-P interval).

C. Ventricular deflections:

1. Rate: slower than the atrial because of the blocked P waves.

2. Rhythm:

   a. Regular: constant A-V conduction ratio.
   b. Regularly irregular: variable conduction ratio or runs of escape rhythm with ventricular captures.
3. Configuration:

   a. Normal.
   b. Wide and bizarre: bundle branch block (incomplete bilateral bundle branch block is likely to be present).

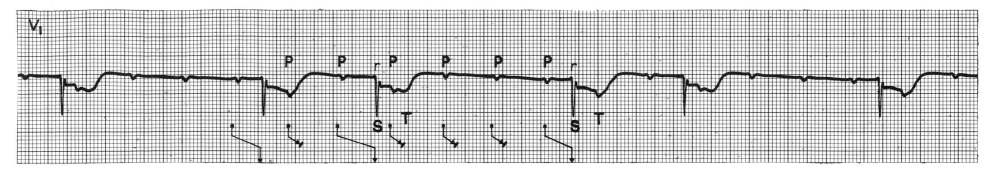

Rhythm 7-4,b. Sinus tachycardia at a rate of 110 per minute with high grade A-V block. The conduction ratio is 4:1 alternating with 2:1. The P-R interval following a long pause is shorter than that of the other conducted beats. The average ventricular rate is 35 per minute.

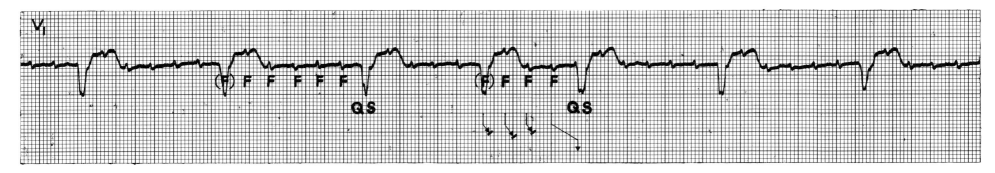

Rhythm 7-4,c. Atrial flutter with high grade A-V block and bundle branch block. The conduction ratio varies between 4:1 and 6:1. The atrial rate is 240 per minute and the average ventricular rate 45 per minute.

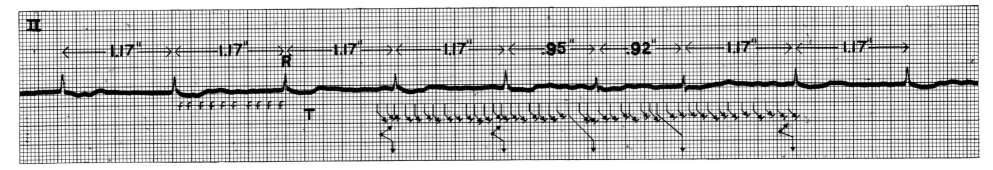

Rhythm 7-4,d. Atrial fibrillation with high grade A-V block and A-V nodal escape rhythm at a rate of 51 per minute. The occurrence of ventricular captures by atrial fibrillation impulses proves that the A-V block is not complete and that A-V dissociation is the mechanism causing atrial and ventricular activity to be transiently independent.

Complete A-V block

Complete interruption of conduction at the level of the A-V node or of both the bundle branches. The atria and the ventricles are activated by separate foci and beat independently of each other.

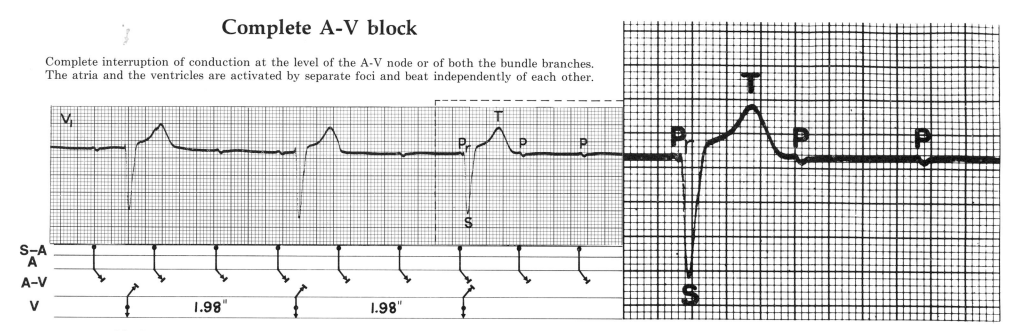

Rhythm 7-5,a. Sinus rhythm at a rate of 85 per minute with complete A-V block. There is idioventricular rhythm at a rate of 30 per minute.

ELECTROCARDIOGRAPHIC CRITERIA

A. Atrial deflections:

1. Rate, rhythm and configuration depend on the atrial mechanism (sinus or ectopic).
2. The P-P interval that includes a QRS complex may be shorter than the P-P interval without a QRS complex (ventriculophasic sinus arrhythmia).

B. A-V conduction:

1. There is no conduction between the atria and ventricles in a forward direction.

2. The atrial deflections bear no constant relationship to the QRS complexes and the "P-R interval" continuously changes in duration.
3. Rarely retrograde conduction to the atria of an idioventricular impulse to the atria occurs in the presence of complete A-V block (unidirectional block).

C. Ventricular deflections:

1. Rate: depends on the ventricular mechanism:
   a. Idioventricular escape rhythm: below 40 per minute.
   b. Idionodal escape rhythm: 40 to 60 per minute.

2. Rhythm: regular or slightly irregular.
3. Configuration:
   a. Normal: rescuing focus located in the A-V node.
   b. Wide and bizarre· rescuing focus located either in the ventricles or in the A-V node with bundle branch block.

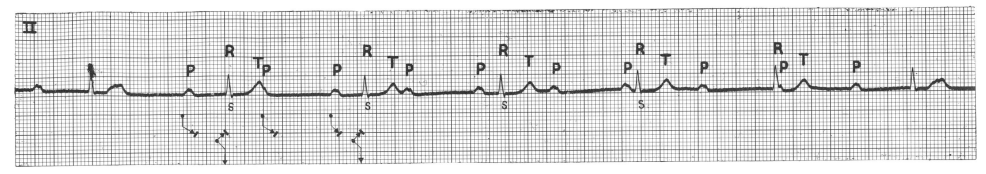

Rhythm 7-5,b. Sinus rhythm at a rate of 75 per minute and complete A-V block. The ventricles are under the control of idionodal escape rhythm at a rate of 42 per minute.

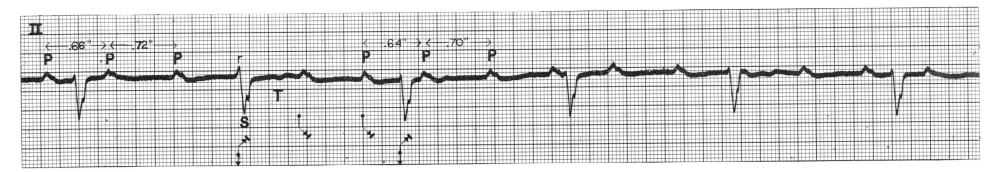

Rhythm 7-5,c. Sinus rhythm at a rate of 90 per minute and complete A-V block. There is ventriculophasic sinus arrhythmia and idioventricular rhythm at a rate of 35 per minute.

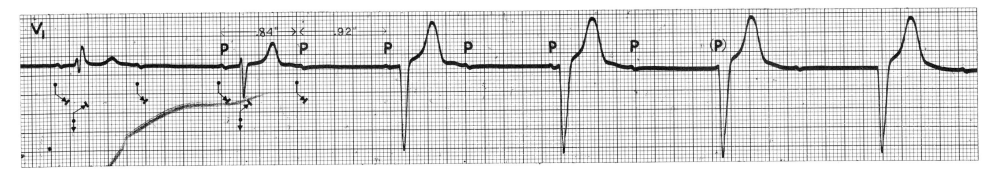

Rhythm 7-5,d. Sinus rhythm at a rate of 75 per minute and complete A-V block. There is ventriculophasic sinus arrhythmia. Idioventricular rhythm is present at a rate of 35 per minute and the QRS configuration varies, probably owing to multifocal ventricular impulses.

Chapter 8

Sino-Atrial (S-A) Block

A conduction disturbance at the junction between the sinus node and the surrounding atrial tissue (S-A junction) can cause delay or block in the transmission of the sinus impulses to the atria. The resulting arrhythmia is called sino-atrial (S-A) block.

Classification of S-A block

S-A block, like A-V block, is divided in two categories, incomplete and complete. Incomplete S-A block is subdivided into first degree and second degree; the latter includes type I (Wenckebach) and type II. Complete S-A block is also called third degree.

First degree S-A block

In first degree S-A block all sinus impulses are conducted to the atria but with delay. This conduction disturbance cannot be recognized on the conventional electrocardiogram. The sinus activity, in fact, does not register any waves on the electrocardiogram and there is no way of detecting how long before each P wave the sinus node has fired.

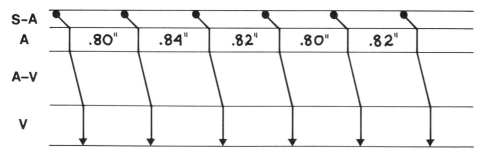

Fig. 8-1. Diagram of first degree S-A block.

Second degree S-A block

In second degree S-A block some sinus impulses are blocked while others are conducted to the atria, with or without delay. This conduction disturbance can be recognized on the electrocardiogram because the intermittent block of the sinus impulses causes sudden pauses, owing to the disappearance of one or more P waves and related QRS-T complexes.

Type I (Wenckebach) second degree S-A block is characterized by a pause which is preceded by progressively shorter P-P intervals and measures less than twice the preceding P-P interval. This phenomenon is analogous to type I (Wenckebach) second degree A-V block and a comparison with the latter can be very helpful in its recognition:

In type I second degree *A-V block* there is progressive delay in conduction from the atria to the ventricles; this causes progressive lengthening of the P-R interval until a P wave is blocked and a pause occurs. In type I second degree *S-A block* the progressive delay in conduction occurs between the sinus node and the atria; because the sinus activity itself does not register any waves on the conventional electrocardiogram, the progressive lengthening of the S-A interval cannot be seen.

In type I second degree *A-V block* the greatest increment in atrioventricular conduction time (P-R interval) occurs between the first and the second conducted beat after the pause, after which the increment becomes progressively smaller; this causes progressive shortening of the *R-R* intervals before the pause. In type I second degree *S-A block* the increment in sino-atrial conduction time behaves in the same manner; as a result there is progressive shortening of the *P-P* interval before the pause.

In type I second degree *A-V block* the duration of the ventricular pause is equal to two P-P cycles minus the difference between the duration of the P-R interval preceding and that of the P-R interval following the pause; the ventricular pause, therefore, measures less than twice the preceding R-R interval. In type I second degree *S-A block* the same mechanism can be invoked; the duration of the sinus cycles and of the S-A intervals cannot be measured but the end result is the same and the atrial pause measures less than twice the preceding P-P interval.

Type II second degree S-A block is characterized by pauses which are preceded by P-P intervals of constant duration (or with slight variations due to sinus arrhythmia). Each pause measures twice, three times, etc. the normal P-P interval. This conduction disturbance is analogous to type II second degree A-V block where the P-R and the R-R intervals preceding the pause are also of constant duration.

Third degree S-A block

In third degree S-A block all the sinus impulses fail to reach the atria, causing the complete disappearance of the sinus P waves and related QRS-T complexes. Ectopic rhythms of atrial, A-V nodal or ventricular origin usually take over the control of the heart, preventing cardiac arrest.

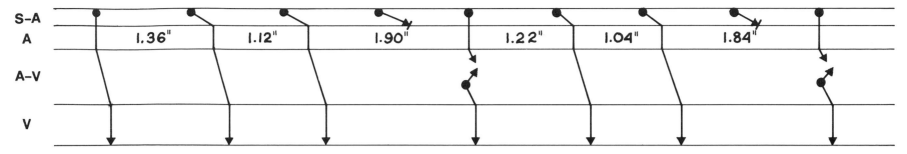

Fig. 8-2. Second degree S-A block type I (Wenckebach). Ladder diagram of Rhythm 8-1,c. Each pause is preceded by progressively shorter P-P intervals and measures less than twice the preceding P-P interval.

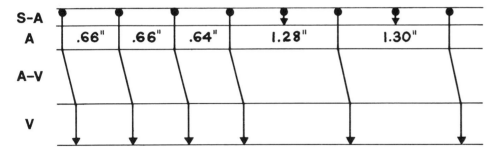

Fig. 8-3. Second degree S-A block type II. Ladder diagram of the first half of Rhythm 8-2,b. The first pause is preceded by P-P intervals which display slight variation in duration owing to sinus arrhythmia but are not progressively shorter as in type I (Wenckebach). Each pause measures about twice the normal P-P interval.

Fig. 8-4. Third degree or complete S-A block. Ladder diagram of the first half of Rhythm 8-2,d. An A-V nodal escape rhythm controls the ventricles and there is retrograde block.

Sinus arrest

Sinus arrest, due to failure of impulse formation within the sinus node, may give the same electrocardiographic manifestations of sino-atrial block. When the sinus arrest is intermittent the arrhythmia resembles second degree S-A block type II; when it is permanent it resembles third degree S-A block. The differential diagnosis between sinus arrest and S-A block may be very difficult. It is believed that, unlike S-A block, sinus arrest is rarely followed by atrial escape beats or rhythm because the same pathological process that causes sinus arrest also causes a general depression of the atrial ectopic activity.[18]

Sick sinus syndrome

Sino-atrial block may be a manifestation of the so-called "sick sinus syndrome."[42] This syndrome, which results from a failing sinus node, also includes other manifestations such as periodic severe sinus bradycardia, periods of sinus arrest with occurrence of atrial or A-V nodal ectopic rhythms, failure of the sinus rhythm to reappear after cardioversion from atrial fibrillation, chronic atrial fibrillation with associated high grade or complete A-V block.

CLINICAL NOTES

Sino-atrial block is usually a transient arrhythmia. Among its frequent causes are coronary heart disease, especially acute inferior wall infarction, hypertensive cardiovascular disease, digitalis and quinidine toxicity, and the use of propranolol.[77]

When sino-atrial block causes marked slowing of the ventricular rate, the associated fall in cardiac output may induce or aggravate hypotension, heart failure, and myocardial or cerebral ischemia, especially in patients with severe cardiovascular disease. Complete interruption of conduction of the sinus impulse to the atria and the ventricles may cause cardiac standstill if a subsidiary focus, located in the atria, A-V node or ventricles, fails to take over the control of the heart.

The treatment of sino-atrial block includes the treatment of the underlying condition, the removal of any causative drug, the use of atropine or isoproterenol and, in selected cases, temporary or permanent artificial pacing.

Second Degree Sino-Atrial Block—Type I (Wenckebach)

Conduction disturbance in the S-A junction causing progressive delay and block in the transmission of sinus impulses to the atria.

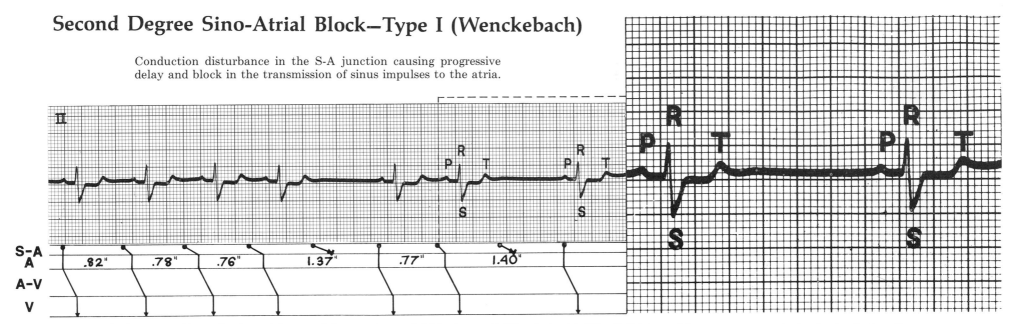

Rhythm 8-1,a. Sinus rhythm with second degree sino-atrial block type I (Wenckebach). The P-P interval becomes progressively shorter before the pause which measures less than twice the preceding P-P interval.

ELECTROCARDIOGRAPHIC CRITERIA

A. Atrial deflections:

1. The atrial rhythm may be sinus bradycardia, normal sinus rhythm or sinus tachycardia.
2. A sinus P wave and related QRS-T complex fail to occur, causing a pause.
3. The P-P intervals become progressively shorter before the pause.
4. The P-P interval that includes a pause measures less than twice the P-P interval preceding the pause.
5. An atrial escape beat may terminate the pause.

B. A-V conduction: may be normal, or various degrees of A-V block may be present.

C. Ventricular deflections:

1. Rate: depends on the atrial rate and the A-V conduction mechanism.
2. Rhythm:
   a. Regularly irregular: one or more QRS-T complexes are missing.
   b. An A-V nodal or ventricular escape beat may terminate the pause.
3. Configuration:
   a. Normal.
   b. Wide and bizarre because of bundle branch block.

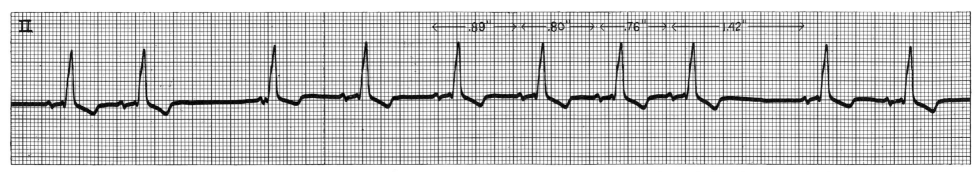

Rhythm 8-1,b. Sinus rhythm with type I second degree sino-atrial block. The P-P intervals become shorter before the pause. The first pause is terminated by an A-V nodal escape.

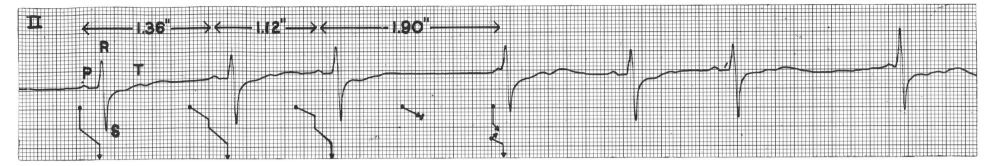

Rhythm 8-1,c. Sinus bradycardia with type I second degree sino-atrial block. Each pause is terminated by an A-V nodal escape.

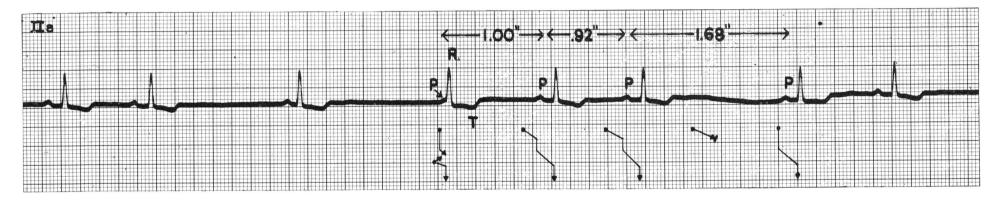

Rhythm 8-1,d. Sinus rhythm with type I second degree sino-atrial block. A sequence with progressively shorter P-P intervals and a pause measuring less than twice the preceding P-P interval confirm the presence of the Wenckebach phenomenon.

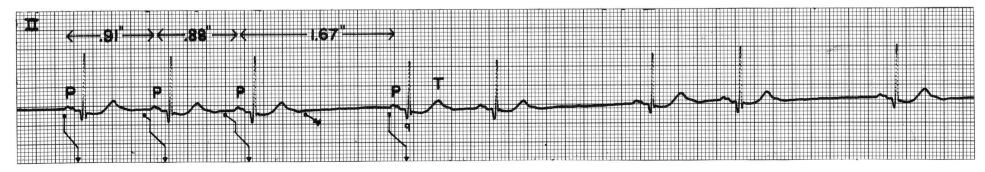

Rhythm 8-1,e. Sinus rhythm with second degree sino-atrial block type I. The P-P intervals become progressively shorter before the pause which measures less than twice the preceding P-P interval.

Second Degree Sino-Atrial Block—Type II

Conduction disturbance in the S-A junction, causing intermittent and sudden block in the transmission of sinus impulses to the atria.

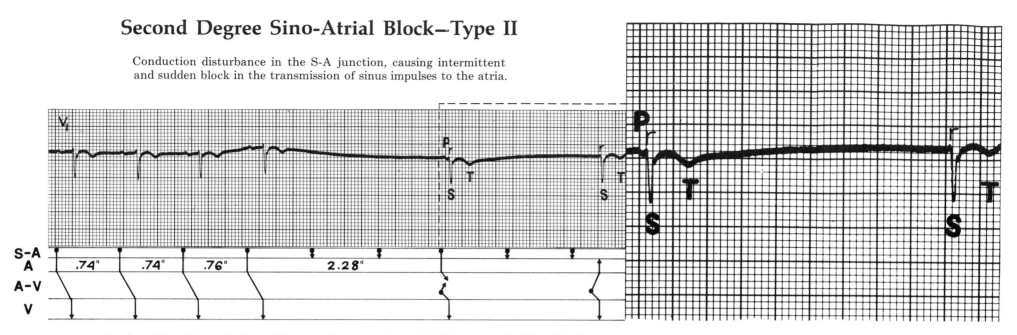

Rhythm 8-2,a. Sinus rhythm with second degree sino-atrial block type II. The P-P intervals preceding the pause vary slightly, owing to sinus arrhythmia, but do not become progressively shorter as in type I. The first pause measures exactly three times the preceding P-P interval. Two A-V nodal escape beats interrupt the long pauses.

ELECTROCARDIOGRAPHIC CRITERIA

A. Atrial deflections:

1. The atrial mechanism may be sinus bradycardia, normal sinus rhythm or sinus tachycardia.
2. One or more sinus P waves and related QRS-T complexes fail to occur, causing a pause.
3. The P-P intervals before the pause are of constant duration.
4. The P-P interval that includes a pause measures twice, three times etc. the P-P interval preceding the pause.
5. Sino-atrial block with constant conduction ratio of 2:1, 3:1 etc. may mimic marked sinus bradycardia.

B. A-V conduction: may be normal, or various degrees of A-V block may be present.

C. Ventricular deflections:

1. Rate: depends on the atrial rate and the A-V conduction mechanism.
2. Rhythm:
   a. Regularly irregular: one or more QRS-T complexes are missing.
   b. An A-V nodal or ventricular escape beat may terminate the pause.
3. Configuration:
   a. Normal.
   b. Wide and bizarre because of bundle branch block.

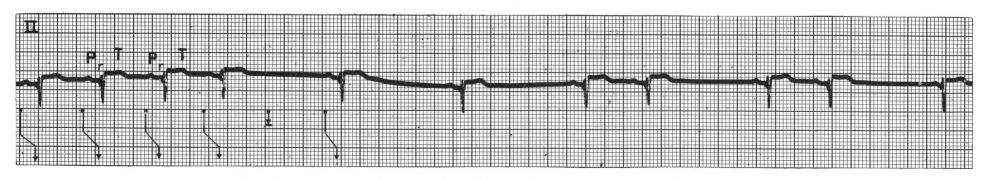

Rhythm 8-2,b. Sinus rhythm with intermittent 2:1 sino-atrial block. Each pause measures twice the preceding P-P interval.

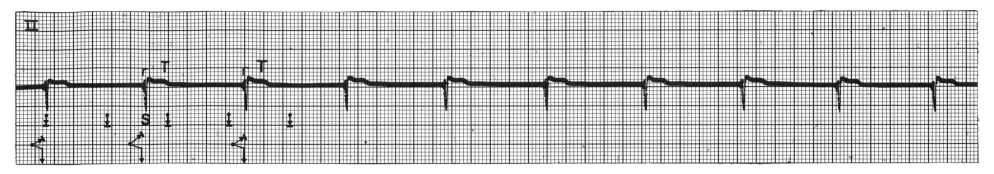

Rhythm 8-2,c. Same patient as in Fig. 8-2,b. Third degree (or complete) sino-atrial block has developed and an idionodal escape rhythm controls the ventricles. Without the previous tracing, the rhythm probably would have been diagnosed simply as "mid" nodal escape rhythm.

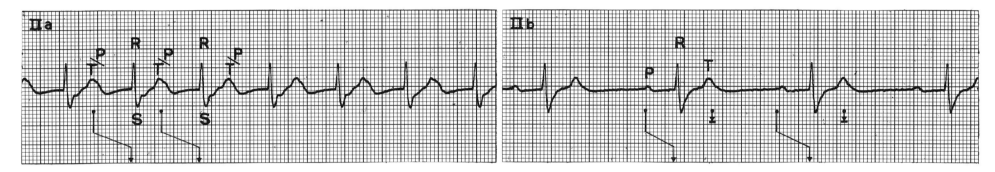

Rhythm 8-2,d. Both strips were recorded from the same patient, a few minutes apart. In IIa: sinus rhythm at a rate of 84 per minute with first degree A-V block. In IIb: 2:1 second degree sino-atrial block has developed and the rate is exactly half of that present in IIa. Without the previous tracing the rhythm in IIb probably would have been diagnosed as simple sinus bradycardia (rate: 42 per minute).

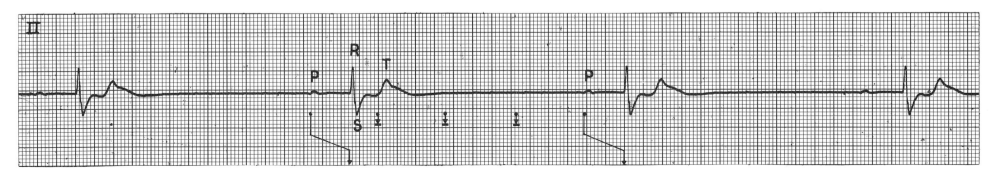

Rhythm 8-3,e. Same patient as in 8-2,e. The sino-atrial block has become 4:1, causing an apparent sinus bradycardia of marked degree (rate: 21 per minute).

Chapter 9

Intraventricular Block

Intraventricular block is caused by delay or block of supraventricular impulses (sinus or ectopic) in the intraventricular conduction pathways.

The His bundle gives origin to two bundle branches, the right and the left. The left bundle branch divides almost immediately into two divisions—the anterior and the posterior. The intraventricular conduction system is therefore composed of three conduction pathways (also called fascicles): (1) the right bundle branch, (2) the anterior division and (3) the posterior division of the left bundle branch.

Conduction delay or block may occur in only one, in two or in all three fascicles at the same time. The following forms of intraventricular block may therefore occur:

Monofascicular block:

Left anterior hemiblock (LAH): conduction delay or block in the anterior division of the left bundle branch.

Left posterior hemiblock (LPH): conduction delay or block in the posterior division of the left bundle branch.

Right bundle branch block (RBBB): conduction delay or block in the right bundle branch.

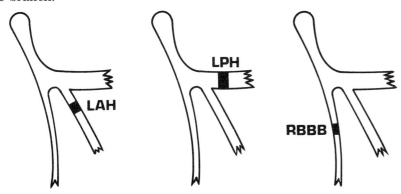

Fig. 9-1. Diagrams illustrating the three forms of monofascicular block.

Left bundle branch block (LBBB) may also be considered a monofascicular block when the delay or block occurs in the main trunk of the left bundle branch, before it bifurcates into its anterior and posterior divisions.

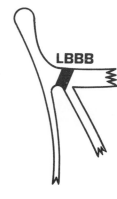

Fig. 9-2. Diagram illustrating left bundle branch block at the level of its main trunk.

Bifascicular block:

Right bundle branch block with left anterior hemiblock (RBBB + LAH): Conduction delay or block in both the right bundle branch and the anterior division of the left bundle branch.

Right bundle branch block with left posterior hemiblock (RBBB + LPH): Conduction delay or block in both the right bundle branch and the posterior division of the left bundle branch.

Left anterior and left posterior hemiblock (LAH + LPH): conduction delay or block in both the anterior and posterior divisions of the left bundle branch.

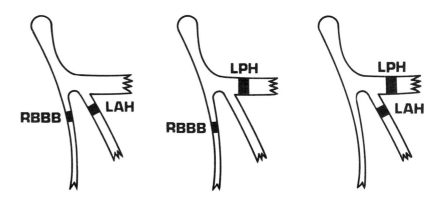

Fig. 9-3. Diagrams illustrating the three forms of bifascicular block.

Trifascicular block

Complete trifascicular block is caused by failure of conduction in all the three intraventricular conduction fascicles and results in complete A-V block.

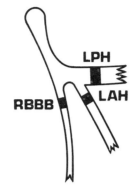

Fig. 9-4. Diagram illustrating complete tri-fascicular block.

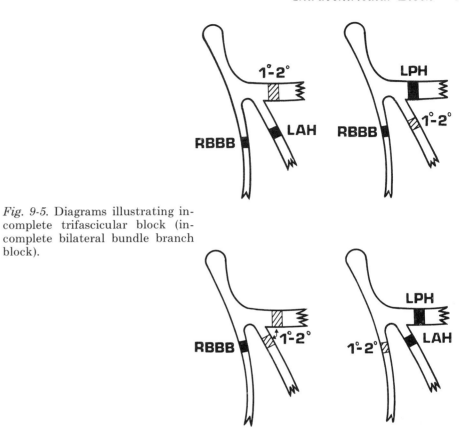

Fig. 9-5. Diagrams illustrating in-complete trifascicular block (in-complete bilateral bundle branch block).

Incomplete trifascicular block includes the following varieties:

Right bundle branch block with left anterior hemiblock and first or second degree A-V block, when the latter is caused by conduction delay or block in the left posterior fascicle.

Right bundle branch block with left posterior hemiblock and first or second degree A-V block, when the latter is caused by conduction delay or block in the left anterior fascicle.

Bilateral bundle branch block

The term complete bilateral bundle branch block is synonymous with the term complete trifascicular block.

The term incomplete bilateral bundle branch block is used by some to designate bifascicular block (with the exception of left anterior plus left posterior hemiblock because the two conduction fascicles are both divisions of the same bundle branch), as well as incomplete trifascicular block. Other varieties of incomplete bilateral bundle branch block are represented by:

Right bundle branch block with first or second degree A-V block, when the latter is caused by conduction delay or block in the left bundle branch (main trunk or both anterior and posterior divisions).

Left bundle branch block with first or second degree A-V block, when the latter is caused by conduction delay or block in the right bundle branch.

Alternating bundle branch block: periods of right bundle branch block alternate with periods of left bundle branch block.

Electrophysiological principles

In right or left bundle branch block the supraventricular impulses (sinus or ectopic) reach one ventricle first, through the conducting bundle branch. The impulses then spread to the opposite ventricle, with delay. The conduction delay needed by the impulses to reach the blocked ventricle is in the order of 0.04 to 0.06 second and, therefore, the QRS complex becomes wide, measuring 0.12 second or more.

In left anterior or left posterior hemiblock the supraventricular impulses reach the right ventricle through the conducting right bundle branch and one wall of the left ventricle through the conducting left fascicle. The impulses spread to the opposite wall of the left ventricle through the Purkinje fibers that furnish extensive connections between the anterior and posterior fascicle.[17] The conduction delay needed by the impulses to reach the blocked left ventricular wall is only 0.01 or 0.02 second and, therefore, the width of the QRS complex increases only slightly, remaining well within normal limits. The asynchronous activation of the anterior and posterior wall of the left ventricle, on the other hand, causes a marked change in the direction of the QRS frontal plane axis—to the left in left anterior hemiblock, and to the right in left posterior hemiblock.

When right bundle branch block is associated with left anterior or left posterior hemiblock, both an increase in QRS width and a marked change in the direction of the QRS frontal plane axis are seen. Right bundle branch block with left anterior hemiblock is characterized by a wide QRS complex with its frontal plane axis shifted to the left, whereas right bundle branch block with left posterior hemiblock produces a wide QRS complex with its frontal plane axis shifted to the right.

Electrocardiographic recognition of intraventricular block

In order to recognize the various forms of intraventricular block one must be familiar with the 12-lead electrocardiogram and be able to determine the electrical axis of the QRS complex in the frontal plane. Several excellent textbooks of electrocardiography are available to the reader seeking detailed information on this subject.

A teaching method utilized by us as well as others[12,16,28] allows the estimation of the electrical axis in a rapid and simple manner, while the different varieties of intraventricular block can be identified by using a minimal number of electrocardiographic leads.[28] In our approach, leads I, II, and III are used to quickly recognize the presence of left anterior and left posterior hemiblock; lead V_1 is used to diagnose right or left bundle branch block.

Electrical axis of the QRS complex in the frontal plane

The electrical axis of the QRS complex in the frontal plane can be determined approximately by becoming familiar with the hexaxial reference system and with three basic principles governing the relationship between the QRS electrical forces and the frontal plane leads.

The *hexaxial reference system* is obtained by superimposing the three sides of the Einthoven's triangle (representing the axes of leads I, II, and III) at their midpoints, while retaining their orientation, and adding the axes of the three unipolar limb leads aVR, aVL and aVF. The six lines meeting at their midpoints form angles of 30° with each other.

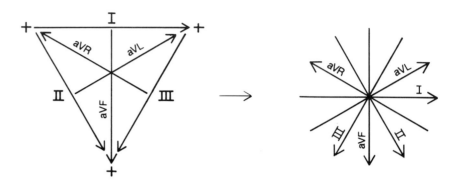

Fig. 9-7. The three limb leads are added to the figure.

The resulting figure is enclosed in a circle and the degrees are marked starting at 3 o'clock with 0°, labeling as positive the degrees in the lower half of the figure and as negative those in the upper half. The six lead signs are placed so as to indicate the positive pole of each lead.

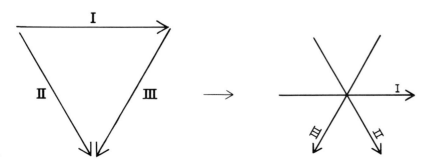

Fig. 9-6. Diagram illustrating the rearranging of the three sides of the Einthoven triangle.

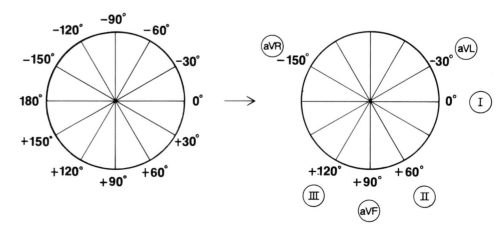

Fig. 9-8. The hexaxial reference system.

The six frontal plane leads will therefore be located as follows:

Lead I at 0°   Lead II at +60°   Lead aVR at −150°
Lead aVL at −30°   Lead aVF at +90°
                      Lead III at +120°

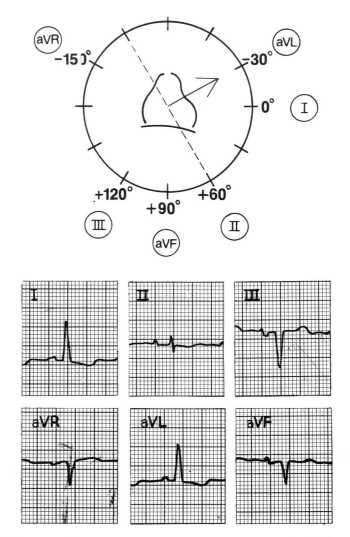

The 3 *basic principles* governing the relationship between the QRS electrical forces and the frontal leads are as follows:

1. The tallest QRS complex is recorded in the lead toward which the electrical forces are directed (*B*, in Fig. 9-9).

2. A QRS complex with R wave and S wave of the same voltage (equiphasic) is recorded in the lead that is perpendicular to the direction of the electrical forces (*C*, in Fig. 9-9).

3. A negative QRS complex is recorded in the lead or leads that "look at the tail" of the electrical forces (*A*, in Fig. 9-9).

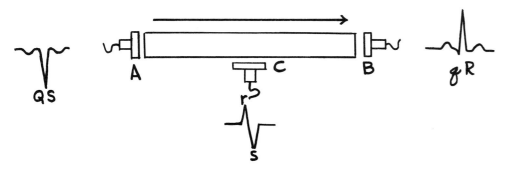

Fig. 9-9. Diagram illustrating the relationship between the QRS electrical forces and the electrocardiographic leads. (Ritota, M. C.: Diagnostic Electrocardiography. Fig. 3-14. Philadelphia, J. B. Lippincott, 1969)

Fig. 9-10. Diagram and tracing illustrating a QRS axis of −30° in the frontal plane.

Applying these basic principles it can be readily understood how electrical forces traveling toward lead aVL (−30°) cause a tall QRS complex in this lead, an equiphasic QRS complex in lead II (which is perpendicular to the direction of the electrical forces), and a negative QRS in leads III, aVF, and aVR (which look at the tail of the same forces); lead I also shows an upright QRS but not as tall as that in lead aVL.

Similarly, electrical forces traveling toward lead aVF (+90°) cause a tall QRS complex in this lead, an equiphasic QRS in lead I (which is perpendicular to the direction of the electrical forces), and a negative QRS in leads aVR and aVL (which look at the tail of the electrical forces); leads II and III also show an upright QRS but not as tall as in lead aVF.

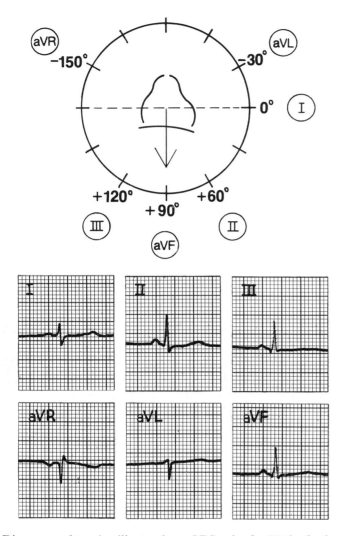

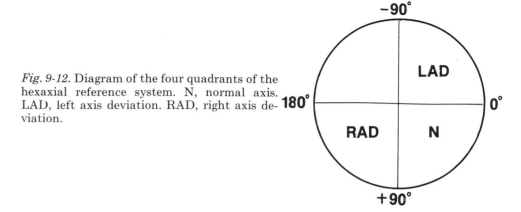

Fig. 9-12. Diagram of the four quadrants of the hexaxial reference system. N, normal axis. LAD, left axis deviation. RAD, right axis deviation.

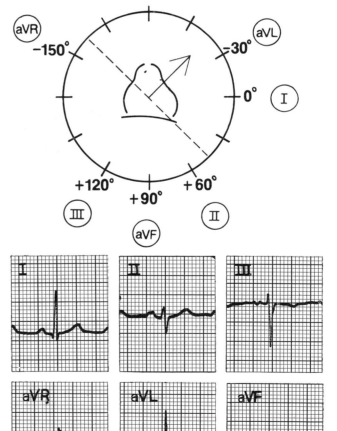

Fig. 9-11. Diagram and tracing illustrating a QRS axis of +90° in the frontal plane.

Fig. 9-13. Diagram and tracing illustrating the QRS axis in left anterior hemiblock.

The approximate direction of the QRS frontal plane axis may also be determined by using leads I, II and III only, instead of all six frontal plane leads.

The normal QRS axis in the frontal plane (N) is directed between 0° and +90°. Left axis deviation (LAD) is present when the axis is oriented between 0° and −90°, whereas right axis deviation (RAD) is diagnosed when the axis is directed between +90° and 180°.

In left anterior hemiblock the QRS electrical axis is markedly shifted to the left, more than −30° and often between −45° and −60°; lead I and aVL therefore show a predominantly positive QRS complex, whereas leads II, III and aVF show a predominantly negative QRS complex.

Conversely, left posterior hemiblock causes a shift of the QRS axis to the right, usually at about $-120°$; leads I and aVL thus show a predominantly negative QRS complex, whereas leads II, III and aVF show a predominantly positive QRS complex.

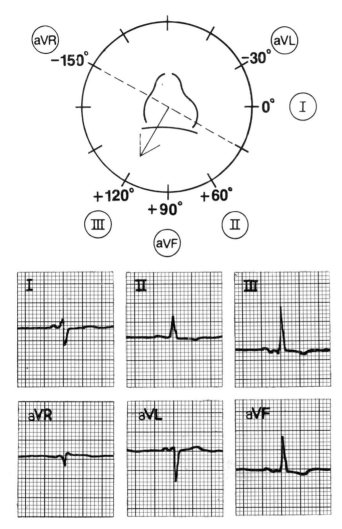

Fig. 9-14. Diagram and tracing illustrating the QRS axis in left posterior hemiblock.

LEFT ANTERIOR HEMIBLOCK

Left anterior hemiblock is caused by conduction delay or block in the anterior division of the left bundle branch. The supraventricular impulses (sinus or ectopic) activate the right ventricle through the right bundle branch and the posterior wall of the left ventricle through the left posterior fascicle. The impulses reach the anterior wall of the left ventricle, supplied by the blocked left anterior fascicle, through the Purkinje fibers that connect the posterior and the anterior fascicle. The resulting asynchronous activation of the left ventricle (the posterior wall is activated first, then the anterior wall) causes a marked shift of the QRS frontal plane axis to the left.

Atrial deflections and A-V conduction

The atrial rate, rhythm and configuration depend on the atrial mechanism, which may be sinus or ectopic. A-V conduction is usually normal.

Ventricular deflections

The QRS width is usually normal. The frontal plane axis of the QRS complex is shifted markedly to the left, beyond $-30°$ and often between $-45°$ and $-60°$.

Left anterior hemiblock can be quickly recognized by examining the QRS pattern in leads I, II, III and V_1. Lead I shows a predominantly positive QRS complex with small q wave and tall R wave; leads II and III show a predominantly negative QRS with small r wave and deep S wave. In lead V_1 the QRS is predominantly negative with no r wave or with small r and deep S wave.

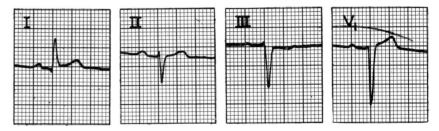

Fig. 9-15. Left anterior hemiblock.

CLINICAL NOTES

Left anterior hemiblock is the most common intraventricular conduction defect.[17] It is frequently associated with coronary heart disease hypertension, cardiomyopathies and aortic valve disease. Often the conduction disturbance appears following an acute anterior wall infarction.

Left anterior hemiblock is asymptomatic and does not cause any hemodynamic abnormality. Treatment is not necessary unless other intraventricular conduction fascicles are involved and the development of symptomatic A-V block can be anticipated.

LEFT POSTERIOR HEMIBLOCK

Left posterior hemiblock results from conduction delay or block in the posterior division of the left bundle branch. The supraventricular impulses (sinus or ectopic) activate the right ventricle through the right bundle branch and the anterior wall of the left ventricle through the left anterior fascicle. The impulses reach the posterior wall of the left ventricle, supplied by the blocked left posterior fascicle, through the Purkinje fibers that connect the anterior and the posterior fascicle. The resulting asynchronous activation of the left ventricle (the anterior wall is activated first, then the posterior wall) causes a shift of the QRS frontal plane axis to the right.

Atrial deflections and A-V conduction

The atrial rate, rhythm and configuration depend on the atrial mechanism, which may be sinus or ectopic. A-V conduction is usually normal.

Ventricular deflections

The QRS width is usually normal. The frontal plane axis of the QRS complex is shifted to the right, often to about $+120°$.

Left posterior hemiblock can be quickly recognized by examining the QRS pattern in leads I, II and III. Lead I shows a predominantly negative QRS complex with small r wave and deep S wave; leads II and III show a predominantly positive QRS complex with small q wave and tall R wave. In lead V_1 the QRS is predominantly negative with no r wave or with small r and deep S wave.

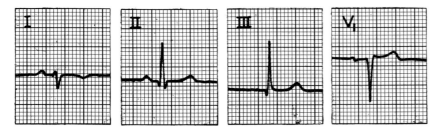

Fig. 9-16. Left posterior hemiblock.

Other conditions may cause right axis deviation and mimic left posterior hemiblock. Among the most frequent are a normal vertical heart in a young, slender individual and right ventricular hypertrophy caused by congenital heart defects, acquired valvular lesions including mitral stenosis and tricuspid insufficiency, and chronic lung disease. Clinical data such as the patient's history, age, height and weight, and other laboratory data such as previous electrocardiograms and a chest x-ray, are needed to rule out these conditions.

CLINICAL NOTES

Left posterior hemiblock is the least common intraventricular conduction

defect. It is rarely seen in the isolated or pure form, being usually associated with right bundle branch block (see below).

Left posterior hemiblock is asymptomatic and does not cause any hemodynamic abnormality. Treatment is not necessary unless other intraventricular conduction fascicles are involved and the occurrence of symptomatic A-V block can be anticipated.

RIGHT BUNDLE BRANCH BLOCK

Right bundle branch block results from conduction delay or block in the right bundle branch. The supraventricular impulses (sinus or ectopic) reach the left ventricle first through the anterior and posterior divisions of the left bundle branch. The right ventricle is activated with delay and, as a result, the QRS complex becomes wide and bizarre.

Atrial deflections

The atrial rate, rhythm and configuration depend on the atrial mechanism, which may be sinus or ectopic.

A-V conduction

May be normal. If first or second degree A-V block is associated with right bundle branch block, the A-V conduction delay or block may be occurring in the left bundle branch rather than in the A-V node (incomplete bilateral bundle branch block).

Ventricular deflections

The QRS width is increased to 0.12 second or more; the widening occurs in the second part of the QRS complex while the first part remains normal. The frontal plane axis of the QRS is essentially the same as before the occurrence of the block.

Right bundle branch block can be quickly recognized by examining the QRS pattern in leads I, II, III and V_1. Leads I and II show a predominantly positive QRS complex with wide S wave. Lead III displays a QRS predominantly positive or negative, according to the direction of the axis. In lead V_1 the QRS is predominantly positive, wide and often M-shaped.

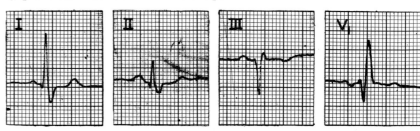

Fig. 9-17. Right bundle branch block.

CLINICAL NOTES

Coronary heart disease and right ventricular hypertrophy are among the most frequent causes of right bundle branch block. This type of intraventricular block is asymptomatic, does not cause any hemodynamic abnormality and usually does not require any treatment. Prophylactic insertion of a temporary transvenous pacemaker electrode has been recommended by some[64] when right bundle branch block complicates anterior wall infarction, in view of the significant incidence of sudden cardiac arrest in such cases. Others, however, have concluded that the prophylactic measure is not warranted.[79] The involvement of other conduction fascicles may make this measure the more necessary.[76]

RIGHT BUNDLE BRANCH BLOCK WITH LEFT ANTERIOR HEMIBLOCK

This form of bifascicular block is caused by conduction delay or block in both the right bundle branch and the anterior division of the left bundle branch. The supraventricular impulses (sinus or ectopic) reach first the posterior wall of the left ventricle through the posterior division of the left bundle branch; the anterior wall of the left ventricle is activated through the Purkinje network situated between the anterior and the posterior fascicles, while the right ventricle is invaded with delay. As a result the QRS complex becomes wide and bizarre and, in addition, the QRS axis in the frontal plane shifts markedly to the left.

Atrial deflections

The atrial rate, rhythm and configuration depend on the atrial mechanism, which may be sinus or ectopic.

A-V conduction

May be normal. If first or second degree A-V block is associated, the A-V conduction delay or block may be occurring in the remaining left posterior fascicle rather than in the A-V node (incomplete trifascicular block).

Ventricular deflections

The QRS width is increased to 0.12 or more; the widening occurs in the second part of the QRS while the first part remains normal. The frontal plane axis of the QRS complex is shifted markedly to the left, usually between −45° and −60°.

Right bundle branch block with left anterior hemiblock can be quickly recognized by examining the QRS complex in leads I, II, III and V_1. Lead I shows a predominantly positive QRS complex with small q wave, tall R and wide S wave. Leads II and III show a predominantly negative QRS complex with small r wave and a deep, wide S wave. In lead V_1 the QRS is predominantly positive, wide and often M-shaped.

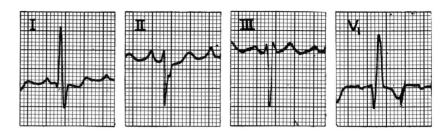

Fig. 9-18. Right bundle branch block with left anterior hemiblock.

CLINICAL NOTES

Hypertension and coronary heart disease are among the most common causes of this type of bifascicular block.[17] Prophylactic use of a temporary transvenous pacemaker has been recommended when right bundle branch block with left anterior hemiblock complicates acute myocardial infarction.[48,76]

RIGHT BUNDLE BRANCH BLOCK WITH LEFT POSTERIOR HEMIBLOCK

This form of bifascicular block results from conduction delay or block in both the right bundle branch and the posterior division of the left bundle branch. The supraventricular impulses (sinus or ectopic) reach first the anterior wall of the left ventricle through the anterior division of the left bundle branch; the posterior wall of the left ventricle is activated through the Purkinje network situated between the anterior and posterior divisions, while the right ventricle is invaded with delay. As a result the QRS complex becomes wide and bizarre and, in addition, its frontal plane axis shifts to the right.

Atrial deflections

The atrial rate, rhythm and configuration depend on the atrial mechanism, which may be sinus or ectopic.

A-V conduction

May be normal. If first or second degree A-V block are associated, the A-V conduction delay or block may be occurring in the remaining left anterior division rather than in the A-V node (incomplete trifascicular block).

Ventricular deflections

The QRS width is increased to 0.12 second or more. The widening occurs in the second part of the QRS while the first part remains normal. The frontal plane axis of the QRS complex is shifted to the right, usually to about +120°.

Right bundle branch block with left posterior hemiblock can be quickly recognized by examining the QRS complex in leads I, II, III and V_1. Lead I shows a wide and predominantly negative QRS complex with small r wave and deep, wide S wave. Leads II and III show a predominantly positive QRS complex with small q wave and tall, wide R wave. In lead V_1 the QRS complex is wide, predominantly positive and often M-shaped.

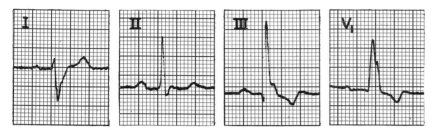

Fig. 9-19. Right bundle branch block with left posterior hemiblock.

In the presence of right bundle branch block, other conditions may cause right axis deviation and mimic associated left posterior hemiblock. As in pure left posterior hemiblock, clinical data such as the patient's history, age, height and weight, and other laboratory data such as previous electrocardiograms and a chest x-ray are needed to rule out these conditions.

CLINICAL NOTES

Coronary heart disease is one of the most common causes of right bundle branch block with left posterior hemiblock. The combination of anterior and inferior myocardial infarctions with septal involvement is frequently associated with this type of bifascicular block.[17] In view of the possible development of sudden complete A-V block some authors recommend the use of artificial pacing as a prophylactic measure.[76]

LEFT BUNDLE BRANCH BLOCK

Left bundle branch block results from conduction delay or block in the left bundle branch, either at the level of the main trunk or at the level of both its anterior and posterior divisions. The supraventricular impulses (sinus or ectopic) reach first the right ventricle through the right bundle branch; the left ventricle is then activated with delay and, as a result, the QRS complex becomes wide and bizarre.

Atrial deflections

The atrial rate, rhythm and configurations depend on the atrial mechanism, which may be sinus or ectopic.

A-V conduction

May be normal. If first degree or second degree A-V block are associated with left bundle branch block, the A-V conduction delay or block may be occurring in the right bundle branch rather than in the A-V node (incomplete bilateral bundle branch block).

Ventricular deflections

The QRS width is increased to 0.12 second or more. The widening involves the first as well as the second part of the QRS complex. The frontal plane axis of the QRS is essentially the same as before the occurrence of the block.

Left bundle branch block can be quickly recognized by examining the QRS pattern in leads I, II, III and V_1. Lead I shows a wide, predominantly positive and often M-shaped QRS complex. Leads II and III display a QRS which is predominantly positive or negative, according to the direction of its frontal plane axis. In lead V_1 the QRS complex is predominantly negative either without r wave or with small r wave followed by wide and deep S wave.

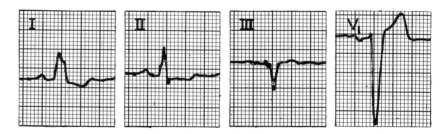

Fig. 9-20. Left bundle branch block.

CLINICAL NOTES

Many patients with left bundle branch block have severe heart disease. Coronary heart disease, hypertensive cardiovascular disease and valvular disease are among the most frequent causes. Myocardial infarction usually cannot be recognized in the presence of left bundle branch block. The intraventricular conduction defect per se does not cause any hemodynamic abnormality and the treatment is that of the underlying condition.

Intraventricular Block

LEFT ANTERIOR HEMIBLOCK (LAH)

A. Atrial deflections: depend on the atrial mechanism.

B. A-V conduction: usually normal.

C. Ventricular deflections:

1. QRS width: usually normal.
2. QRS axis shifted markedly to the left.
3. Lead I: QRS predominantly positive with small q wave and tall R wave.
4. Leads II and III: QRS predominantly negative with small r and deep S wave.
5. Lead V_1: QRS predominantly negative with no r wave or with small r and deep S wave.

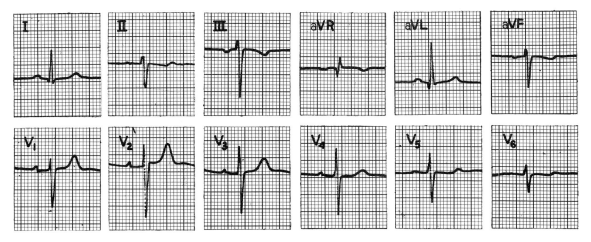

Rhythm 9-1,a. Normal sinus rhythm with left anterior hemiblock.

LEFT POSTERIOR HEMIBLOCK (LPH)

A. Atrial deflections: depend upon the atrial mechanism.

B. A-V conduction: usually normal.

C. Ventricular deflections:

1. QRS width: usually normal.
2. QRS axis shifted to the right.
3. Lead I: QRS predominantly negative with small r wave and deep S wave.
4. Leads II and III: QRS predominantly positive with small q wave and tall R wave.
5. Lead V_1: QRS predominantly negative with no r wave or with small r and deep S wave.

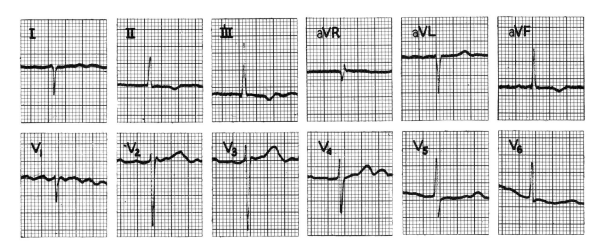

Rhythm 9-1,b. Atrial fibrillation with left posterior hemiblock.

Intraventricular Block

RIGHT BUNDLE BRANCH BLOCK (RBBB)

A. Atrial deflections: depend upon the atrial mechanism.

B. A-V conduction:

1. Normal.
2. First or second degree A-V block (may be due to incomplete bilateral bundle branch block).

C. Ventricular deflections:

1. QRS width: increased to 0.12 second or more.
2. QRS axis: essentially the same as before the occurrence of the block.
3. Leads I and II: QRS predominantly positive with wide S wave.
4. Lead III: QRS predominantly positive or negative according to direction of axis.
5. Lead V_1: QRS predominantly positive, wide and often M-shaped.

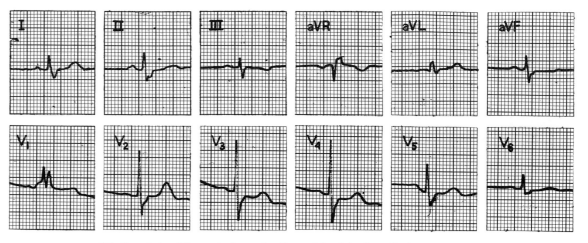

Rhythm 9-1,c. Normal sinus rhythm with right bundle branch block.

RIGHT BUNDLE BRANCH BLOCK WITH LEFT ANTERIOR HEMIBLOCK

A. Atrial deflections: depend upon the atrial mechanism.

B. A-V conduction:

1. Normal.
2. First or second degree A-V block (may be due to incomplete trifascicular block).

C. Ventricular deflections:

1. QRS width: increased to 0.12 second or more.
2. QRS axis: shifted markedly to the left.
3. Lead I: QRS predominantly positive with small q wave, tall R wave and wide S wave.
4. Leads II and III: QRS predominantly negative with small r wave and deep, wide S wave.
5. Lead V_1: QRS predominantly positive, wide and often M-shaped.

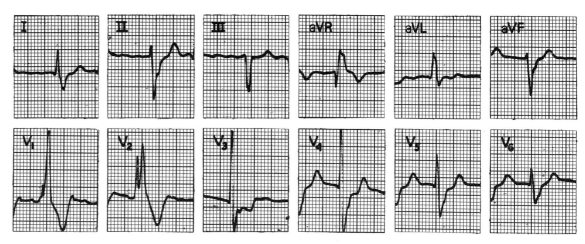

Rhythm 9-1,d. Atrial fibrillation with right bundle branch block and left anterior hemiblock.

Intraventricular Block

RIGHT BUNDLE BRANCH BLOCK WITH LEFT POSTERIOR HEMIBLOCK

A. Atrial deflections: depend upon the atrial mechanism.

B. A-V conduction:

1. Normal.
2. First or second degree A-V block (may be due to incomplete trifascicular block).

C. Ventricular deflections:

1. QRS width: increased to 0.12 second or more.
2. QRS axis: shifted to the right.
3. Lead I: QRS predominantly negative with small r wave and deep, wide S wave.
4. Leads II and III: QRS predominantly positive with small q wave and tall, wide R wave.
5. Lead V_1: QRS predominantly positive, wide and often M-shaped.

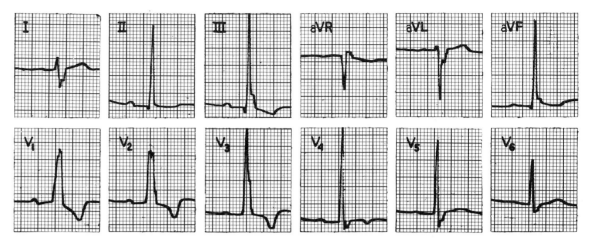

Rhythm 9-1,e. Normal sinus rhythm, first degree A-V block, right bundle branch block and left posterior hemiblock.

LEFT BUNDLE BRANCH BLOCK

A. Atrial deflections: depend upon the atrial mechanism.

B. A-V conduction:

1. Normal.
2. First or second degree A-V block (may be due to incomplete bilateral bundle branch block).

C. Ventricular deflections:

1. QRS width: increased to 0.12 second or more.
2. QRS axis: essentially the same as before the occurrence of the block.
3. Lead I: QRS predominantly positive and often M-shaped.
4. Leads II and III: QRS predominantly positive or negative according to direction of axis.
5. Lead V_1: QRS predominantly negative either without r wave or with small r wave and deep, wide S wave.

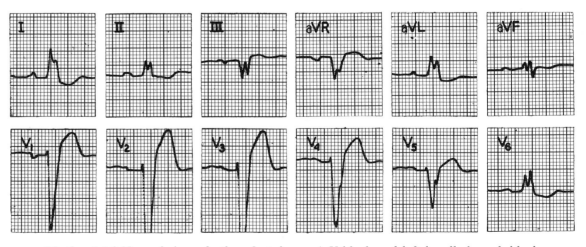

Rhythm 9-1,f. Normal sinus rhythm, first degree A-V block and left bundle branch block.

Chapter 10

Ventricular Ectopic Rhythms

Ventricular ectopic rhythms are caused by the repetitive firing of one or more ectopic foci located in the ventricles. They consist of six or more consecutive ventricular ectopic beats which temporarily seize control of the ventricles and, if the impulses can be conducted retrogradely, of the atria as well.

Classification and mechanism of production

Ventricular foci have an inherent or natural rate below 40 per minute and, under normal circumstances, they are continuously discharged by the faster sinus or ectopic supraventricular impulses. When the atrial rate becomes too slow and when the supraventricular impulses fail to reach the ventricles, a ventricular focus can manifest its activity in a repetitive fashion. The resulting "passive" rhythm is called *idioventricular escape rhythm*.

A ventricular focus may also acquire enhanced automaticity, produce impulses at a rate faster than 40 per minute and temporarily seize control of the ventricles with an "active" mechanism. "Active" ventricular ectopic rhythms include *nonparoxysmal ventricular tachycardia, paroxysmal ventricular tachycardia, ventricular flutter* and *ventricular fibrillation*.

The most important factor which determines the occurrence of one ventricular ectopic rhythm instead of another is the discharge rate of the ectopic focus or foci. For convenience and didactic reasons arbitrary rates have been set in the classification of the various ventricular rhythms. These rates provide a useful guide although it should be remembered that there is overlapping and that exceptions may occur.

Ventricular Rates

Idioventricular escape rhythm	below 40 per minute
Nonparoxysmal ventricular tachycardia	40 to 100 per minute
Paroxysmal ventricular tachycardia	100 to 250 per minute
Ventricular flutter	150 to 300 per minute
Ventricular fibrillation	150 to 500 per minute (chaotic)

In ventricular ectopic rhythms the atria and the ventricles beat independently of each other because of A-V dissociation or A-V block.

A-V dissociation during ventricular tachycardia usually results from differential refractoriness in the A-V node. This means that there are two areas in the A-V node with different refractory periods: a high area with a longer refractory period (penetrated by the sinus or ectopic supraventricular impulses) and a low area with a shorter refractory period (penetrated retrogradely by the ventricular impulses). Differential refractoriness in the A-V node is illustrated in Figure 10-1.

Occasionally a sinus or ectopic supraventricular impulse may reach the ventricles at an opportune time, causing a ventricular capture or fusion beat. Conversely, a ventricular impulse may reach the atria, causing an atrial capture or fusion beat. Ventricular fusion beats are often referred to as Dressler beats.[39]

The ventricular impulses first invade the ventricle in which they originate, then spread to the opposite ventricle with delay. The resulting QRS complexes are wide and bizarre; their configuration resembles that of right bundle branch

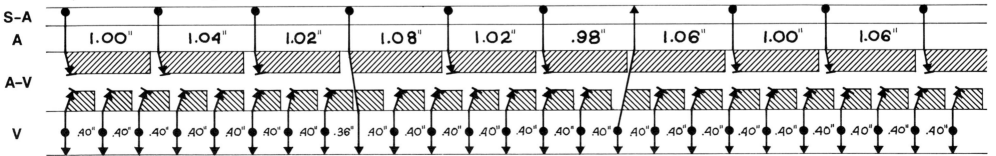

Fig. 10-1. Ladder diagram of ventricular tachycardia during sinus rhythm illustrating the occurrence of differential refractoriness in the A-V node. A sinus impulse arrives at an opportune time, causing a ventricular capture, and a ventricular impulse is retroconducted to the atria, causing an atrial capture.

block if the impulses originate in the left ventricle, and that of left bundle branch block if the impulses originate in the right ventricle. When the ventricular impulses are multifocal or when unifocal impulses change their direction of propagation in the ventricular myocardium, the QRS configuration varies.

The QRS width in ventricular ectopic rhythms may occasionally remain within normal limits. His bundle electrography has shown that this occurs when the pacemaking focus is located in one of the intraventricular conduction fascicles and its impulses simultaneously travel distally to reach the ventricle and centrally to reach the His bundle and the opposite bundle branch.[33,62] Another explanation for this apparent paradox is that, in the lead used for monitoring, the initial or terminal portion of the QRS complex happens to be isoelectric; if this is the case, a rhythm strip recorded in a different lead will show that the QRS complex is actually wide.

IDIOVENTRICULAR ESCAPE RHYTHM

Idioventricular escape rhythm is a "passive" rhythm resulting from the repetitive firing of a ventricular focus at its inherent or natural rate of below 40 per minute. The rhythm occurs as a safety mechanism whenever impulses from a higher focus, including the sinus node, fail to occur or are prevented from reaching the ventricles by A-V dissociation or A-V block.

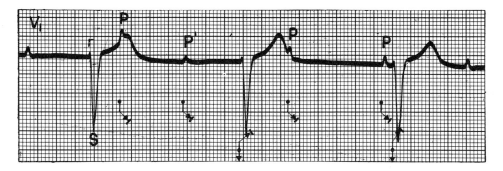

Fig. 10-2. Idioventricular escape rhythm during sinus rhythm with atrial extrasystoles and complete A-V block. The QRS complexes resemble left bundle branch block and, therefore, the ectopic focus is located in the right ventricle.

Atrial deflections

The rate, rhythm and configuration of the atrial deflections depend on the atrial mechanism, which may be sinus or ectopic. The sinus or ectopic atrial waves precede, are hidden within or follow the QRS complexes. An inverted P' wave (atrial capture) rarely follows a QRS complex of ventricular origin. The P-P interval which includes a QRS complex may be shorter than the P-P interval without a QRS complex (ventriculophasic sinus arrhythmia).

A-V conduction

When visible, the sinus or ectopic atrial waves "travel" toward, inside and away from the QRS complexes (A-V dissociation): they bear no constant relationship to the QRS so that the "P-P interval" continuously changes in duration. Ventricular captures and fusion beats are often preceded by a P wave and normal or prolonged P-R interval.

Ventricular deflections

The ventricular rate in idioventricular escape rhythm is below 40 per minute. At the onset of the escape rhythm the ventricular rate may gradually increase for a few beats: this is called the Treppe phenomenon and is due to a "warming up" of the dormant ventricular focus. The ventricular rhythm is usually regular.

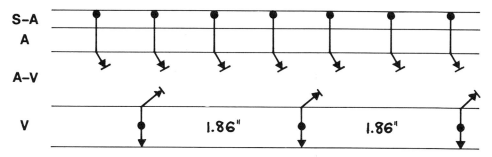

Fig. 10-3. Idioventricular escape rhythm during sinus rhythm with complete A-V block. Ladder diagram of the first half of Rhythm 10-1,b.

The QRS complexes are wide and bizarre. Their configuration resembles right bundle branch block when the ectopic impulses originate in the left ventricle and left bundle branch block when they originate in the right ventricle.

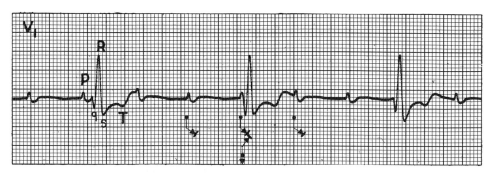

Fig. 10-4. Idioventricular escape rhythm during sinus tachycardia and complete A-V block. The QRS complexes resemble right bundle branch block and, therefore, the ectopic focus is located in the left ventricle.

The QRS rate, rhythm and configuration may vary owing either to unifocal ventricular impulses with changes in discharge rate and direction of myocardial propagation or to multifocal ventricular impulses.

Ventricular captures cause premature QRS complexes, often of normal configuration. Ventricular fusion beats are also premature but their configuration is intermediate between that of a capture and that of an idioventricular beat.

CLINICAL NOTES

The most frequent cause of idioventricular escape rhythm is high grade or complete A-V block. Marked sinus bradycardia, sinus arrest and sino-atrial block may also cause the appearance of idioventricular escape rhythm when the A-V node, which has a faster natural rate, is unable to fire or its impulses are unable to reach the ventricles.

Idioventricular escape rhythm is almost always symptomatic, especially in the presence of advanced cardiovascular disease. Stokes-Adams attacks may occur, owing either to ventricular standstill or to superimposed ventricular tachycardia and ventricular fibrillation.

The treatment of idioventricular escape rhythm usually consists of artificial pacing, especially in symptomatic patients, since drugs needed to control heart failure and other associated arrhythmias may then be used with impunity. Isoproterenol I.V. drip may be needed as a temporary measure. When the cause is digitalis toxicity, discontinuation of the drug is mandatory.

VENTRICULAR TACHYCARDIA

Ventricular tachycardia is an "active" rhythm resulting from the repetitive firing of one or more ectopic ventricular foci at a rate faster than 40 per minute. Ventricular tachycardia is classified into two forms, according to the discharge rate of the ectopic ventricular focus: *nonparoxysmal* when the ventricular rate is between 40 and 100 per minute, and *paroxysmal* when the rate is between 100 and 250 per minute.

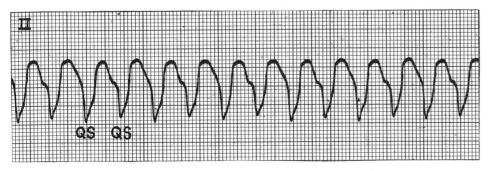

Fig. 10-5. Paroxysmal ventricular tachycardia.

Nonparoxysmal ventricular tachycardia is also called idioventricular tachycardia,[18] slow ventricular tachycardia,[26] or accelerated idioventricular rhythm.[12]

Atrial deflections

The rate, rhythm and configuration of the atrial deflections depend on the atrial mechanism, which may be sinus or ectopic. Identification of the atrial mechanism may be difficult when the ventricular rate is fast. Sinus or ectopic atrial waves may precede, be hidden within or follow the QRS complexes. When there is retrograde conduction to the atria the inverted P' waves (atrial captures) follow the QRS complexes of ventricular origin.

A-V conduction

When visible, the sinus or ectopic atrial waves "travel" toward, inside and away from the QRS complexes (A-V dissociation): they bear no constant relationship to the QRS so that the "P-R interval" continuously changes in duration.

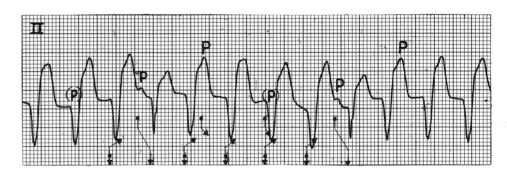

Fig. 10-6. Paroxysmal ventricular tachycardia with two ventricular capture by the sinus impulses. The QRS complexes resemble left bundle branch block and, therefore, the ectopic focus is located in the right ventricle.

Ventricular tachycardia may be superimposed on first, second or third degree A-V block. The presence of A-V block, however, can be diagnosed with certainty only when the ventricular tachycardia is intermittent.

Ventricular deflections

In nonparoxysmal ventricular tachycardia the ventricular rate is between 40 and 100 per minute whereas in the paroxysmal form the rate is between 100 and 250 per minute. The ventricular rhythm is regular or slightly irregular. A variety of the paroxysmal form, characterized by short runs of ventricular tachycardia separated by normal beats, is called repetitive ventricular tachycardia.

The QRS complexes are wide and bizarre. Their configuration resembles right bundle branch block when the ectopic impulses originate in the left ventricle

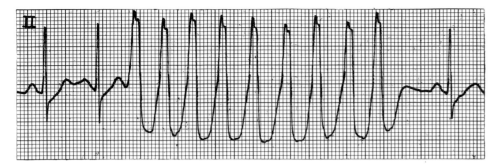

Fig. 10-7. Repetitive ventricular tachycardia during sinus rhythm.

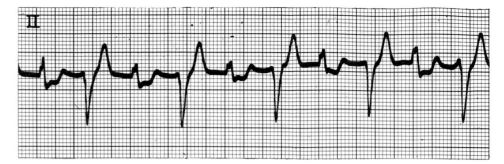

Fig. 10-9. Bidirectional ventricular tachycardia.

and left bundle branch block when the ectopic impulses originate in the right ventricle. The contour of some QRS complexes, ST segments, or T waves may vary because of superimposed P waves.

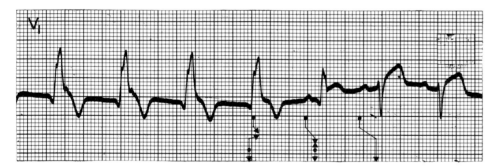

Fig. 10-8. Nonparoxysmal ventricular tachycardia during sinus rhythm. A ventricular fusion beat and two ventricular captures can be seen. The QRS complexes resemble right bundle branch block and, therefore, the ectopic focus is located in the left ventricle.

Ventricular captures appear as premature QRS complexes, often of normal configuration and preceded by a P wave. The QRS complex of the ventricular fusion beats has a configuration intermediate to that of a ventricular capture and that of a ventricular tachycardia beat.

The QRS rate, rhythm and configuration may vary, owing either to unifocal ventricular impulses with changes in discharge rate and direction of myocardial propagation or to multifocal ventricular impulse. *Bidirectional ventricular tachycardia* is characterized by wide and bizarre QRS complexes of two different configurations which are opposite in direction and frequently alternate.

CLINICAL NOTES

Ventricular tachycardia may occasionally occur in apparently normal individuals. Most frequently, however, it is associated with coronary heart disease,

especially acute myocardial infarction, or hypertensive or rheumatic heart disease. Bidirectional ventricular tachycardia is often associated with digitalis toxicity.

Nonparoxysmal ventricular tachycardia may be asymptomatic and cause no circulatory abnormality. Paroxysmal ventricular tachycardia, on the other hand, is almost always symptomatic, and its fast ventricular rate frequently causes a fall in the cardiac output which, in turn, produces or aggravates hypotension, heart failure, and myocardial and cerebral ischemia. Ventricular flutter and fibrillation may rapidly ensue. The sudden termination of a ventricular tachycardia episode may be followed by ventricular standstill.

Nonparoxysmal ventricular tachycardia often does not require any active treatment. Atropine may be used to accelerate the sinus rhythm and override the ectopic ventricular rhythm. The use of suppressive cardiac drugs such as lidocaine or procainamide has been discouraged by some.[74]

Paroxysmal ventricular tachycardia should be treated as soon as possible. Drugs used include lidocaine, procainamide, quinidine, propranolol and, in congestive heart failure, digitalis. Diphenylhydantoin or propranolol may be effective in treating ventricular tachycardia caused by digitalis toxicity. Electrical cardioversion may be indicated when the arrhythmia causes hemodynamic deterioration. In cases resistant to drug treatment artificial pacing may be needed to "overdrive" the ectopic ventricular rhythm.

VENTRICULAR FLUTTER AND FIBRILLATION

Ventricular flutter is caused by the repetitive and rapid firing of one or more ectopic ventricular foci at a rate usually between 150 and 300 per minute and with a fairly regular rhythm. Ventricular flutter may rapidly deteriorate into ventricular fibrillation.

Ventricular fibrillation results from the repetitive and rapid firing of multiple ectopic ventricular foci (theory of multifocal impulse formation) at a very fast rate and with a chaotic rhythm. Coordinated electrical and mechanical activity of the ventricles is no longer present. The rate of the chaotic waves ranges between 150 and 500 per minute. There are two varieties of ventricular fibrillation: the "coarse" type and the "fine" or anoxic type.

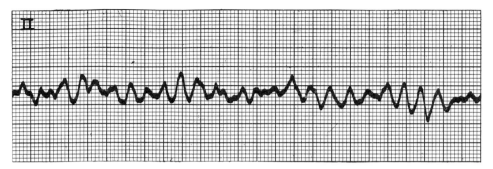

Fig. 10-10. "Coarse" ventricular fibrillation.

Atrial deflections and A-V conduction

The atrial deflections cannot be recognized and there is no A-V conduction.

Ventricular deflections

In ventricular flutter the ventricular rate is usually between 150 and 300 per minute and therefore, at least in some cases, in the ventricular tachycardia range. The distinctive characteristic of ventricular flutter is that the QRS complexes are wider, more bizarre, and tall, one merging into the other; the ST segments and the T waves cannot be recognized.

In ventricular fibrillation the ventricular waves are irregular and chaotic, with continuously changing rate and configuration. P, QRS and T deflections cannot be recognized. There are two types of ventricular fibrillation: the "coarse" type with prominent ventricular waves and the "fine" or anoxic type with shallow waves.

CLINICAL NOTES

Ventricular flutter and ventricular fibrillation are the most common causes of sudden death and are frequently associated with acute myocardial infarction and digitalis toxicity.

In ventricular flutter cardiac contraction is still present but the cardiac output becomes extremely low and the arrhythmia is always symptomatic. In ventricular fibrillation the heart loses its pumping action completely and circulatory arrest occurs.

Treatment must be instituted as quickly as possible. Electrical precordial shock may be successful in restoring an effective cardiac rhythm. When the defibrillator is not immediately available, cardiopulmonary resuscitation maneuvers should be carried out until electrical defibrillation can be applied. Once effective cardiac rhythm is restored, drugs used in the treatment of paroxysmal ventricular tachycardia should be employed to prevent recurrences.

Idioventricular Escape Rhythm

Ectopic rhythm due to the repetitive firing of an ectopic ventricular focus at a rate below 40 per minute.

Rhythm 10-1,a. Idioventricular escape rhythm at a rate of 31 per minute. There is sinus tachycardia at a rate of 105 per minute and complete A-V block.

ELECTROCARDIOGRAPHIC CRITERIA

A. Atrial deflections:

1. Rate, rhythm and configuration depend on the atrial mechanism (sinus or ectopic).
2. The sinus or ectopic atrial waves precede, are hidden within or follow the QRS complexes.
3. An inverted P' wave rarely follows a QRS complex (atrial capture).
4. The P-P interval that includes a QRS complex may be shorter than the P-P interval without a QRS complex (ventriculophasic sinus arrhythmia).

B. A-V conduction:

1. The sinus or ectopic atrial waves bear no constant relationship to the QRS complexes and the "P-R interval" continuously changes in duration (A-V dissociation).
2. Ventricular captures and fusion beats are often preceded by a P wave with normal or prolonged P-R interval.

C. Ventricular deflections:

1. Rate: below 40 per minute.
2. Rhythm: usually regular.
3. QRS configuration: wide and bizarre.
   a. Resembling right bundle branch block: ectopic focus located in the left ventricle.
   b. Resembling left bundle branch block: ectopic focus located in the right ventricle.
4. Ventricular captures: premature QRS complexes, often of normal configuration. Ventricular fusion beats: premature QRS complexes with configuration intermediate to that of a capture and that of an idioventricular beat.
5. The QRS rate, rhythm and configuration may vary:
   a. Unifocal ventricular impulses with changes in discharge rate and direction of myocardial propagation.
   b. Multifocal ventricular impulses.

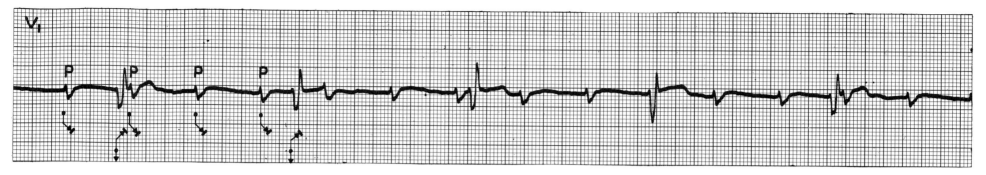

Rhythm 10-1,b. Idioventricular escape rhythm at a rate of 33 per minute. There is sinus rhythm at a rate of 88 per minute and complete A-V block.

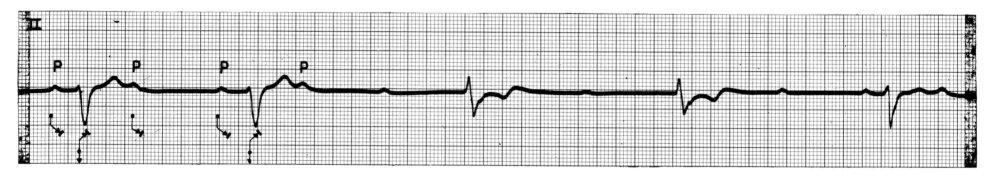

Rhythm 10-1,c. Idioventricular escape rhythm with QRS complexes of varying rate, rhythm and configuration probably due to multifocal ventricular impulses. There is sinus rhythm at a rate of 68 per minute, shifting pacemaker with the sinus node and complete A-V block.

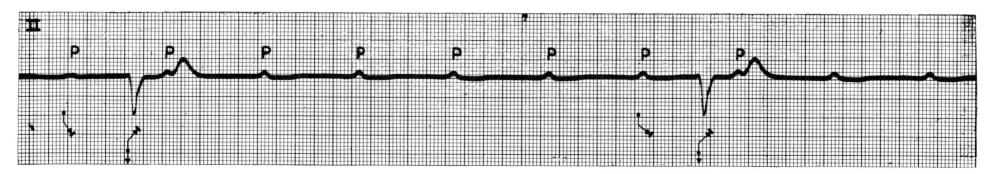

Rhythm 10-1,d. Idioventricular escape rhythm at the unusually slow rate of 10 beats per minute. The atria are under the control of sinus bradycardia at a rate of 59 per minute and there is complete A-V block.

Ventricular Tachycardia

Ectopic rhythm due to the repetitive firing of an ectopic ventricular focus at a rate of 40 to 100 per minute (nonparoxysmal form) or of 100 to 250 per minute (paroxysmal form).

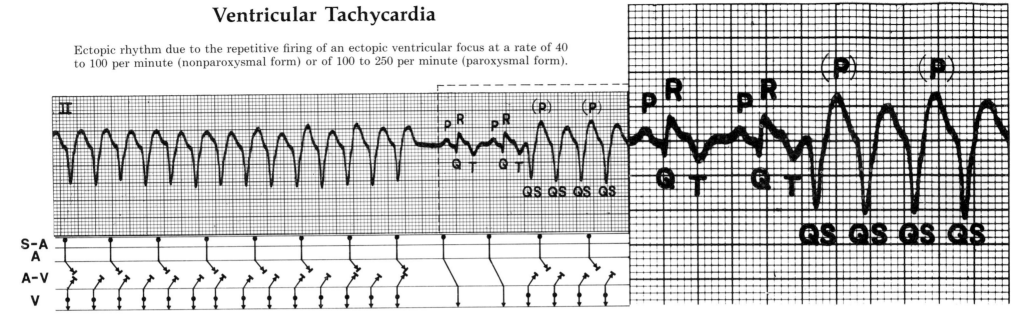

Rhythm 10-2,a. Paroxysmal ventricular tachycardia at a rate of 200 per minute. The paroxysm ends spontaneously and two ventricular captures by sinus impulses occur before the ventricular tachycardia begins again.

ELECTROCARDIOGRAPHIC CRITERIA

A. Atrial deflections:

1. Rate, rhythm and configuration depend on the atrial mechanism (sinus or ectopic). Identification of the atrial mechanism may be difficult.
2. The sinus or ectopic atrial waves precede, are hidden within or follow the QRS complexes.
3. An inverted P' wave rarely follows a QRS complex (atrial capture).

B. A-V conduction:

1. The sinus or ectopic atrial waves bear no constant relationship to the QRS complexes and the "P-R interval" continuously changes in duration (A-V dissociation).
2. Ventricular captures and fusion beats are often preceded by a P wave with normal or prolonged P-R interval.
3. Ventricular tachycardia may be superimposed on first, second, or third degree A-V block. The presence of A-V block can be diagnosed only when the ventricular tachycardia is intermittent.

C. Ventricular deflections:

1. Rate:
   a. Nonparoxysmal ventricular tachycardia: between 40 and 100 per minute.
   b. Paroxysmal ventricular tachycardia: between 100 and 250 per minute.
2. Rhythm: regular or slightly irregular.
3. QRS configuration: wide and bizarre.
   a. Resembling right bundle branch block: ectopic focus located in the left ventricle.
   b. Resembling left bundle branch block: ectopic focus located in the right ventricle.
4. Ventricular captures: premature QRS complexes, often of normal configuration. Ventricular fusion beats: premature QRS complexes with configuration intermediate between that of a capture and that of a ventricular tachycardia beat.
5. The QRS rate, rhythm and configuration may vary:
   a. Unifocal ventricular impulses with changes in discharge rate and direction of myocardial propagation.
   b. Multifocal ventricular impulses.

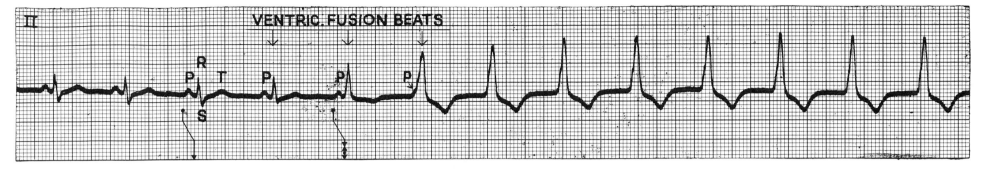

Rhythm 10-2,b. Sinus rhythm at a rate of 75 per minute followed by a run of nonparoxysmal ventricular tachycardia that begins with three ventricular fusion beats. The ectopic ventricular focus has a rate very similar to that of the sinus node and the sinus P waves become buried within the QRS complexes.

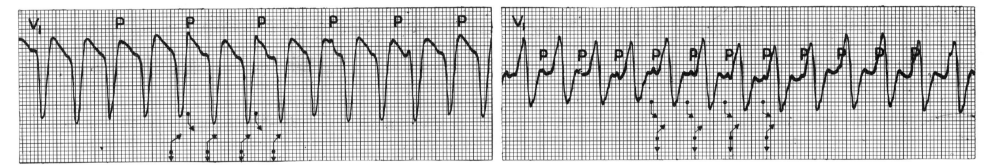

Rhythm 10-2,c. Paroxysmal ventricular tachycardia at a rate of 165 per minute. A-V dissociation is easily spotted. There are no captures or fusion beats.

Rhythm 10-2,d. Paroxysmal ventricular tachycardia at a rate of 160 per minute. The atria are under the control of either sinus tachycardia or atrial tachycardia impulses. The P (or P') waves "travel" toward and inside the QRS complex, confirming the presence of A-V dissociation.

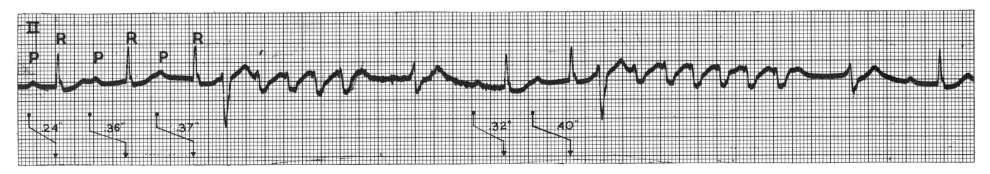

Rhythm 10-2,e. Sinus rhythm at a rate of 88 per minute and repetitive paroxysmal ventricular tachycardia superimposed on second degree A-V block type I (Wenckebach). Each paroxysm is followed by a ventricular escape beat.

Ventricular Flutter and Fibrillation

Rapid ectopic rhythms originating in the ventricles. Ventricular flutter has a rate of 150 to 300 per minute. Ventricular fibrillation consists of chaotic activity.

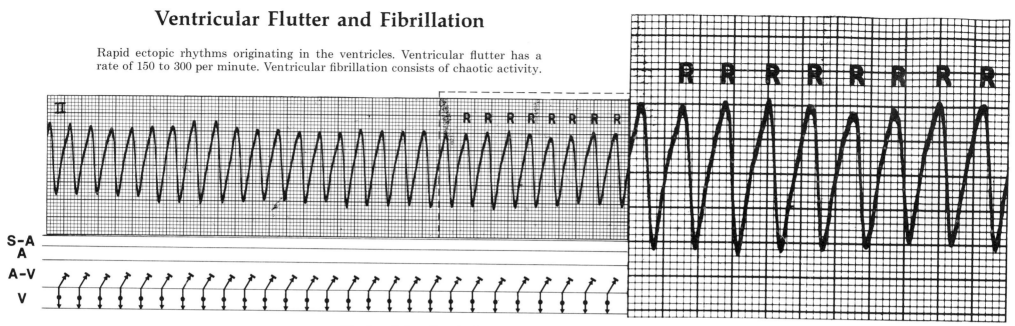

Rhythm 10-3,a. Ventricular flutter at a rate of 200 per minute.

ELECTROCARDIOGRAPHIC CRITERIA

A. Atrial deflections: cannot be recognized.

B. A-V conduction: none.

C. Ventricular deflections:

1. Ventricular flutter:
   a. Rate: 150–300 per minute.
   b. Rhythm: regular.
   c. Configuration: very wide, bizarre and tall QRS complexes, one merging into the other. ST segments and T waves cannot be recognized.

2. Ventricular fibrillation:
   a. Rate 150–500 per minute.
   b. Irregular, chaotic and bizarre waves. P, QRS and T deflections cannot be recognized.
   c. Two types: "coarse" ventricular fibrillation and "fine" or anoxic ventricular fibrillation.

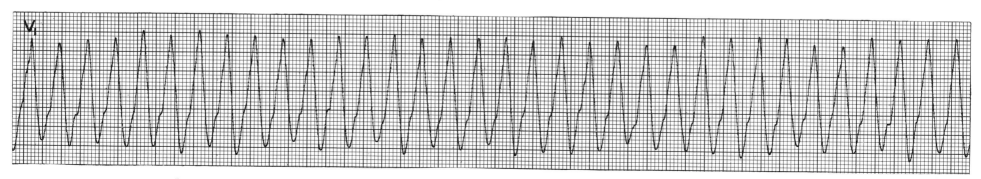

Rhythm 10-3,b. Ventricular flutter at the rate of 200 per minute.

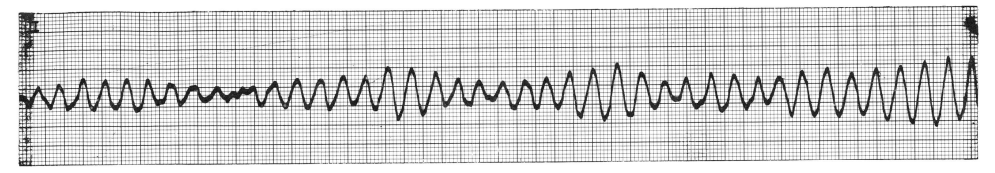

Rhythm 10-3,c. "Coarse" ventricular fibrillation.

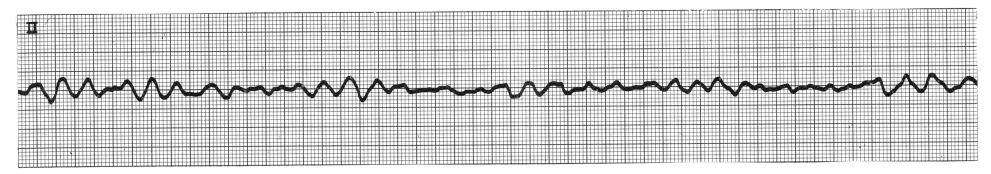

Rhythm 10-3,d. "Coarse" ventricular fibrillation.

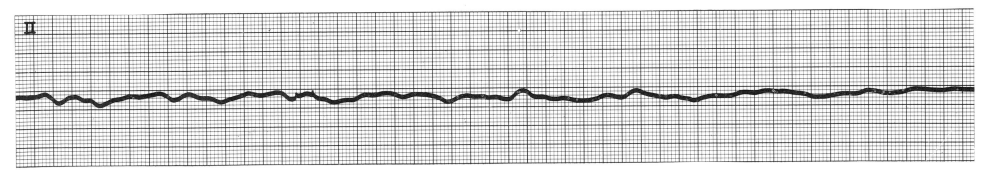

Rhythm 10-3,e. "Fine" ventricular fibrillation.

Chapter 11

Parasystole

Parasystole is a dual rhythm caused by the repetitive firing of an ectopic (parasystolic) focus which competes with the dominant cardiac rhythm. The parasystolic focus is commonly located in the ventricles, less commonly in the A-V node and rarely in the atria. The dominant cardiac rhythm may be sinus rhythm, atrial tachycardia, atrial flutter, atrial fibrillation or A-V nodal tachycardia.

Mechanism of production

In parasystole the ectopic focus is completely protected from outside interference. This protection, called entrance block, represents a form of unidirectional block which prevents outside impulses from reaching and discharging the parasystolic focus, while allowing its impulses to spread to the surrounding myocardium. The area of unidirectional block is situated in the immediate vicinity of the parasystolic focus and does not represent a form of atrioventricular conduction disturbance.

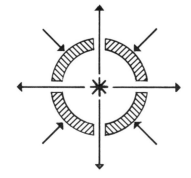

Fig. 11-1. Diagram illustrating the theory of entrance block in parasystole. The pacemaking focus is located in the center of the circle.

The parasystolic focus fires regular impulses, undisturbed by the dominant cardiac rhythm. Only those impulses that fall outside the refractory period induced by the dominant rhythm can spread to the surrounding myocardium

and produce ectopic beats. A fusion beat occurs whenever a parasystolic impulse activates only part of the myocardium while an impulse of the dominant cardiac rhythm activates the remainder.

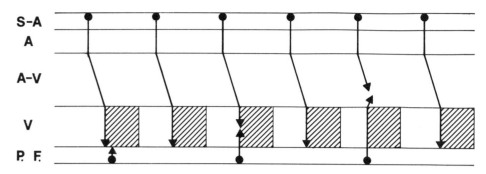

Fig. 11-2. Ladder diagram showing ventricular parasystole during sinus rhythm. The first parasystolic impulse finds the myocardium refractory, the second causes a ventricular fusion beat, the third produces a pure parasystolic beat. The sinus impulses activating the ventricles cannot reach the parasystolic focus (P.F.) because of entrance block.

Electrocardiographic manifestations

The following features are typical of parasystole:

1. The parasystolic beats appear as ectopic beats with variable coupling interval and similar configuration.

2. There is a mathematical relationship between the inter-ectopic intervals (the distance separating the parasystolic beats): the longer inter-ectopic intervals are multiples of the shorter ones. The shortest inter-ectopic interval may represent the rate of the parasystolic focus.

3. Fusion beats appear as ectopic beats having a configuration intermediate to that of the pure parasystolic beats and that of the dominant rhythm beats.

The rate of the parasystolic focus may range between 20 and 400 per minute[5,14] and may vary in the same tracing, usually by not more than a few hundredths of a second. Parasystole therefore occurs as a slow rhythm, as well as a fast rhythm called parasystolic tachycardia. An apparently slow parasystolic rhythm may be recorded although the actual rate of the parasystolic focus is twice, three times, etc. faster; this is due to 2:1, 3:1, etc. exit block from the parasystolic focus. Exit block is described in Chapter 14.

Ventricular parasystole is not a rare arrhythmia; A-V nodal parasystole is uncommon, and atrial parasystole is very rare.

VENTRICULAR PARASYSTOLE

The parasystolic focus is located in the ventricles. Its impulses (1) may find the myocardium refractory and are thus prevented from spreading to the surrounding tissue, or (2) may activate only part of the ventricles while the remainder is activated by the dominant cardiac impulses (ventricular fusion beats), or (3) may find the myocardium outside its refractory period and activate both ventricles (pure parasystolic beats).

Ventricular parasystole may be intermittent and, very seldom, may originate from more than one ventricular focus (double ventricular parasystole[31]). It has been reported that the same ectopic ventricular focus may at times cause ventricular extrasystoles and at other times cause ventricular parasystole.[78,81]

Atrial deflections

The rate, rhythm and configuration depend on the atrial mechanism, which may be sinus or ectopic. An inverted P′ wave may follow a ventricular parasystolic beat when its impulse is conducted retrogradely to the atria (atrial capture).

A-V conduction

A-V conduction is usually normal. Parasystole associated with varying degrees of A-V block has been reported.[5,29]

Ventricular deflections

The ventricular rate is below 40 per minute. When the rate is faster than 40 per minute the rhythm is called parasystolic ventricular tachycardia and, if all the parasystolic impulses activate the ventricles, the rhythm then resembles nonparoxysmal or paroxysmal ventricular tachycardia. In such a case, the parasystolic nature of the arrhythmia becomes evident only when the tachycardia is intermittent.

Isolated ventricular parasystolic beats appear as ectopic ventricular beats with variable coupling interval and similar configuration. The longer inter-ectopic intervals are multiples of the shorter inter-ectopic intervals. Ventricular fusion beats appear as QRS complexes having a configuration intermediate to that of the pure parasystolic beats and that of the dominant rhythm beats.

CLINICAL NOTES

Parasystole may occur in apparently healthy individuals as well as in cardiac patients, especially those affected by coronary heart disease and hypertensive cardiovascular disease. It is usually a transient arrhythmia but, in some cases, it may persist for years. The symptoms, if any, are similar to those caused by ectopic beats or rhythms of nonparasystolic nature.

The treatment of parasystole should be directed toward the underlying condition. Antiarrhythmic agents such as lidocaine, propranolol and procainamide may be indicated in some cases, particularly when a rapid parasystolic rhythm is present.

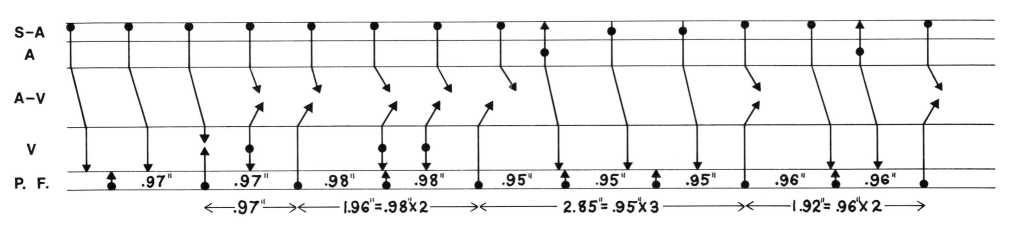

Fig. 11-3. Parasystolic ventricular tachycardia during sinus rhythm. Multifocal ventricular extrasystoles and one atrial extrasystole are also present. Ladder diagram of Rhythm 11-1,b.

Ventricular Parasystole

Ectopic rhythm due to the repetitive firing of an ectopic (parasystolic) ventricular focus at a rate usually below 40 per minute.

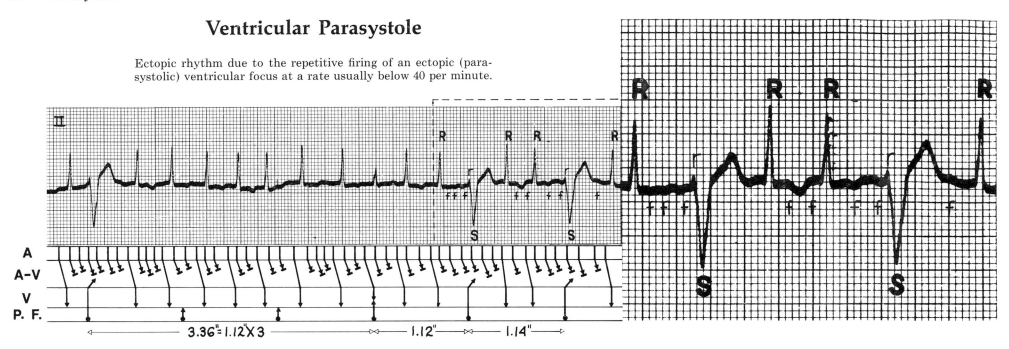

Rhythm 11-1,a. Atrial fibrillation with average ventricular rate 150 per minute. The isolated ectopic beats are the manifestation of a parasystolic ventricular tachycardia at a rate of 53 per minute. A ventricular fusion beat is present.

ELECTROCARDIOGRAPHIC CRITERIA

A. Atrial deflections:

1. The atrial mechanism may be sinus or ectopic.
2. When there is retroconduction to the atria an inverted P′ wave follows the parasystolic QRS complex.

B. A-V conduction: usually normal.

C. Ventricular deflections:

1. Rate:
   a. Below 40 per minute: ventricular parasystole or parasystolic ventricular tachycardia with exit block.
   b. Above 40 per minute: parasystolic ventricular tachycardia.
   c. The shortest inter-ectopic interval may represent the rate of the parasystolic focus. This rate usually varies by not more than a few hundredths of a second in the same tracing.

2. Rhythm and configuration:
   a. Ectopic ventricular beats with variable coupling interval and similar configuration.
   b. The longer inter-ectopic intervals are multiples of the shorter inter-ectopic intervals.
   c. Ventricular fusion beats appear as QRS complexes having a configuration intermediate to that of the pure parasystolic beats and that of the dominant rhythm beats.

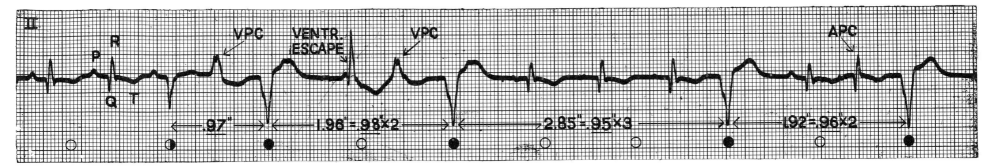

Rhythm 11-1,b. Sinus rhythm at a rate of 95 per minute with shifting pacemaker in the S-A node, one atrial extrasystole, multifocal ventricular extrasystoles, one ventricular escape, and parasystolic ventricular tachycardia at a rate of 108 per minute. The position of the parasystolic impulses is indicated by black dots (pure parasystolic beats), open circles (non-manifest parasystolic discharges) and half-shaded circles (fusion beats). The ladder diagram of this strip is shown in Figure 11-3.

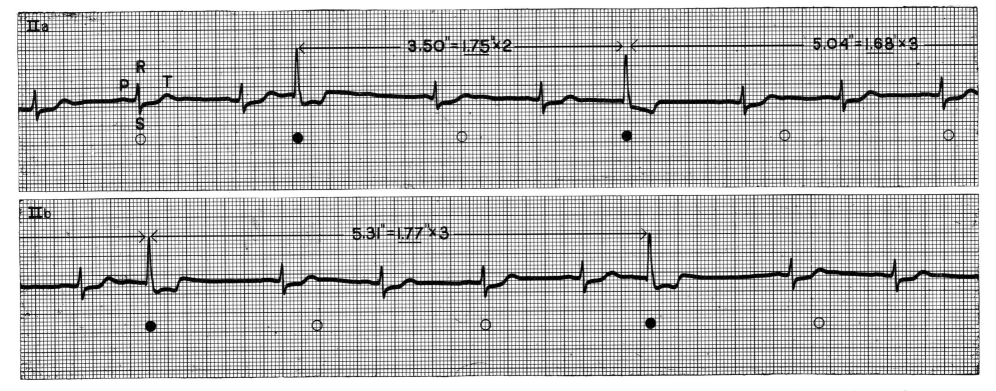

Rhythm 11-1,c. Sinus bradycardia at a rate of 58 per minute and ventricular parasystole. The rate of the parasystolic focus is 34 per minute and there are no fusion beats. The two strips IIa and IIb are continuous.

Chapter 12

Reciprocal Beats and Rhythm

Ectopic beats and rhythms may be caused by a re-entry mechanism as well as by enhanced automaticity of the specialized fibers in the conduction tissue of the heart.

There are two types of re-entry mechanism: local re-entry, and circus movement re-entry.[49]

Local re-entry occurs when myocardial fibers still being excited are in the immediate vicinity of other fibers which have already regained their excitability. Focal re-excitation of the latter fibers can occur, giving rise to isolated ectopic beats or, if the phenomenon is repetitive, to ectopic rhythms.

Circus movement re-entry occurs when a propagating impulse finds a pathway that initially fails to conduct in one direction (unidirectional block). While the impulse spreads through other fibers, the pathway recovers its excitability and becomes capable of conducting the same impulse in the opposite direction. Repeated circulation of the impulse along the same route creates a circus movement. This mechanism can also be established when conduction is delayed in an area of the re-entry circuit; the delay allows other areas to recover from the initial activation and to conduct the impulses in the opposite direction.

A specific form of re-entry is responsible for the production of so-called reciprocal beats and rhythm.

Mechanism of production of reciprocal conduction sequences

An impulse originating in the sinus node, the atria, the A-V node or the ventricles can be conducted first in one direction through a pathway and then return in the opposite direction through another pathway, causing a reciprocal conduction sequence and the appearance on the electrocardiogram of a reciprocal beat.

Reciprocal conduction sequences between the atria and the ventricles can occur only when the following conditions are met:

1. There are two pathways of conduction. Both pathways are situated in the A-V node or His bundle (longitudinal dissociation), or one pathway is the normal A-V conduction tissue and the other an accessory pathway.
2. There is unidirectional block in one of the two pathways.
3. The conduction time is prolonged within the re-entry circuit.

An *A-V nodal* impulse is usually conducted in two directions—forward to the ventricles and retrogradely to the atria. When the impulse finds two pathways of retrograde conduction it may be blocked in one and conducted slowly in the other. Once the impulse reaches the upper part of the A-V node it may find the previously blocked pathway recovered and, while continuing its retrograde journey to activate the atria, the same impulse may be conducted down again to the ventricles (see Fig. 12-1). The second ventricular excitation is called *reciprocal beat.*

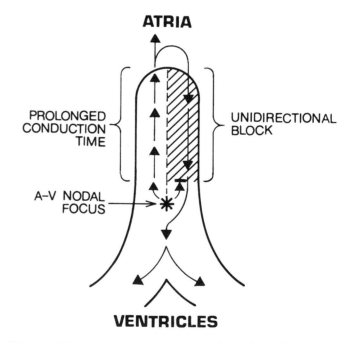

Fig. 12-1. Diagram illustrating the mechanism of a reciprocal sequence originating in the A-V node. Longitudinal dissociation is present and results in two different pathways within the A-V node. In the right pathway there is unidirectional block; in the left the conduction time is prolonged.

Through an analogous mechanism a *sinus* impulse (or an ectopic atrial impulse) can first spread forward to activate the atria and the ventricles and then travel back to reactivate the atria. The second atrial activation is called *reversed reciprocal beat* or atrial echo.

Similarly, a *ventricular* impulse that activates the ventricles and succeeds in spreading to the atria in a retrograde fashion can return in a forward direction to re-excite the ventricles. The second ventricular excitation is called *return extrasystole.*

A sinus, atrial, A-V nodal or ventricular impulse may spread to the ventricles and then back to the atria, down again to the ventricles and back up to the atria once more. If this sequence keeps repeating itself, a continuous circus movement is created between the atria and the ventricles and an initial reciprocal beat is followed by a run of *reciprocal rhythm.* A circus movement between

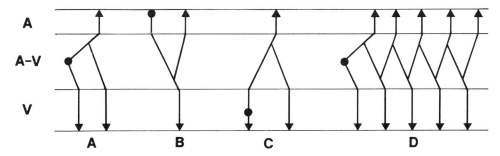

Fig. 12-2. Ladder diagram illustrating reciprocal beats and rhythm. A, reciprocal beat; B, reversed reciprocal beat or atrial echo; C, return extrasystole; D, reciprocal rhythm.

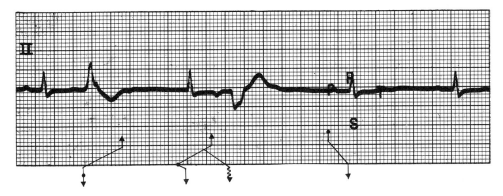

Fig. 12-3. Sinus bradycardia at a rate of 55 per minute. A ventricular extrasystole is followed by retrograde conduction and its postextrasystolic pause is terminated by an A-V nodal escape beat. The escape beat is in turn followed by a reciprocal beat with aberrant ventricular conduction.

the normal pathways and an accessory pathway is responsible for the reciprocal tachycardias frequently associated with the Wolff-Parkinson-White syndrome.

Electrocardiographic manifestations of the reciprocal sequences

A reciprocal impulse originating in the A-V node causes the appearance of an inverted P′ wave sandwiched between a QRS of A-V nodal origin and another QRS complex. A reciprocal impulse originating in the sinus node or in the atria produces a QRS complex sandwiched between a P (or P′) wave and an inverted P′ wave. When the reciprocal impulse originates in the ventricles it creates an inverted P′ wave sandwiched between a QRS of ventricular origin and another QRS complex. A train of reciprocal impulses causes a run of QRS complexes with inverted P′ waves sandwiched between them.

In each reciprocal sequence a conduction delay is present, causing the prolongation of either the P-R or the R-P′ interval. The reciprocal QRS complexes may be normal in configuration or may be wide and bizarre because of aberrant ventricular conduction.

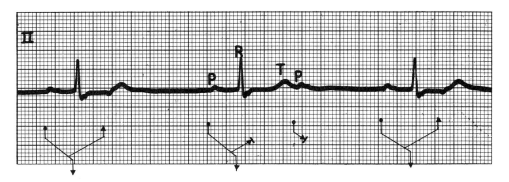

Fig. 12-4. Sinus rhythm with first degree A-V block and reversed reciprocal beats.

CLINICAL NOTES

The clinical significance of reciprocal beats and rhythm is similar to that of ectopic beats and rhythm not due to re-entry mechanism. Digitalis is a frequent cause of reciprocal beating.

Reciprocal Beats and Rhythm

Reciprocal conduction sequences between the atria
and the ventricles caused by a re-entry mechanism.

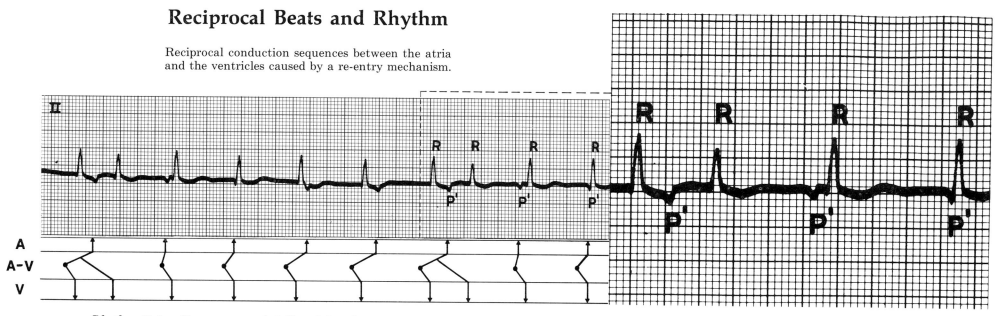

Rhythm 12-1,a. Nonparoxysmal A-V nodal tachycardia with progressively decreasing conduction velocity above the A-V nodal focus (retrograde Wenckebach phenomenon). When the R-P interval exceeds 0.20 second a reciprocal beat occurs.

ELECTROCARDIOGRAPHIC CRITERIA

A. Reciprocal beat originating in the A-V node:

1. Inverted P' wave sandwiched between a QRS complex of A-V nodal origin and another (reciprocal) QRS complex.
2. The R-P' interval is usually longer than 0.20 second.
3. The configuration of the reciprocal QRS complex may be:
   a. Normal.
   b. Wide and bizarre because of aberrant ventricular conduction.

B. Reciprocal beat originating in the sinus node or in the atria (reversed reciprocal beat):

1. QRS complex sandwiched between a P (or P') wave and an inverted P' wave (reciprocal).
2. The P-R interval may be:
   a. Prolonged.
   b. Normal. In this case the R-P' interval is the one that is prolonged.

C. Reciprocal beat originating in the ventricles (return extrasystole):

1. Inverted P' wave sandwiched between a QRS complex of ventricular origin and another (reciprocal) QRS complex.
2. The R-P' interval is usually longer than 0.20 second.
3. The configuration of the reciprocal QRS complex may be:
   a. Normal.
   b. Wide and bizarre because of aberrant ventricular conduction.

D. Reciprocal rhythm:

1. Run of QRS complexes with inverted P' waves sandwiched between them.
2. The ventricular rate is similar to that of ectopic atrial, A-V nodal and ventricular rhythms without re-entry.
3. The QRS configuration may be:
   a. Normal.
   b. Wide and bizarre because of aberrant ventricular conduction.

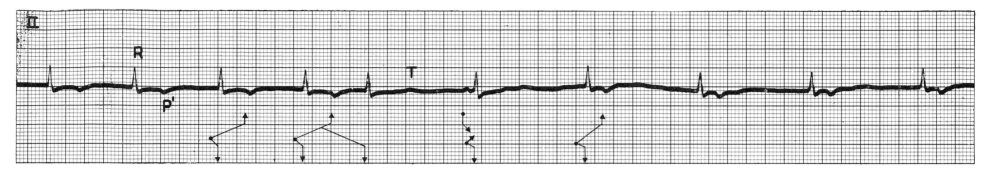

Rhythm 12-1,b. "Low" nodal ectopic rhythm with one reciprocal beat.

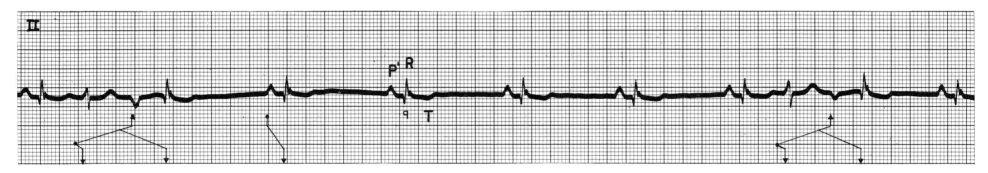

Rhythm 12-1,c. Sinus bradycardia at a rate of 48 per minute with reciprocal beats originating in the A-V node. Both the R-P′ and the P′-R intervals are prolonged.

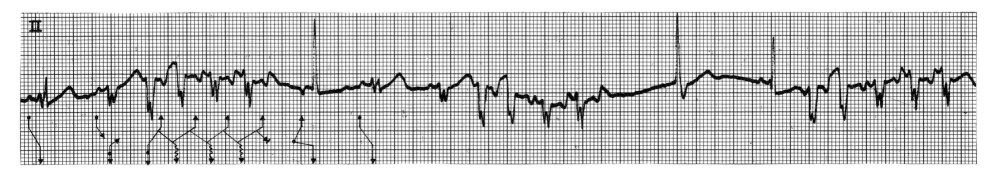

Rhythm 12-1,d. Sinus rhythm interrupted by runs of reciprocal rhythm probably originating in the ventricles. The pause after each run is terminated by an A-V nodal escape beat.

Chapter 13

Ventricular Pre-excitation and the Wolff-Parkinson-White Syndrome

Ventricular pre-excitation occurs when sinus impulses activate some part of the ventricles through an accessory pathway, earlier than through the normal conduction pathways.

The *Wolff-Parkinson-White* (W-P-W) syndrome consists of ventricular pre-excitation associated with paroxysmal supraventricular tachycardias.

Accessory conduction pathways

Three accessory conduction pathways are believed to play a role in ventricular pre-excitation. They are:

The Kent bundle: a muscular connection in the atrioventricular groove, capable of conducting impulses from the atria to either ventricle.

The Mahaim bundle: A conduction pathway connecting the upper part of the His bundle to the ventricles.

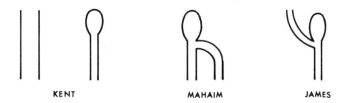

Fig. 13-1. Diagram of the three accessory conduction pathways believed to play a role in ventricular pre-excitation. (Castellanos, A., et al.: Pre-excitation and the Wolff-Parkinson-White syndrome. *In:* Schlant, R. C., and Hurst, J. W. (eds.): Advances in Electrocardiography. p. 249. New York, Grune & Stratton, 1972)

The James bundle: a conduction pathway connecting the atria to the distal portion of the A-V node or the His bundle.

Basic mechanism

The sinus or atrial impulses propagate to the ventricles simultaneously through both the accessory pathway and the normal A-V conduction pathways.

Each impulse spreads more rapidly through the accessory pathway and reaches the ventricles earlier than the same impulse traveling through the normal conduction pathways. Hence, a portion of the ventricles is prematurely stimulated or *pre-excited*, causing a short P-R interval and a wide QRS complex that begins with an abnormal wave called delta wave. While the pre-excitation impulse attempts to activate the surrounding tissue through common myocardium it is "overtaken" by the impulse conducted through the normal pathways; as a result, the remaining ventricular myocardium is activated normally and the remainder of the QRS complex is inscribed normally.

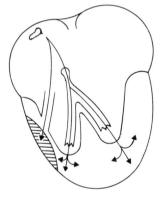

Fig. 13-2. Diagram showing the propagation of a sinus impulse through both an accessory pathway (Kent bundle) and the normal A-V conduction pathways.

The QRS complex of ventricular pre-excitation can therefore be considered a fusion complex due to the recombination in the ventricles of an impulse that has reached them through two different conduction pathways.

The degree of pre-excitation may vary in the same patient and, at times, conduction to the ventricles may be entirely normal, resulting in normal P-R intervals and normal QRS complexes. At other times conduction to the whole ventricular myocardium occurs through the accessory pathway only, causing very short P-R intervals and pure pre-excitation QRS complexes which are very wide and bizarre.

The P-R interval

The P-R interval in ventricular pre-excitation is usually short and measures less than 0.12 second. As a rule it is shortened by as much as the QRS is widened.

Cases of pre-excitation syndrome with normal or even prolonged P-R interval have been reported[44,67] and therefore the lack of short P-R in the presence of

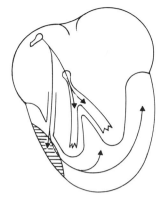

Fig. 13-3. Diagram showing the propagation to the ventricles of a sinus impulse through an accessory pathway only.

The delta wave appears as an initial slurring with the shape of the Greek letter delta (Δ). It is usually positive when the QRS is predominantly positive and negative when the QRS is predominantly negative. At times, a negative delta wave may be associated with a predominantly positive QRS complex and mimic the pathological Q wave caused by myocardial infarction.

When the ventricles are entirely activated by the pre-excitation impulse the QRS complex becomes very wide and bizarre.

Types of ventricular pre-excitation

There are two types of ventricular pre-excitation, type A and type B. In type A the QRS complex is predominantly positive in leads V_1 and V_2, as in right bundle branch block. In type B the QRS is predominantly negative in the same leads, as in left bundle branch block.

The Wolff-Parkinson-White (W-P-W) syndrome

Ventricular pre-excitation associated with paroxysmal tachycardias is called the W-P-W syndrome. Patients without paroxysmal tachycardias may have ventricular pre-excitation but they do not have the W-P-W syndrome.[20]

The paroxysmal tachycardias of the W-P-W syndrome are usually supraventricular and include atrial tachycardia, A-V nodal tachycardia, atrial flutter (rare) and atrial fibrillation. Atrial and A-V nodal tachycardia are generally considered as caused by a reciprocal mechanism.[18,40]

The ventricular rate during a paroxysm of tachycardia is usually very rapid, often faster than 180 to 200 per minute. The QRS configuration is normal when conduction to the ventricles occurs only through the normal pathways. When conduction occurs through both the normal and the accessory pathways, the QRS complexes are widened, usually with an easily identifiable delta wave. Very

wide QRS complex with delta wave does not exclude the diagnosis of pre-excitation.

At times the P-R duration varies in association with changes in magnitude of the delta wave; when this variation occurs progressively it is called the "concertina effect": the P-R interval gradually becomes shorter with more prominent delta waves, and then longer, with less prominent delta waves (see Fig. 13-7).

The QRS complex

In ventricular pre-excitation the QRS complex is widened and consists of an abnormal first portion (delta wave) inscribed by the impulse conducted through the accessory pathway, and a normal second portion inscribed by the impulse conducted through the normal conduction pathways.

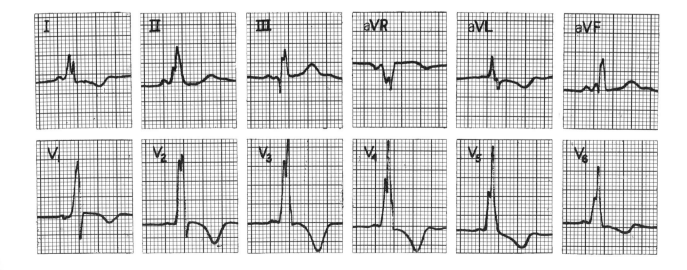

Fig. 13-4. Ventricular pre-excitation, type A.

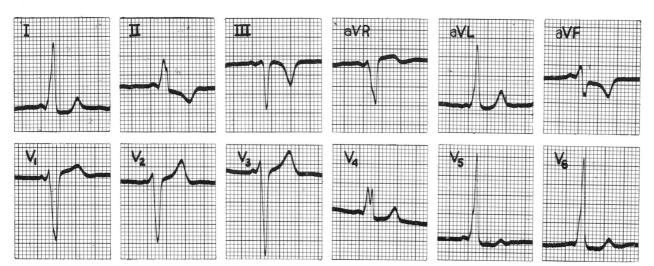

Fig. 13-5. Ventricular pre-excitation, type B.

wide and bizarre QRS complexes are recorded when conduction occurs solely through the accessory pathway. The aberrant QRS complexes in the W-P-W syndrome mimic ventricular extrasystoles and ventricular tachycardia.

The Lown-Ganong-Levine syndrome

Lown, Ganong and Levine described a syndrome consisting of normal P waves and QRS complexes, short P-R interval and tendency to develop paroxysmal tachycardias.[59]

This syndrome is considered a variant of the W-P-W syndrome and probably results from the presence of an accessory pathway of conduction. This pathway, probably the James bundle, bypasses the A-V node and allows the sinus or supraventricular ectopic impulses to reach the ventricles earlier, causing a short P-R interval. Unlike the W-P-W syndrome, however, activation of the ventricles occurs entirely through the bundle of His and the bundle branches so that the QRS complex remains normal in configuration.

CLINICAL NOTES

Ventricular pre-excitation probably results from a congenital anomaly and its familial origin has been postulated. It has been reported that 60 to 70 per cent of adults with the W-P-W syndrome show no evidence of heart disease.[39] The syndrome, however, may be associated with congenital heart defects, particularly the Ebstein anomaly of the tricuspid valve, or with acquired heart disease.

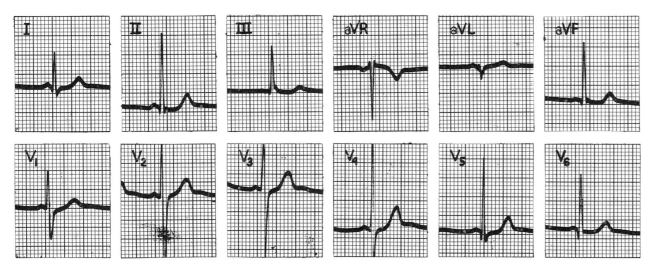

Fig. 13-6. Lown-Ganong-Levine syndrome.

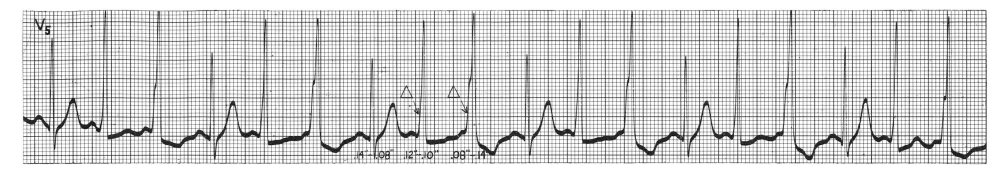

Fig. 13-7. Sinus tachycardia and ventricular pre-excitation. The "concertina effect" is clearly visible.

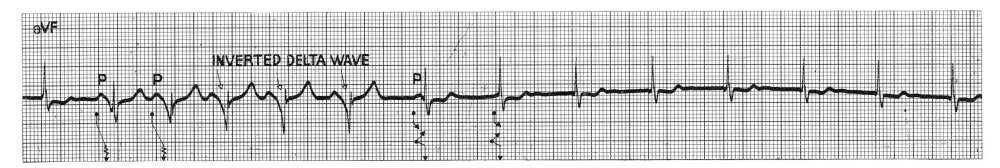

Fig. 13-8. Sinus rhythm with ventricular pre-excitation is preceded and followed by A-V dissociation between the sinus and the A-V node. The QRS complexes of sinus origin show an inverted delta wave which mimics the pathological Q wave of myocardial infarction; the A-V nodal beats display normal intraventricular conduction. (Same patient as in Fig. 13-1,c)

Ventricular pre-excitation causes no symptoms and is often identified when a routine electrocardiogram is recorded. The paroxysmal tachycardias of the W-P-W syndrome may cause palpitations and, in patients with underlying heart disease, may induce or aggravate hypotension, heart failure, myocardial and cerebral ischemia. Sudden death during or after an episode of paroxysmal tachycardia has been reported, presumably caused by ventricular fibrillation.[6,36]

In most cases the paroxysmal tachycardias of the W-P-W syndrome convert spontaneously to normal sinus rhythm.[50] Simple measures such as breath holding, Valsalva maneuver or carotid sinus massage may terminate the episode. Direct current (DC) shock is considered the most effective treatment of any type of tachyarrhythmia caused by the W-P-W syndrome.[5] Various drugs have been employed to terminate the paroxysmal episodes; propranolol and quinidine sulfate, alone or in combination with digitalis, are usually effective.[5,6] Other drugs such as procainamide and lidocaine have been used. The best results in the prophylaxis of paroxysmal tachycardias are given by propranolol or by a combination of propranolol and quinidine.[20] Surgical division of the A-V bundle or of the accessory pathway has been performed successfully in patients with drug-resistant and life-threatening recurrent tachycardias associated with the W-P-W syndrome.[24,32,37,41]

Ventricular Pre-excitation and the Wolff-Parkinson-White Syndrome

Ventricular pre-excitation occurs when sinus impulses activate some part of the ventricles through an accessory pathway, earlier than through the normal conduction pathways. When associated with paroxysmal tachycardias it is called the Wolff-Parkinson-White syndrome.

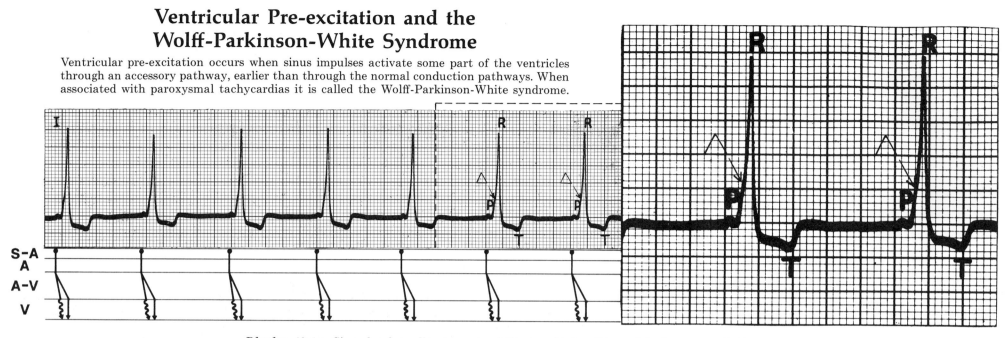

Rhythm 13-1,a. Sinus bradycardia at a rate of 59 per minute with ventricular pre-excitation.

ELECTROCARDIOGRAPHIC CRITERIA

VENTRICULAR PRE-EXCITATION

A. Atrial deflections: normal sinus P waves.

B. A-V conduction:

1. Short P-R interval, measuring less than 0.12 second.
2. The P-R interval may be normal or even prolonged.
3. "Concertina effect:" the P-R interval becomes gradually shorter with more prominent delta waves and longer with less prominent delta waves.

C. Ventricular deflections:

1. Widened QRS complexes with an initial slurring or delta wave.

a. Type A pre-excitation: QRS complexes predominantly positive in V_1 and V_2, as in right bundle branch block.
b. Type B pre-excitation: QRS complexes predominantly negative in V_1 and V_2, as in left bundle branch block.
2. QRS complexes of normal width and configuration (Lown-Ganong-Levine syndrome).

WOLFF-PARKINSON-WHITE-SYNDROME

A. Atrial deflections: the atrial waves are usually difficult to recognize because of the rapid ventricular rate.

B. A-V conduction: in atrial tachycardia, A-V nodal tachycardia and atrial flutter there is frequently 1:1 conduction.

C. Ventricular deflections:

1. Rate: Very rapid, often faster than 180–200 per minute.
2. Rhythm:
   a. Usually regular in atrial tachycardia, A-V nodal tachycardia and atrial flutter.
   b. Irregularly irregular in atrial fibrillation.
3. Configuration:
   a. Normal QRS complexes with no delta wave, when conduction occurs through the normal pathway only.
   b. Wide QRS complexes, usually with an easily identifiable delta wave, when conduction occurs through both the normal and the accessory pathways.
   c. Very wide and bizarre QRS complexes, when conduction occurs through the accessory pathway only.

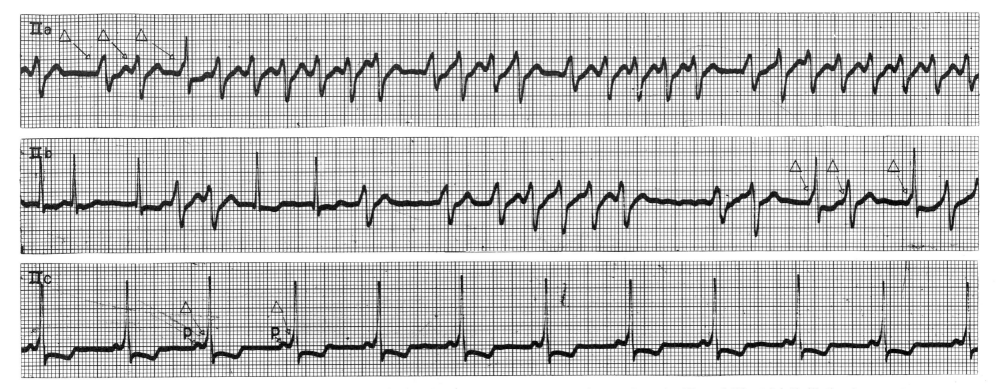

Rhythm 13-1,b. The three strips were recorded from the same patient and are not continuous. In strips IIa and IIb atrial fibrillation is present, with ventricular rate often as fast as 200 per minute. Most QRS complexes are wide and bizarre; but some show less aberration and a clear delta wave; others are of normal width and configuration. Strip IIc, recorded after conversion to sinus rhythm, confirms the presence of ventricular pre-excitation and the diagnosis of Wolff-Parkinson-White syndrome.

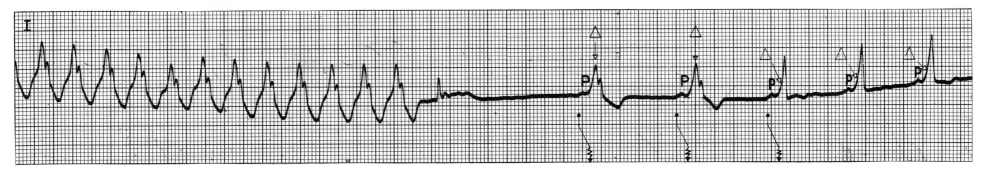

Rhythm 13-1,c. Wolff-Parkinson-White syndrome. A run of supraventricular tachycardia with wide and bizarre QRS complexes is followed by resumption of sinus rhythm with varying degrees of pre-excitation. (Same patient as in Fig. 13-8.)

Chapter 14

Exit Block

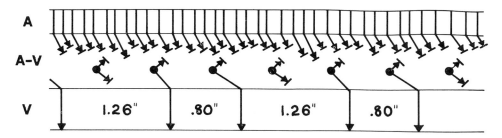

Fig. 14-2. Atrial fibrillation with high grade or complete A-V block and nonparoxysmal A-V nodal tachycardia. There is intermittent exit block, and the conducted A-V nodal impulses reach the ventricle with second degree A-V block Wenckebach type I. This is the ladder diagram of Rhythm 4-4,f.

Exit block is defined as the failure of a natural or artificial impulse to spread to the surrounding myocardium at a time when the myocardium has recovered from its refractory period.

Basic mechanism

Exit block of a natural or artificial impulse may be caused by either (1) a conduction depression surrounding the pacemaker focus, or (2) a decrease in intensity of the impulse.

The most frequent cause of exit block appears to be a conduction depression[43] which prevents some of the impulses from spreading to the surrounding myocardium while outside impulses may reach the pacemaking focus (unidirectional block).

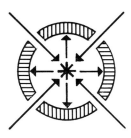

Fig. 14-1. Diagram illustrating the theory of exit block. The pacemaking focus is located in the center of the circle.

Exit block may occur as a type I (Wenckebach) conduction disturbance, causing the impulses to emerge from the pacemaking focus with progressively greater difficulty until they are blocked. It may also occur as a type II (Mobitz) disturbance, with sudden failure of conduction to the surrounding myocardium.

Exit block is a phenomenon common to all cardiac tissues with pacemaking or latent pacemaking properties[46] as well as to artificial pacemakers. The site of origin of impulses which may show exit block therefore can be the sinus node,

the atria, the A-V node, the ventricles, or an artificial pacemaker. Exit block also can be a feature of re-entry rhythms.

Electrocardiographic manifestations

Exit block of natural cardiac impulses. A natural cardiac impulse produces a wave on the electrocardiogram only when it succeeds in activating the surrounding myocardium. Exit block from a natural pacemaking focus therefore does not cause direct electrocardiographic manifestations. It can be recognized only indirectly, based on the changes in rate and rhythm of the P waves or QRS complexes resulting from the sudden or progressive failure of conduction of the impulses to the surrounding myocardium.

The occurrence or the disappearance of type II (Mobitz) exit block produces sudden changes in the manifest rate of the pacemaking focus. For example, the rate of the P waves is suddenly reduced to half when 2:1 sino-atrial exit block occurs and suddenly doubles when a previously present 2:1 sino-atrial exit block disappears. The Wenckebach type of sino-atrial exit block, on the other hand, causes progressive shortening of the P-P intervals, followed by a long pause, owing to the blocked sinus impulse.

The following varieties of exit block of natural cardiac impulses are known to occur:

1. Exit block from the sinus node (better known as sino-atrial block)
2. Atrial tachycardia or atrial flutter with exit block[54]
3. A-V nodal exit block during A-V nodal ectopic rhythms
4. Ventricular exit block during ventricular ectopic rhythms
5. Exit block in parasystole
6. Exit block in re-entry rhythms[43,56]

Exit block of artificial pacemaker impulses. On the electrocardiogram the impulse from an artificial pacemaker produces a sharp and narrow deflection called spike, regardless of whether the myocardium is activated or not. On the electrocardiogram, exit block from an artificial pacemaker can therefore be recognized directly, based on the failure of pacemaker spikes to activate the heart when the myocardium has recovered from its refractory period.

CLINICAL NOTES

The clinical significance of exit block from a natural focus is that of the underlying arrhythmia. Exit block from an artificial pacemaker is evidence of pacemaker malfunction and its causes include inadequate positioning or displacement of the electrode tip, increase in threshold above the output of the battery, and battery depletion; the treatment may require repositioning or replacement of the pacemaker electrode and replacement of the battery pack.

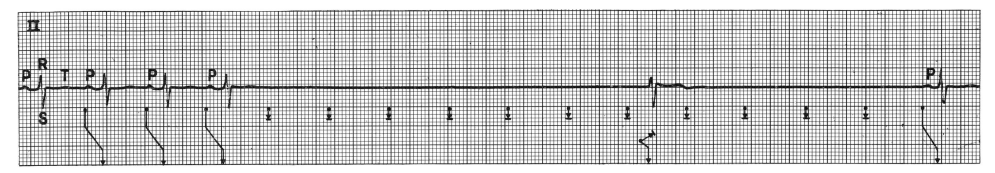

Rhythm 14-1,a. Sinus rhythm with second degree sino-atrial block type II. There is sudden exit block of 11 consecutive sinus impulses, causing atrial standstill for 7½ seconds. An A-V nodal escape beat interrupts the long ventricular pause.

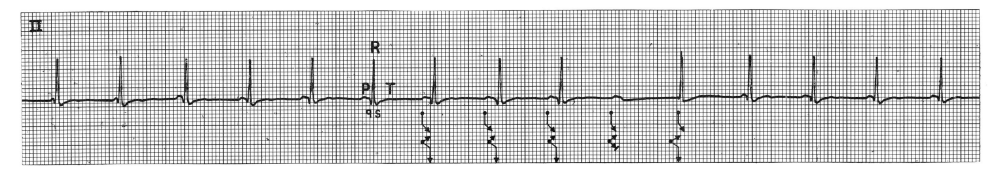

Rhythm 14-1,b. A-V dissociation between the sinus node and the A-V node. The atria are in sinus rhythm while the ventricles are under the control of a nonparoxysmal A-V nodal tachycardia. Note the sudden ventricular pause due to exit block of one A-V nodal impulse.

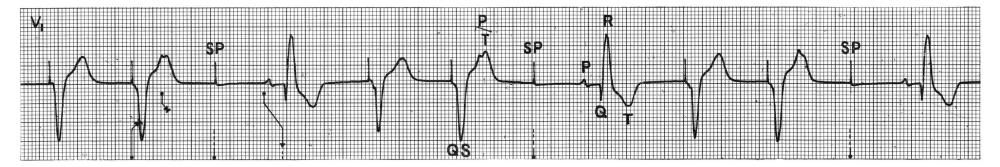

Rhythm 14-1,c. Malfunctioning ventricular-inhibited pacemaker. Three isolated spikes (SP) show exit block failing to activate the ventricles at a time when the myocardium has recovered from its refractory period. The spontaneous rhythm is sinus bradycardia with right bundle branch block.

Chapter 15

Concealed Conduction

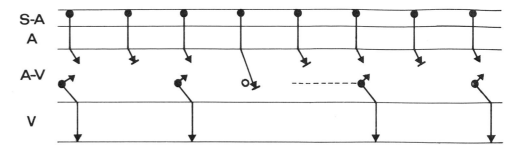

Concealed conduction is defined as the incomplete penetration of a cardiac impulse (sinus or ectopic) in an area of conducting tissue.

Effects of concealed conduction

An impulse that travels along a conducting pathway in a forward or retrograde fashion but fails to traverse it completely (incomplete penetration) may cause:

1. Delay or block in the *conduction* of a subsequent impulse.

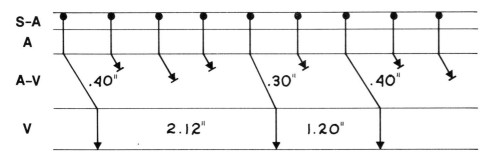

Fig. 15-1. Sinus tachycardia with high grade A-V block. The third sinus impulse penetrates the A-V nodal region incompletely, rendering it refractory and causing the block of the following sinus impulse. Ladder diagram of the first half of Rhythm 7-4,b.

2. Delay in the *expected discharge* of a subsequent impulse.

Electrocardiographic manifestations

Incomplete penetration of an impulse in a conducting pathway does not produce any waves on the electrocardiogram. The recognition of concealed conduction therefore can only be made indirectly and is based on its effect on the rhythm and conduction of subsequent impulses.

Concealed conduction may occur anywhere in the heart; most frequently it occurs in the A-V node. Common electrocardiographic manifestations are:

1. A prolonged P-R interval or the block of a sinus P wave following an A-V nodal or ventricular ectopic beat: the ectopic impulse penetrates the A-V node in a retrograde fashion, rendering it partially or completely refractory; the subsequent sinus impulse is thus conducted to the ventricles with delay or is completely blocked (concealed retrograde conduction).

2. A long ventricular pause following a ventricular extrasystole during atrial tachycardia, atrial flutter or atrial fibrillation: incomplete retrograde penetration of the ventricular impulse in the A-V node causes the block of a number of subsequent atrial impulses.

3. A 3:1 or higher degree of block during sinus or ectopic supraventricular rhythms, particularly atrial flutter: the supraventricular impulses penetrate the A-V node incompletely, rendering it refractory and causing the block of one or more subsequent impulses.

4. The irregularly irregular ventricular rhythm in atrial fibrillation: the time interval between QRS complexes changes continuously, owing to conduction delay and block of fibrillatory impulses at different levels in the A-V node.

5. Change in rhythm of an ectopic A-V nodal focus: sinus or atrial impulses penetrate the A-V node incompletely, disturb the ectopic focus and postpone its discharge.

6. Failure of A-V nodal escape beats to appear when high grade A-V block causes slow ventricular rates (a ventricular escape beat may occur instead): sinus or atrial impulses penetrate the A-V node incompletely and discharge its escape foci. An alternate explanation for the failure of A-V nodal escape beats to occur under these circumstances is the presence of significant damage in the A-V nodal tissue.

Less common manifestation of concealed conduction have been reported, including concealed extrasystoles, concealed reciprocal captures, concealed Wenckebach sequences in the bundle branches[72] and in the anterior division of the left bundle branch.[60]

CLINICAL NOTES

Concealed conduction may occur in the normal heart or, more frequently, in patients with heart disease and A-V conduction disturbances. Digitalis toxicity is a frequent cause of concealed conduction.

Slow ventricular rates due to concealed conduction of supraventricular im-pulses in the A-V node can cause or aggravate myocardial and cerebral ischemia or congestive heart failure. Long ventricular pauses due to repetitive concealed A-V conduction may produce Stokes-Adams attacks.

The treatment of concealed conduction is that of the underlying condition.

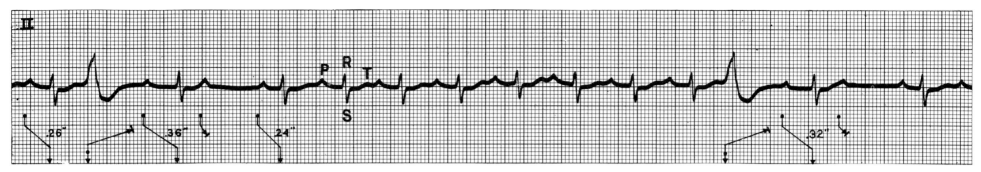

Rhythm 15-1,a. Sinus rhythm with first degree A-V block and unifocal ventricular extrasystoles. The ectopic ventricular impulses penetrate the A-V node in a retrograde fashion, causing further lengthening of the subsequent P-R interval (concealed retrograde conduction). The second P wave after each ventricular extrasystole is not conducted because it lands on the T wave of the preceding beat.

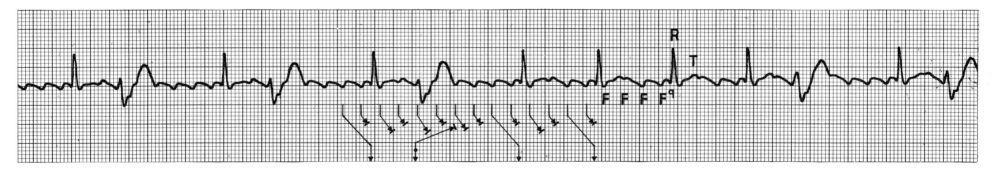

Rhythm 15-1,b. Atrial flutter with 4:1 A-V block and unifocal ventricular extrasystoles, often in bigeminy. Concealed retrograde conduction of the ventricular impulse in the A-V node is responsible for the pause following each extrasystole.

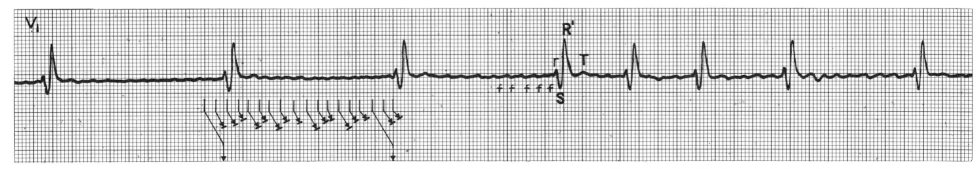

Rhythm 15-1,c. Atrial fibrillation with high grade A-V block and ventricular rate averaging 45 per minute. The irregularly irregular ventricular response results from concealed conduction of the atrial fibrillation impulses in the A-V node. The same explanation can be invoked for the failure of A-V nodal escape beats to occur in spite of the slow ventricular rate.

Chapter 16

Aberrant Ventricular Conduction

Sinus or ectopic supraventricular impulses activate the ventricles in an abnormal fashion when:

1. there is *transient failure* of conduction in one of the bundle branches;
2. there is *permanent failure* of conduction in one of the bundle branches;
3. there is *more rapid* conduction to some part of the ventricles through an accessory pathway.

The term aberrant ventricular conduction (or aberration) is most often applied to transient failure of conduction in the right or the left bundle branch; permanent failure of conduction in either bundle branch is called bundle branch block, and the more rapid conduction to the ventricles is referred to as ventricular pre-excitation.

Mechanism of production

Aberrant ventricular conduction occurs when a sinus or ectopic supraventricular impulse, after traversing the A-V node, reaches the bifurcation of the His bundle at a time when only one of the bundle branches can conduct, while the other has not yet fully recovered from its refractory period. Under these circumstances the impulse spreads first to one ventricle through the conducting bundle branch and then to the opposite ventricle with delay, causing a wide and bizarre QRS complex.

The occurrence of aberrant ventricular conduction is favored by:

1. *A short coupling interval:* The shorter the time interval between the supraventricular impulse and the preceding beat, the greater the likelihood that the former will reach one of the bundle branches during its refractory period.

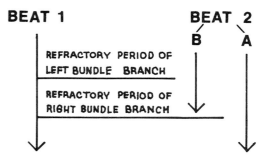

Fig. 16-1. The effect of a short coupling interval on the appearance of aberrant ventricular conduction. Beat 2 is conducted normally in position A. In position B the coupling interval is shorter so that beat 2 reaches the right bundle branch when the latter is still refractory.

2. *A long preceding ventricular cycle:* The duration of the refractory period of the conduction tissues of the heart, including the bundle branches, is not constant and is influenced by the heart rate. Within limits, acceleration of the

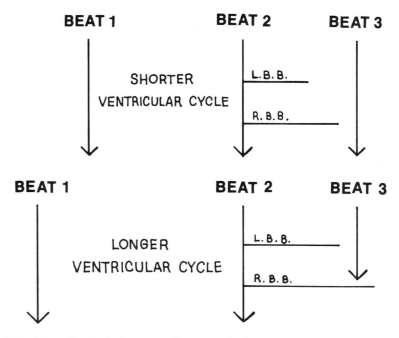

Fig. 16-2. The effect of the preceding ventricular cycle on the appearance of aberrant conduction. When the preceding ventricular cycle is longer, the refractory period of both bundle branches lengthens so that beat 3 reaches the right bundle branch when the latter is still refractory.

heart rate shortens the refractory period, whereas slowing has the reverse effect. When the rhythm is irregular, a long ventricular cycle results in a longer refractory period; the following impulse is therefore more likely to be conducted with aberration.

Aberrant ventricular conduction may occur during sinus rhythm, with atrial and A-V nodal extrasystoles, or during any supraventricular ectopic rhythm such as atrial and A-V nodal tachycardia, atrial flutter and atrial fibrillation. In atrial fibrillation aberrant ventricular conduction tends to occur more frequently when the ventricular response is rapid.

When the heart accelerates, aberrant conduction may occur for a number of beats in a row. The phenomenon is then called *rate-related* aberrant ventricular conduction (some use the term rate-related bundle branch block) and the rate at which aberration appears is called the *critical rate.*

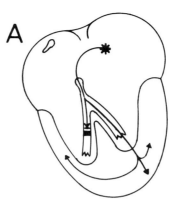

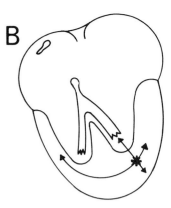

Fig. 16-4. Diagrams showing (*A*) an atrial ectopic impulse with aberrant ventricular conduction, right bundle branch type, and (*B*) a left ventricular ectopic impulse. Both spread to the right ventricle with delay.

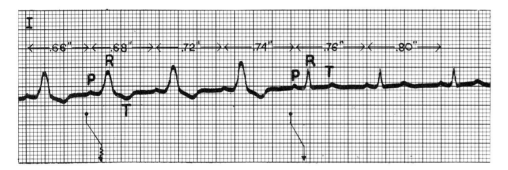

Fig. 16-3. Rate-related aberrant ventricular conduction. As the sinus rate becomes slower the conduction disturbance disappears.

Electrocardiographic manifestations

Wide and bizarre QRS complexes may be due to either of the following:

1. Aberrant ventricular conduction of supraventricular beats (sinus or ectopic): The impulses originate in the sinus node, the atria or the A-V node and activate one ventricle first through the conducting bundle branch; then they spread to the opposite ventricle with delay.

2. Ventricular ectopic beats: the impulses originate in one ventricle, which is activated first; then they spread to the opposite ventricle with delay.

Supraventricular beats with aberrant ventricular conduction thus closely resemble ventricular ectopic beats. The differential diagnosis between the two phenomena is very important; aberrant ventricular conduction, in fact, usually has little clinical significance whereas ventricular ectopic activity often has serious clinical and therapeutic implications.

The following electrocardiographic manifestations may be helpful in the recognition of aberrant ventricular conduction:

1. *Right bundle branch block configuration:* The right bundle branch is more prone to transmission failure than the left bundle branch. Aberrantly conducted beats display a QRS configuration of right bundle branch block in 75 to 85 percent of the cases.[75]

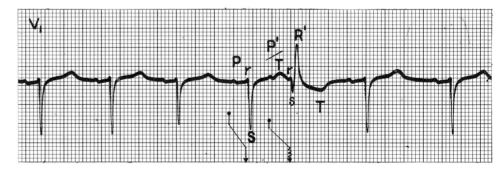

Fig. 16-5. Atrial extrasystole with aberrant ventricular conduction. The aberrant QRS complex has the configuration of right bundle branch block.

The QRS complex may show marked left axis deviation, owing to aberrant conduction in the left anterior division of the left bundle branch, or right axis deviation, owing to aberrant conduction in the posterior division. Aberrantly conducted beats may also display a QRS configuration of left bundle branch block.

2. *The initial vector* (or initial portion of the QRS complex) has usually the same direction in the aberrant beats as in the normally conducted beats.

3. *Varying degrees of aberration* are frequently seen, with fine gradations from slightly abnormal to more abnormal QRS complexes.

4. *The presence of atrial activity:* An atrial deflection often precedes each

aberrantly conducted beat, confirming the supraventricular origin of the QRS complex.

5. *The coupling interval:* The coupling interval (the time interval between an aberrant beat and the preceding beat) is of variable duration and is often shorter than the interval between nonaberrant beats in the same tracing.

6. *The preceding ventricular cycle:* An aberrantly conducted beat may occur when a short ventricular cycle is preceded by a long one. This long–short sequence terminated by aberration is not infrequently seen in atrial fibrillation and is called the *Ashman phenomenon.* The long–short sequence is responsible for the aberration of the second beat of a run of fast supraventricular rhythm and for the aberrant beats occurring in some cases of variable second degree A-V block.

7. *The pairing interval:* If aberrantly conducted beats occur in pairs the interval between the two beats of each pair is variable.

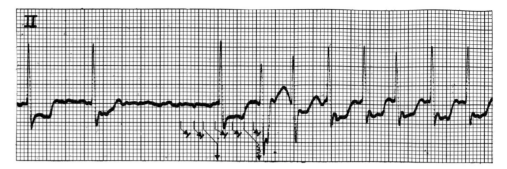

Fig. 16-6. A long–short sequence is terminated by an aberrant beat in atrial fibrillation (Ashman phenomenon). Note that the aberrant beat is the second of a run of rapid rate.

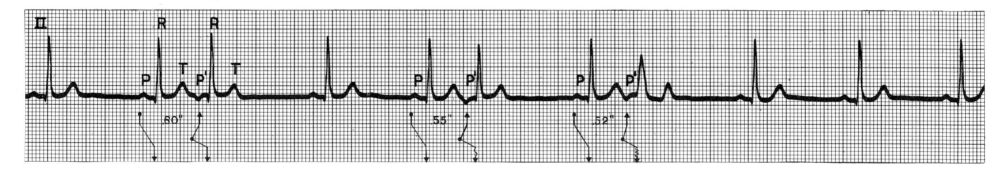

Fig. 16-7. Sinus bradycardia at a rate of 55 per minute and "high" A-V nodal extrasystoles with and without aberrant ventricular conduction. As the inverted P′ wave becomes closer to the previous beat, the QRS complex becomes more aberrant.

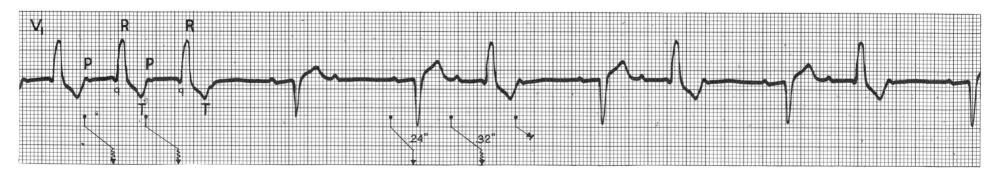

Fig. 16-8. Sinus rhythm with second degree A-V block type I (Wenckebach). During runs of 1:1 conduction the QRS complex shows right bundle branch block configuration. When A-V conduction becomes 3:2, only the second P wave of each sequence is followed by aberrant ventricular conduction.

8. *The postaberrancy pause:* Aberrantly conducted beats are usually followed by a noncompensatory pause. During atrial fibrillation there is generally no significant pause following each beat conducted with aberration.

Bradycardia-dependent aberrancy

Aberrant ventricular conduction may occur in supraventricular *escape* beats or upon *slowing* of the heart rate. Among the theories postulated to explain this apparent paradox are the following:

1. Supraventricular impulses can spread along the accessory pathways described by Mahaim and thus invade the ventricles in an abnormal fashion.[66]

2. Impulses originating in the distal portion of the A-V node can be conducted down only part of the His bundle and thus reach a certain portion of the ventricles first.[66]

3. Latent pacemaking cells in the bundle branches may undergo spontaneous diastolic (phase 4) depolarization. This results in slowing of conduction in the involved area and therefore in aberrant ventricular conduction.[82,83]

CLINICAL NOTES

The clinical and prognostic significance of aberrant ventricular conduction is still controversial. Aberrant conduction occurring with very premature supraventricular beats or during supraventricular ectopic tachycardias with rapid ventricular rates is probably physiological and of no clinical importance. When it occurs with relatively long coupling and slow ventricular rates it is probably a pathological event and the expression of an abnormal conduction system.[5]

The differentiation between aberrant beats and ventricular ectopic beats can be of major importance in the treatment of a supraventricular arrhythmia with fast ventricular rate, when digitalis is the treatment of choice. The occurrence of aberrant ventricular conduction under these circumstances is usually an indication to increase the digitalis dosage. An incorrect diagnosis of ventricular ectopic beats, on the other hand, may preclude the use of digitalis and lead to the administration of drugs, such as procainamide and quinidine, which may be potentially harmful by further depressing intraventricular conduction.

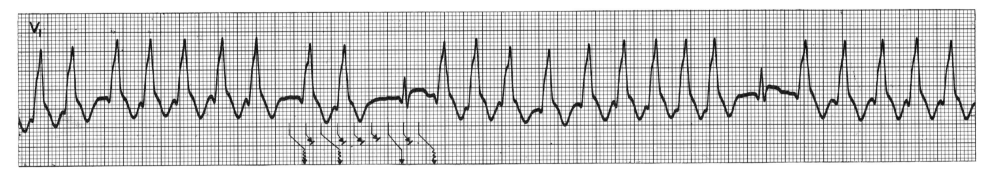

Fig. 16-9. Atrial fibrillation with rapid ventricular rate averaging 140 per minute and aberrant ventricular conduction. Longer ventricular pauses are followed by less aberrant beats.

Aberrant Ventricular Conduction Mimicking
Ventricular Extrasystoles

Sinus or ectopic supraventricular impulses conducted to the ventricles with aberration may closely resemble ventricular extrasystoles.

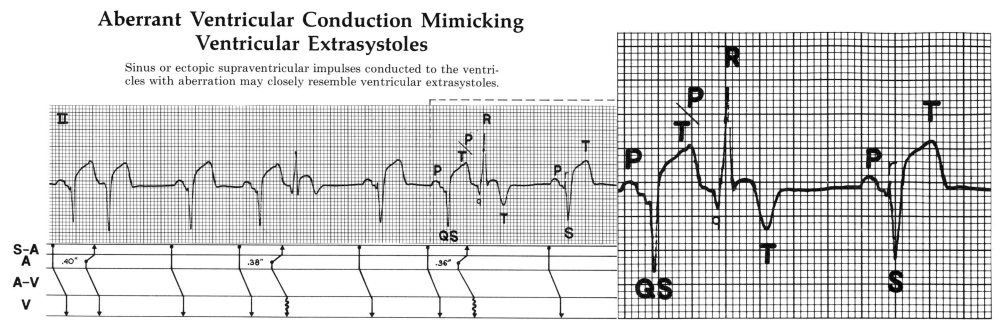

Rhythm 16-1,a. Sinus rhythm with atrial extrasystoles in trigeminy. The first ectopic atrial impulse is conducted to the ventricles normally; the other two with different degrees of aberration.

ELECTROCARDIOGRAPHIC CRITERIA

A. Atrial deflections:

1. During sinus rhythm:
   a. Atrial extrasystole with aberrant conduction: premature P′ wave preceding a wide and bizarre QRS complex.
   b. A-V nodal extrasystole with aberrant conduction: premature and inverted P′ wave preceding a wide and bizarre QRS complex. When the P′ wave is hidden within or follows the QRS complex, the A-V nodal extrasystole with aberrant conduction often cannot be differentiated from a ventricular extrasystole.

2. The atrial mechanism may be atrial tachycardia, atrial flutter, atrial fibrillation or A-V nodal tachycardia.

B. A-V conduction: aberrant ventricular conduction is more likely to occur when there is variable A-V block causing long-short sequences.

C. Ventricular deflections:

1. QRS configuration:
   a. Right bundle branch block pattern is much more frequent than left bundle branch block pattern.
   b. Initial vector often the same as in normally conducted beats.
   c. Various degrees of aberration.
2. Coupling interval:
   a. Short coupling interval.
   b. Short coupling interval preceded by a long ventricular cycle (Ashman phenomenon).
   c. Variable coupling interval.
3. When pairs occur, there is variable pairing interval.
4. Postextrasystolic pause:
   a. Usually noncompensatory.
   b. In atrial fibrillation there is frequently no significant pause following each aberrantly conducted beat.

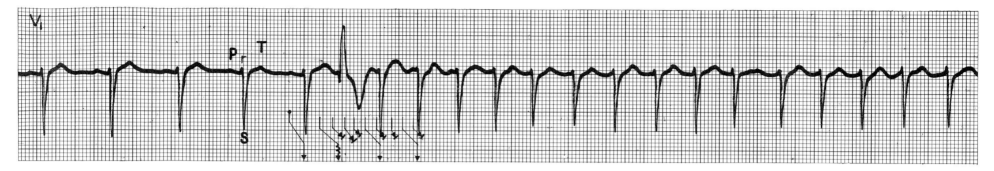

Rhythm 16-1,b. Sinus rhythm followed by atrial fibrillation at a rapid ventricular rate averaging 150 per minute. The second beat of the run of rapid rate occurs after a long–short sequence and is aberrant (Ashman phenomenon).

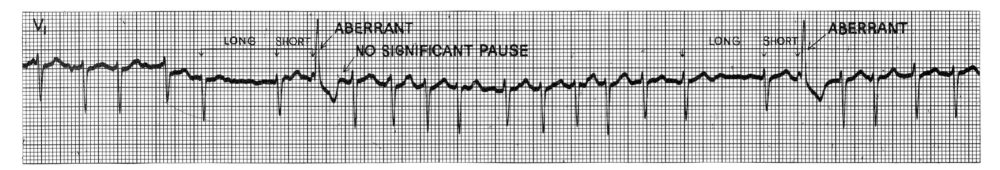

Rhythm 16-1,c. Atrial fibrillation with rapid ventricular rate averaging 140 per minute. There are two aberrantly conducted beats which follow long-short sequences and mimic ventricular extrasystoles.

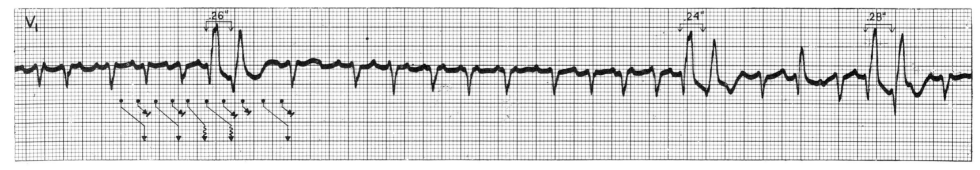

Rhythm 16-1,d. Atrial flutter with variable A-V block and intermittent aberrant ventricular conduction mimicking ventricular extrasystoles, isolated or in pairs. There are varying degrees of aberration and variable pairing interval.

Aberrant Ventricular Conduction Mimicking Ventricular Tachycardia

Ectopic supraventricular tachycardia with aberrant ventricular conduction may closely resemble ventricular tachycardia.

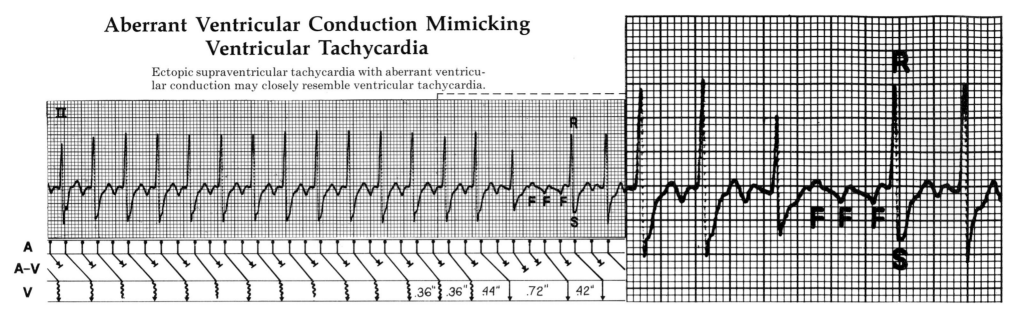

Rhythm 16-2,a. Atrial flutter with variable A-V block and aberrant ventricular conduction. When 2:1 conduction is present, the arrhythmia mimics ventricular tachycardia.

ELECTROCARDIOGRAPHIC CRITERIA

A. Atrial deflections:

1. Rate, rhythm and configuration depend upon the atrial mechanism (sinus or ectopic).
2. Identification of the atrial mechanism may be difficult.

B. A-V conduction: There is no evidence of A-V dissociation: the P waves do not "travel" toward,

inside and away from the QRS complexes like in ventricular tachycardia.

C. Ventricular deflections:

1. Rate: depends upon the type of supraventricular rhythm.
   a. Aberrant conduction is usually rate-related.
   b. In atrial fibrillation aberrant conduction tends to occur more frequently when the ventricular response is rapid.

2. Rhythm:
   a. Regular or slightly irregular.
   b. Irregularly irregular in atrial fibrillation.
3. Configuration:
   a. Right bundle branch block pattern much more frequent than left bundle branch block pattern.
   b. Initial vector often the same as in normally conducted beats.
   c. Varying degrees of aberration.

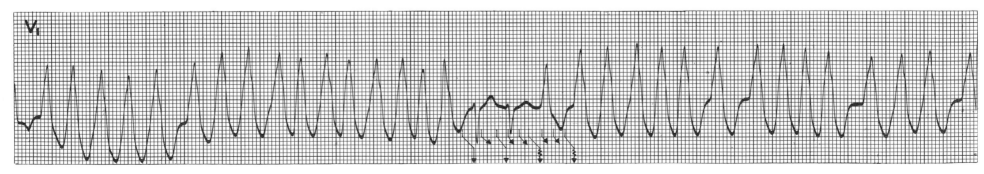

Rhythm 16-2,b. Atrial fibrillation with rapid ventricular rate averaging 200 per minute. All QRS complexes, except two, show aberrant ventricular conduction, right bundle branch block type. Note the irregularly irregular ventricular rhythm.

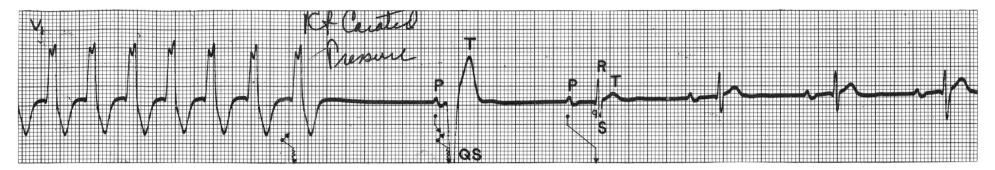

Rhythm 16-2,c. Episode of supraventricular tachycardia at a rate of 150 per minute, with aberrant ventricular conduction, terminated by carotid sinus pressure. Following an escape beat, the rhythm becomes sinus bradycardia and sinus arrhythmia with first degree A-V block.

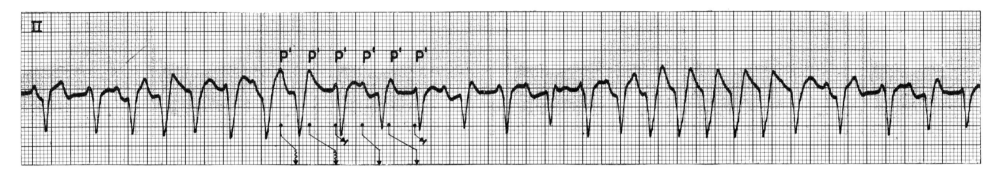

Rhythm 16-2,d. Atrial tachycardia with variable A-V block and intermittent aberrant ventricular conduction. The atrial rate is 200 per minute and the average ventricular rate 150 per minute.

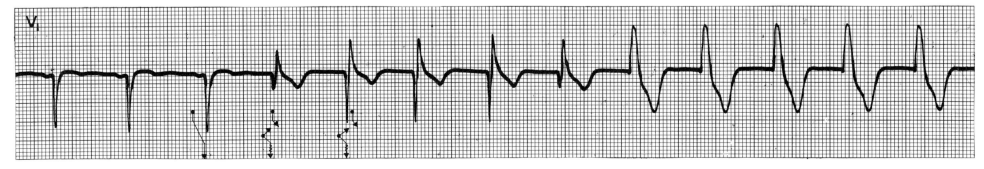

Rhythm 16-2,e. Sinus rhythm interrupted by nonparoxysmal A-V nodal tachycardia with varying degrees of aberrant ventricular conduction.

Chapter 17

Artificial Pacemaker Rhythms

Artificial pacemaker rhythms are produced by a variety of electronic pacemakers used on a temporary or permanent basis to control certain disturbances of the cardiac rate and rhythm.

Pacemaker electrode

The function of the pacemaker electrode is to deliver electrical impulses from the pacemaker to the myocardium and, in some units, also to carry information to the sensing circuits of the pacemaker concerning the spontaneous electrical activity of the heart.

A unipolar or bipolar pacemaker electrode may be introduced transvenously into the right atrium, the coronary sinus and its tributaries, the right ventricle, or may be attached directly to the myocardium through a thoracotomy or mediastinotomy approach. In an emergency, an electrode may be introduced into a cardiac chamber percutaneously via a transthoracic needle. External electrodes may be applied directly to the chest wall.

Pacemaker spike

On the electrocardiogram the electrical impulse delivered by an artificial pacemaker causes a sharp and narrow deflection called pacemaker spike. The spike, which may be positive or negative, immediately precedes the P wave when the atria are paced and the QRS complex when the ventricles are paced.

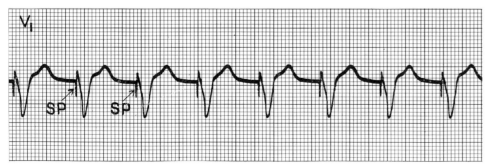

Fig. 17-1. Ventricular pacing. There is no evidence of spontaneous atrial or ventricular activity. SP, pacemaker spike.

Three types of pacemakers are commonly used. They require a single unipolar or bipolar electrode to stimulate the ventricles.

Continuous-asynchronous (or fixed-rate) ventricular pacemaker

This type of unit paces the heart at a preselected rate in a continuous manner and has no sensing circuits.

When there are spontaneous ventricular beats the pacemaker ignores them and continues to fire at the expected time. *Competition* between the pacemaker and the spontaneous ventricular activity results and pacemaker spikes may fall anywhere on the QRS, ST segment and T wave of the spontaneous beats. Spikes that fall on the T wave, during the vulnerable period of the heart, may cause repetitive firing with resulting ventricular tachycardia or ventricular fibrillation. Spikes that fall during the absolute refractory period of the ventricles merely produce an electrical artifact and do not cause any arrhythmia.

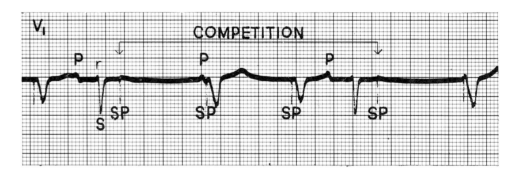

Fig. 17-2. Continuous-asynchronous pacemaker. Spontaneous beats of sinus origin are ignored by the pacemaker and ineffective spikes fall on their T wave (competition). SP, pacemaker spike.

A continuous-asynchronous pacemaker behaves like a parasystolic focus. The lack of a sensing circuit prevents spontaneous cardiac activity from inhibiting the pacemaker. The pacemaker impulses are delivered at regular intervals and spread to the surrounding myocardium whenever they fall outside the ventricular refractory period induced by spontaneous beats. The pacemaker rhythm thus duplicates the electrocardiographic features of a naturally occurring ventricular parasystole.

Ventricular-inhibited (or demand) pacemaker

This type of unit paces the heart at a preselected rate but possesses a sensing circuit which responds to electrical information received through the pacemaker electrode.

Spontaneous ventricular beats occurring after a preset interval from the preceding spike, called refractory period of the pacemaker, are sensed and temporarily inhibit the pacemaker activity (the refractory period of a ventricular-inhibited pacemaker ranges between 0.05 and 0.40 second, depending on the model). The pacemaker fires again only when spontaneous ventricular activity fails to occur within an interval of preset duration, called pacemaker escape interval. When the rate of the spontaneous ventricular beats becomes faster than its pacing rate, the pacemaker does not fire at all.

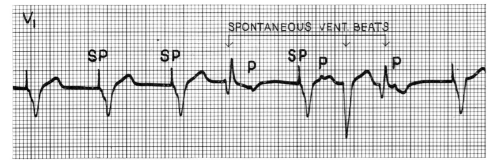

Fig. 17-3. Ventricular-inhibited pacemaker. Spontaneous ventricular beats are sensed and the pacemaker output is temporarily suppressed. The atria are under the control of the sinus node. SP, pacemaker spike.

In the absence of spontaneous ventricular activity (and thus when there is no opportunity for sensing), a ventricular-inhibited pacemaker fires regularly and continuously and therefore cannot be distinguished from a continuous-asynchronous or from a ventricular-triggered unit.

The ventricular-inhibited pacemaker behaves like a ventricular escape focus: its spikes occur as a safety mechanism whenever impulses from a higher focus, including the sinus node, fail to occur or are prevented by A-V dissociation or A-V block from reaching the ventricles. The pacemaker rhythm therefore duplicates the electrocardiographic features of a naturally occurring escape rhythm.

Ventricular-triggered (or ventricular-synchronous) pacemaker

This type of unit paces the heart at a preselected rate and, like the ventricular-inhibited pacemaker, possesses a sensing circuit which responds to electrical information received through the pacemaker electrode.

Spontaneous ventricular beats occurring after a preset interval from the preceding spike, called refractory period of the pacemaker, are sensed. The refractory period of a ventricular-triggered pacemaker has a duration of 0.40 or 0.50 second, depending on the model. Instead of inhibiting the pacemaker, as in the ventricular-inhibited unit, each spontaneous beat causes the occurrence of a "sensing" spike which is delivered shortly after the beginning of the QRS complex. The sensing spikes are completely ineffective because they fall during the absolute refractory period of the heart; their only purpose is to show that the pacemaker is working and that its sensing mechanism is functioning properly.

The pacemaker delivers a "pacing" spike whenever spontaneous ventricular

activity fails to occur within an interval of preset duration, called pacemaker escape interval. When the rate of the spontaneous ventricular beats becomes faster than its pacing rate, the pacemaker delivers only sensing spikes and no pacing spikes at all.

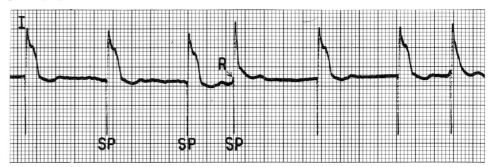

Fig. 17-4. Ventricular-triggered pacing during atrial fibrillation. A spontaneous ventricular beat is sensed and a sensing spike delivered shortly after the beginning of the QRS complex. SP, pacemaker spike.

In the absence of spontaneous ventricular activity (and thus when there is no opportunity for sensing), a ventricular-triggered pacemaker continuously fires only pacing spikes and therefore cannot be differentiated from a continuous-asynchronous or from a ventricular-inhibited unit.

Pacemaker types less commonly used

Atrial-triggered (or atrial-synchronous) pacemaker. This type of unit has more complex circuitry and requires two electrodes. One electrode is placed in the atrium and the other in the ventricle.

Spontaneous atrial activity is *sensed* by the atrial electrode and, after a delay similar to the normal P-R interval, the ventricles are paced through the ventricular electrode. The pacemaker, therefore, preserves the normal sequence of atrioventricular electrical activity while bypassing the A-V conduction pathways.

If an atrial tachyarrhythmia occurs and the atrial rate becomes too rapid, a built-in pacemaker refractory period prevents the sensing of every atrial

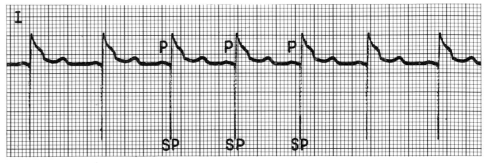

Fig. 17-5. Atrial-triggered pacemaker. A spike (SP) activates the ventricles at a constant interval after each sinus P wave.

impulse. Thus, the pacemaker cannot induce, through a 1:1 response, a dangerously rapid ventricular rate and paces the heart at a rate half that of the atria or slower.

An escape mechanism activates the ventricles through the ventricular electrode whenever atrial activity fails to occur or is not sensed by the pacemaker. Spontaneous ventricular beats falling outside the pacemaker refractory period are sensed and cause a spike which is delivered shortly after the beginning of the QRS complex. This pacemaker, therefore, is in reality both an atrial-triggered and a ventricular-triggered unit.[4]

Bifocal (or A-V sequential demand) pacemaker. This type of unit also requires two electrodes, one placed in the atrium and the other in the ventricle. Both electrodes deliver spikes, but only the ventricular electrode is connected to a sensing circuit; spontaneous ventricular activity is sensed while spontaneous atrial activity is ignored.

The atrial electrode delivers the initial spike to the atria and, after a delay similar to the normal P-R interval, the ventricles are paced via the ventricular electrode. Thus the bifocal pacemaker stimulates the atria and the ventricles in a sequential fashion while bypassing the A-V conduction pathways.

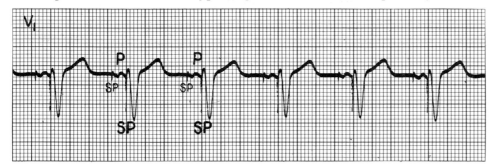

Fig. 17-6. Bifocal pacemaker. There are two spikes (SP) for each cardiac cycle: one spike precedes the P wave, the other precedes the QRS complex.

The pacemaker is of the ventricular-inhibited type and both the atrial and the ventricular spikes can be inhibited by spontaneous QRS complexes. Depending on the spontaneous ventricular activity, the bifocal pacemaker may remain dormant, may stimulate only the atria or may stimulate both the atria and ventricles in sequence, with a "P-R interval" of preset duration.

Atrial deflections

During artificial pacemaker rhythms the atria may be under control of either the sinus node or an ectopic focus. When the atria are paced, a spike precedes the P wave. Paced ventricular beats may be followed by a retrograde inverted P′ wave.

Ventricular deflections: Paced beats

Each pacemaker spike activating the ventricles is followed by a wide and bizarre QRS complex. The pattern of the QRS complex depends on the location of the pacing electrode.

In *right* ventricular stimulation, usually achieved through a transvenous (or endocardial) electrode, the left ventricle is stimulated with delay. The resulting wide QRS complex resembles *left* bundle branch block and appears predominantly negative in lead V_1. When the electrode tip is located at the apex of the right ventricle, the QRS complex in the frontal plane leads shows marked left axis deviation and appears predominantly positive in lead I and predominantly negative in leads II and III. A normal QRS axis, on the other hand, is present when the electrode tip stimulates the outflow tract of the right ventricle.

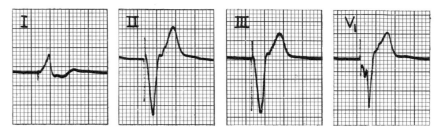

Fig. 17-7. Right ventricular stimulation from the apex.

Left ventricular stimulation can occur (1) through an epicardial electrode implanted on the surface of the left ventricle, (2) through a transvenous electrode which was accidentally introduced into the coronary sinus and stimulates the posterior or lateral aspects of the left ventricle, or (3) through a transvenous electrode which has perforated the myocardium and stimulates the endocardial or epicardial surface of the left ventricle. In *left* ventricular stimulation the right ventricle is stimulated with delay. The resulting wide QRS complex resembles *right* bundle branch block and appears predominantly positive and often M-shaped in lead V_1. In the frontal plane leads the QRS complex usually shows right axis deviation and appears predominantly negative in I and predominantly positive in leads II and III.

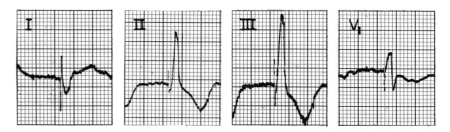

Fig. 17-8. Left ventricular stimulation.

In some cases *right* ventricular stimulation can paradoxically produce a QRS pattern of *right* bundle branch block.[4] Two explanations are given for this phenomenon. According to some authors,[63] the pacemaker impulses delivered to the right ventricular cavity may enter the right bundle branch, travel retrogradely to the A-V node and down to the left bundle branch, producing initial stimulation of the left ventricular septum. Others suggest that in some hearts the anatomical left septum can extend to the right ventricular endocardial surface; when a pacemaker electrode stimulates this right ventricular area it can produce a QRS complex similar to that obtained from stimulation of the anterior left septal surface.[21]

The electrocardiogram cannot be used as an infallible criterion[4] for the diagnosis of right or left ventricular stimulation and the position of the pacing electrode should be confirmed by frontal and lateral x-ray films of the chest.

Ventricular deflections: Fusion and pseudofusion beats

A pacemaker spike may succeed in activating only part of the ventricles while a spontaneous impulse activates the remainder. The resulting *fusion* beat dupli-

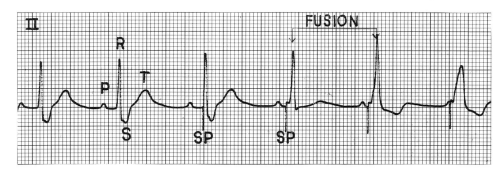

Fig. 17-9. Ventricular-inhibited pacemaker. The first two QRS complexes are pure spontaneous beats. The third QRS is a pseudofusion beat; the fourth and the fifth are both fusion beats. The last one is a pure paced beat. SP, pacemaker spike.

cates the electrocardiographic features of a naturally occurring fusion beat (Chapter 6) and consists of a pacemaker spike followed by a QRS complex having a configuration intermediate to that of a pure paced beat and that of a pure spontaneous beat.

A pseudofusion beat is a spontaneous QRS complex with a superimposed pacemaker spike. The pacemaker impulse does not participate in the activation of the ventricles and the QRS complex has a configuration identical to that of a pure spontaneous beat without a superimposed spike.

Ventricular deflections: Spontaneous beats

During artificial pacemaker rhythms spontaneous ventricular beats may occur. The spontaneous beats may be of sinus origin, or of atrial, A-V nodal or ventricular origin.

Electrocardiographic evidence of ventricular pacemaker malfunction

The electrocardiogram is the simplest and probably the most valuable method of detecting pacemaker failure.[15] Electronic analysis of the pacemaker spike, testing of the sensing circuit with carotid sinus pressure, external magnet, drugs and external overdrive, and x-ray analysis of the pacemaker batteries are also used to detect pacemaker failure.

A malfunctioning ventricular pacemaker may display changes in its predetermined *rate,* which becomes slower in the newer models and faster in the older models. When rapid discharge rates develop, the pacemaker is called a "runaway."

Changes in the 1:1 *sensing* function may occur in a malfunctioning ventricular-inhibited or ventricular-triggered pacemaker and, as a result, spontaneous ventricular beats occurring after the end of the pacemaker refractory period are not sensed; a pacing spike may thus fall during the heart's vulnerable period and cause repetitive firing. A malfunctioning ventricular-triggered unit may sense the T wave and deliver a sensing spike on top of it.

Changes in the 1:1 *pacing* function may result in spikes which are ineffective when they fall outside the refractory period of the ventricles. This is a form of exit block (Chapter 14).

Other manifestations of pacemaker malfunction include irregular pacing *rhythm,* changes in *amplitude* of the spike, and changes in the pacemaker *refractory period.*

CLINICAL NOTES

Artificial cardiac pacing may be performed as a temporary or permanent measure in the treatment of existing arrhythmias or the prophylaxis of anticipated arrhythmias.

The most common indication for cardiac pacing is the control of *slow* cardiac rhythms (bradyarrhythmias) due to second or third degree A-V block, to bilateral bundle branch block, or to sino-atrial block and other manifestations of the sick sinus syndrome. These arrhythmias are often complicated by congestive heart failure, angina, mental confusion, azotemia. By increasing the ventricular rate with a pacemaker, in addition to appropriate drug treatment, the complications listed above are often lessened or eliminated.

Patients with *normal* heart rates may require prophylactic insertion of a cardiac pacemaker when they have a history of Stokes-Adams attacks. Their electrocardiogram often shows evidence of bifascicular or incomplete trifascicular block.

Another indication for artificial cardiac pacing is the "overdrive" suppression of *fast* cardiac rhythms (tachyarrhythmias) due to ventricular or even supraventricular tachycardias that are refractory to drug treatment alone.

Continuous-Asynchronous Ventricular Pacemaker

Artificial pacemaker stimulating the ventricles in a
continuous manner and possessing no sensing circuits.

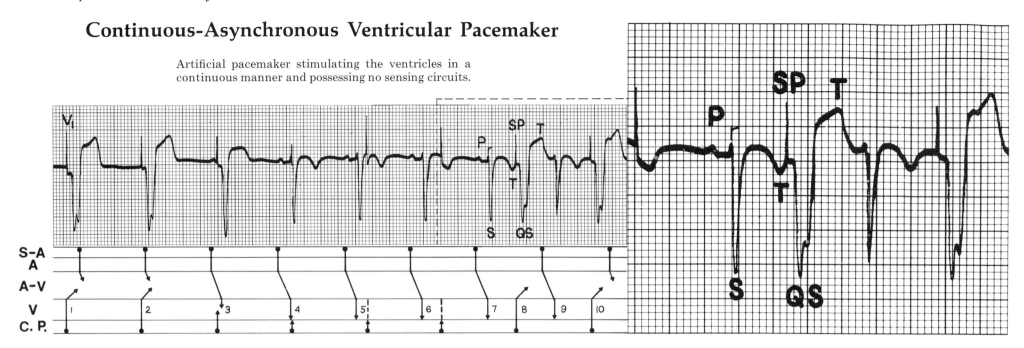

Rhythm 17-1,a. Continuous-asynchronous pacemaker at a rate of 70 per minute, competing with normal sinus rhythm at approximately the same rate. Beats 1, 2, 8, and 10 are pure pacemaker beats; beat 3 is a fusion beat and beat 4 a pseudofusion beat. The spikes landing on beats 4, 5 and 6 are ineffective because they occur during the absolute refractory period of the ventricles. SP, pacemaker spike. C.P., continuous-asynchronous pacemaker.

ELECTROCARDIOGRAPHIC CRITERIA

A. Pacemaker spikes:

1. Rate: preselected, usually 70 per minute.
2. Rhythm: regular.

B. Relationship between spikes and QRS complexes:

1. Competition: when there are spontaneous ventricular beats the pacemaker ignores them and spikes may fall on the QRS, ST segment or T wave of the spontaneous beats. Spikes that fall on the T wave may cause repetitive firing.
2. 1:1 pacing: each spike falling outside the refractory period of the ventricles is followed by a QRS complex.

C. QRS complexes:

1. Paced beats:
   a. *Left* bundle branch block pattern with predominantly negative QRS in lead V_1: right ventricular stimulation.
   b. *Right* bundle branch block pattern with predominantly positive QRS in lead V_1: left ventricular stimulation (probable).

2. Fusion beats: QRS complexes with configuration intermediate to that of a pure paced beat and that of a pure spontaneous beat.
3. Pseudofusion beats: pure spontaneous beats with a superimposed spike.
4. Spontaneous beats: sinus or ectopic. In the absence of spontaneous ventricular beats, a continuous-asynchronous pacemaker cannot be distinguished from a ventricular-inhibited or from a ventricular-triggered unit.

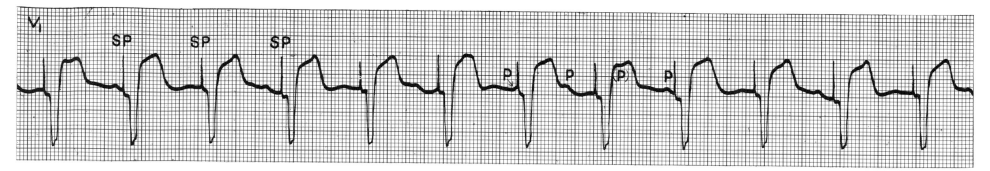

Rhythm 17-1,b. Ventricular pacing at 70 per minute. This is a continuous-asynchronous pacemaker but, in the absence of spontaneous ventricular activity, the pacemaker cannot be distinguished from either a ventricular-inhibited or a ventricular-triggered unit.

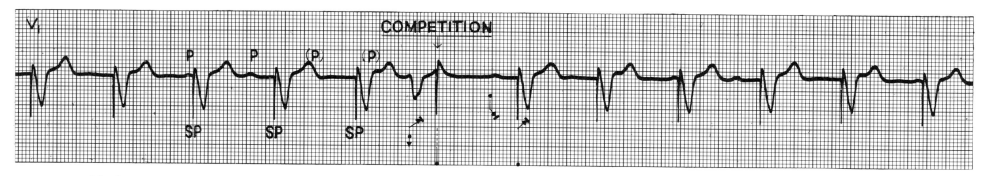

Rhythm 17-1,c. Continuous-asynchronous pacing at a rate of 70 per minute during sinus rhythm with complete A-V block and one ventricular extrasystole. The pacemaker ignores the spontaneous ventricular beat and fires at the expected time. Its spike lands on the T wave of the extrasystole (competition).

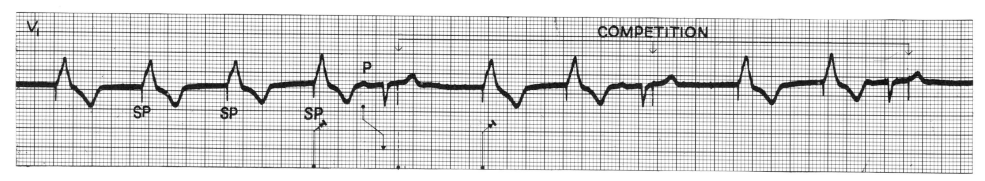

Rhythm 17-1,d. Continuous-asynchronous pacing in a patient with sinus bradycardia and intermittent sino-atrial block. The pacemaker ignores all three spontaneous beats of sinus origin. Its spikes, landing on the ST segment, remain ineffective because they occur during the absolute refractory period of the ventricles; this does not represent pacemaker malfunction but only competition. The QRS complex of the paced beats has right bundle branch block configuration, suggesting left ventricular stimulation.

Ventricular-Inhibited Pacemaker

Artificial pacemaker stimulating the ventricles and possessing sensing circuits that respond to electrical information received through the pacing electrode. The pacemaker is inhibited by spontaneous ventricular activity.

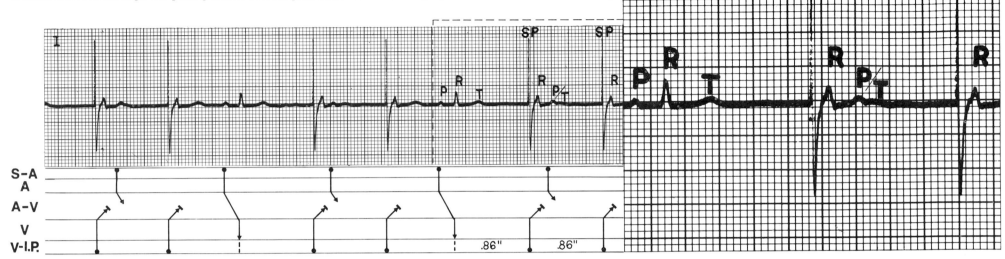

Rhythm 17-2,a. Ventricular-inhibited pacing at a rate of 70 per minute during sinus bradycardia. Spontaneous ventricular beats of sinus origin are sensed and temporarily inhibit the pacemaker activity. The unit fires again whenever spontaneous ventricular beats fail to occur for 0.86 second (pacemaker escape interval). SP, pacemaker spike. V-I.P., ventricular-inhibited pacemaker.

ELECTROCARDIOGRAPHIC CRITERIA

A. Pacemaker spikes:

1. Pacing rate (measured between two consecutive spikes): preselected, usually 70 per minute.
2. Rhythm:
   a. Irregular when there are spontaneous beats.
   b. Regular when there are no spontaneous beats.

B. Relationship between spikes and QRS complexes:

1. 1:1 sensing: spontaneous ventricular beats occurring after the end of the refractory period of the pacemaker are sensed and temporarily inhibit the pacemaker activity. The unit fires again when a spontaneous ventricular beat fails to occur within an interval of preset duration (pacemaker escape interval).
2. 1:1 pacing: each spike is followed by a QRS complex.

C. QRS complexes:

1. Paced beats:
   a. *Left* bundle branch block pattern with predominantly negative QRS in lead V_1: right ventricular stimulation.
   b. *Right* bundle branch block pattern with predominantly positive QRS in lead V_1: left ventricular stimulation (probable).
2. Fusion beats: QRS complexes with configuration intermediate to that of a pure paced beat and that of a pure spontaneous beat.
3. Pseudofusion beats: pure spontaneous beats with a superimposed spike.
4. Spontaneous beats: sinus or ectopic. In the absence of spontaneous ventricular beats, a ventricular-inhibited pacemaker cannot be distinguished from a continuous-asynchronous or from a ventricular-triggered unit.

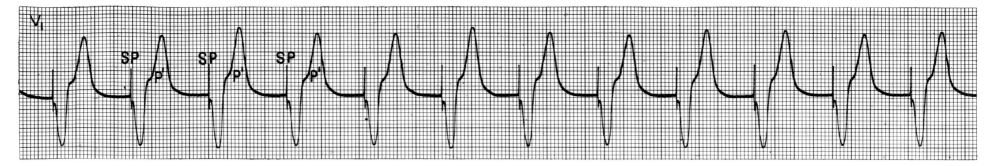

Rhythm 17-2,b. Ventricular pacing at 72 per minute. This is a ventricular-inhibited unit but, in the absence of spontaneous ventricular activity, the pacemaker cannot be distinguished from either a continuous-asynchronous or a ventricular-triggered unit. Note the retroconducted P' wave following each paced beat.

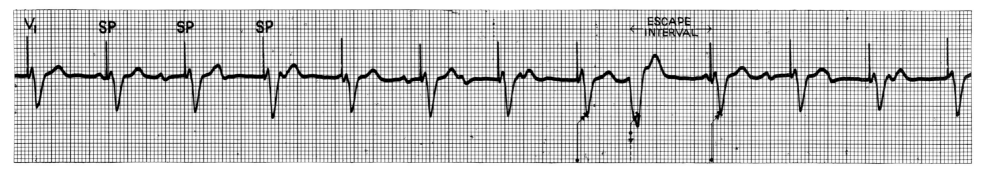

Rhythm 17-2,c. Ventricular-inhibited pacing at 70 per minute in a patient with sinus rhythm and complete A-V block. The pacemaker senses the spontaneous ventricular premature beats, then fires again after an escape interval of 0.86 second.

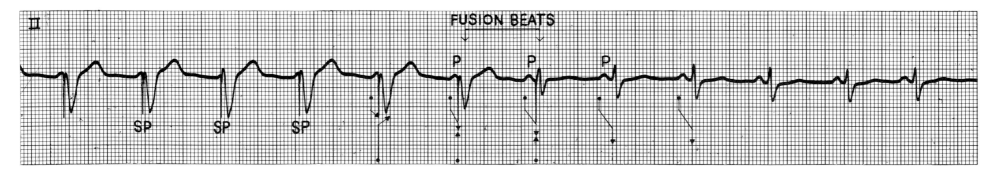

Rhythm 17-2,d. Ventricular-inhibited pacing at 70 per minute in a patient with normal sinus rhythm. The pacemaker stops firing when the rate of the spontaneous beats becomes faster than its pacing rate. There are two fusion beats.

Ventricular-Triggered Pacemaker

Artificial pacemaker stimulating the ventricles and possessing sensing circuits
that respond to electrical information received through the pacing electrode.
The pacemaker delivers a "sensing" spike on the spontaneous ventricular beats.

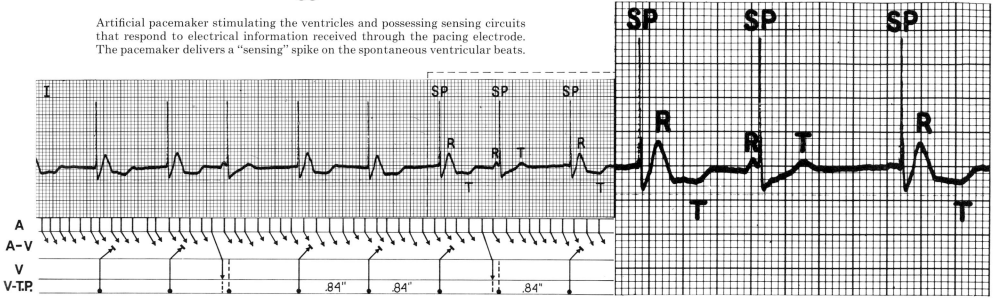

Rhythm 17-3,a. Ventricular-triggered pacing at a rate of 70 per minute during atrial fibrillation. The pacemaker senses two spontaneous beats, delivers
a sensing spike 0.08 second after the beginning of the QRS complex then fires again, after an escape interval of 0.84 second. SP, pacemaker spike;
V-T.P., ventricular-triggered pacemaker.

ELECTROCARDIOGRAPHIC CRITERIA

A. Pacemaker spikes:

1. Sensing spikes: rate and rhythm depend on the
   spontaneous ventricular activity.
2. Pacing spikes:
   a. Rate (measured between two consecutive
      pacing spikes): preselected, usually 70 per
      minute.
   b. Rhythm: regular.

B. Relationship between spikes and QRS complexes:

1. 1:1 sensing: spontaneous ventricular beats
   occurring after the end of the refractory period
   of the pacemaker are sensed and trigger a sensing spike which is delivered shortly after the
   beginning of the QRS complex. A pacing spike
   is fired when spontaneous ventricular activity
   fails to occur within an interval of preset duration (pacemaker escape interval).
2. 1:1 pacing: each pacing spike is followed by a
   QRS complex.

C. QRS complexes:

1. Paced beats:
   a. *Left* bundle branch block pattern with pre-
      dominantly negative QRS in lead V_1: right
      ventricular stimulation.
   b. *Right* bundle branch block pattern with
      predominantly positive QRS in lead V_1: left
      ventricular stimulation (probable).
2. Fusion beats: QRS complexes with configuration intermediate to that of a pure paced beat
   and that of a pure spontaneous beat.
3. Pseudofusion beats: pure spontaneous beats
   with a superimposed spike.
4. Spontaneous beats: sinus or ectopic. In the
   absence of spontaneous ventricular beats, a
   ventricular-triggered pacemaker cannot be distinguished from a continuous-asynchronous or
   from a ventricular-inhibited unit.

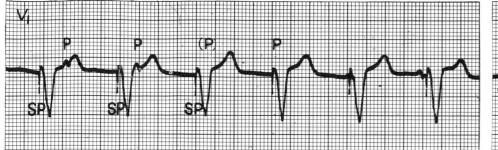

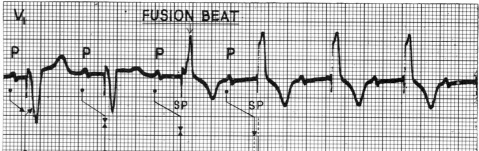

Rhythm 17-3,b. Ventricular pacing at a rate of 73 per minute. This is a ventricular-triggered unit but, in the absence of spontaneous ventricular activity, the pacemaker cannot be distinguished from either a continuous-asynchronous or a ventricular-inhibited unit.

Rhythm 17-3,c. Same patient as in 17-3,b. Sinus beats with first degree A-V block and right bundle branch block occur at a rate slightly faster than that of the pacemaker. Sensing spikes, delivered right after the beginning of each spontaneous QRS complex, identify the pacemaker as a ventricular-triggered unit. The second and third QRS complexes are fusion beats.

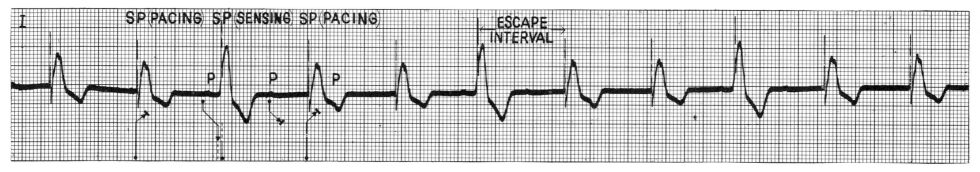

Rhythm 17-3,d. Ventricular-triggered pacing at a rate of 68 per minute during sinus rhythm with second degree A-V block and left bundle branch block. Note the pacing spikes occurring before the beginning of the QRS complex and the sensing spikes occurring shortly after the beginning of the QRS complex.

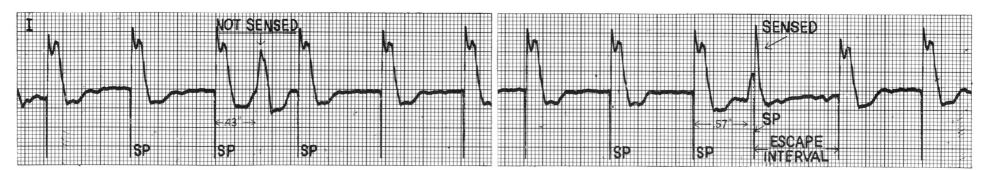

Rhythm 17-3,e. Ventricular-triggered pacing at a rate of 68 per minute during atrial fibrillation. A spontaneous beat is not sensed because it occurs during the refractory period of the pacemaker which, in this unit, has a duration of 0.50 second.

Rhythm 17-3,f. Same patient as in 17-3,e. A spontaneous beat occurring after the end of the pacemaker refractory period is sensed and a sensing spike delivered on its QRS complex.

Electrocardiographic Manifestations of Pacemaker Malfunction

A malfunctioning pacemaker may display changes in discharge rate, sensing function, pacing function, pacing rhythm, amplitude of the pacemaker spikes and duration of its refractory period.

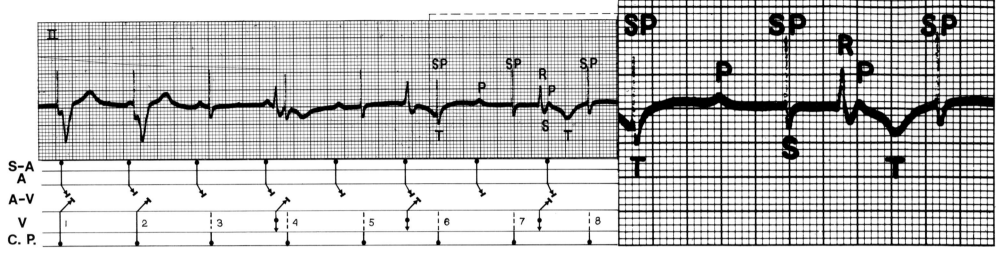

Rhythm 17-4,a. Malfunctioning continuous-asynchronous pacemaker in a patient with sinus rhythm and complete A-V block. Aside from the first two, all the other spikes (SP) are ineffective. Spikes number 3, 5, 7, and 8 fail to activate the ventricles at a time when the myocardium has recovered from its refractory period (exit block). Spikes 4 and 6 show competition. C.P., continuous-asynchronous pacemaker.

ELECTROCARDIOGRAPHIC EVIDENCE OF VENTRICULAR PACEMAKER MALFUNCTION

A. Changes in preselected **rate:** pacing rate becomes slower (newer models) or faster (older models). When rapid discharge rates develop the pacemaker is called a "runaway."

B. Changes in 1:1 **sensing** function:
   1. Ventricular-inhibited pacemaker: spontaneous ventricular beats falling outside the pacemaker refractory period are not sensed.
   2. Ventricular-triggered pacemaker:
      a. Spontaneous ventricular beats falling outside the pacemaker refractory period are not sensed.
      b. The pacemaker senses the T waves.

C. Changes in 1:1 **pacing** function: spikes that fall outside the refractory period of the ventricles re-main ineffective (exit block).

D. Changes in pacing **rhythm,** which becomes irregular.

E. Changes in **amplitude** of the spikes.

F. Changes in duration of the pacemaker **refractory period.**

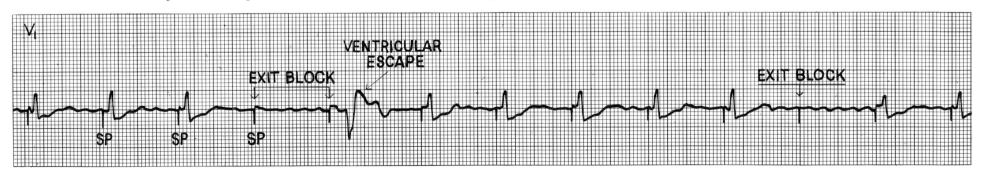

Rhythm 17-4,b. Malfunctioning ventricular-inhibited pacemaker during atrial fibrillation. The pacemaker fails at times to stimulate the ventricles when the myocardium has recovered from its refractory period (exit block). A ventricular escape beat occurs after two consecutive ineffective spikes. The QRS complex of the paced beats shows right bundle branch block configuration, suggesting left ventricular stimulation.

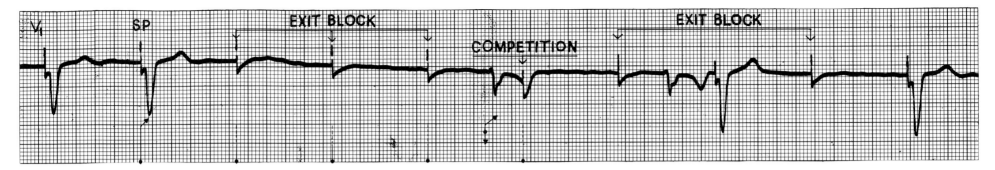

Rhythm 17-4,c. Malfunctioning ventricular-inhibited pacemaker in a patient with atrial fibrillation. The pacing rate has become slower (60 per minute); the unit shows exit block and also fails to sense two spontaneous ventricular escape beats.

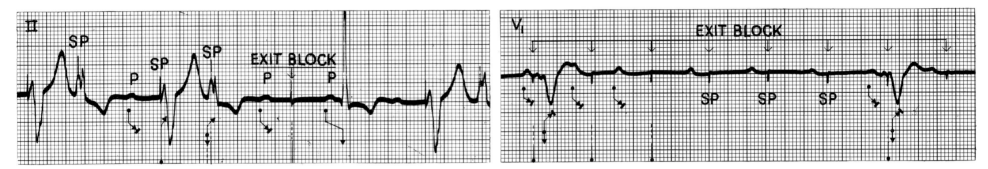

Rhythm 17-4,d. Malfunctioning ventricular-triggered pacemaker in a patient with sinus rhythm and second degree A-V block. The pacemaker senses each ventricular extrasystole and fires a sensing spike after the beginning of the QRS complex. One pacing spike fails to activate the ventricles at a time when the myocardium has recovered from its refractory period (exit block).

Rhythm 17-4,e. Malfunctioning pacemaker firing ineffective spikes at a rapid rate ("runaway" pacemaker) in a patient with sinus rhythm and complete A-V block.

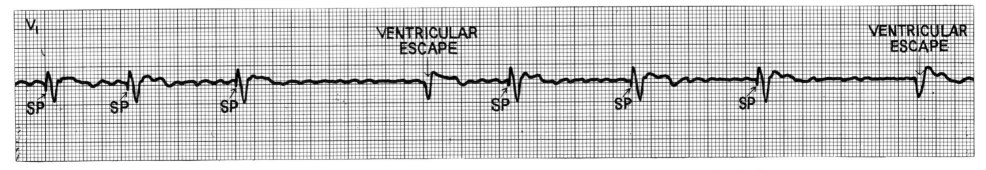

Rhythm 17-4,f. Malfunctioning ventricular-inhibited pacemaker with grossly irregular pacing rhythm.

Chapter 18

Artifacts

Extracardiac signals may become superimposed on the normal cardiac potentials and cause distortions of the electrocardiogram known as artifacts. Some artifacts are immediately obvious; other mimic cardiac arrhythmias and their occurrence may lead to incorrect diagnosis and treatment.[2,3,9,10,19,61,70]

Common artifacts

Three artifacts are fairly common and, in general, easy to recognize:

Muscle tremor: Contraction of the skeletal muscles produces *rapid and irregular* vibrations of the baseline, markedly unequal in shape and amplitude.

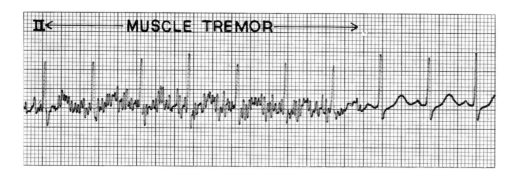

Fig. 18-1. Sinus tachycardia at a rate of 120 per minute. Muscle tremor causes rapid and irregular vibration of the baseline, markedly unequal in amplitude. The last three beats are free of artifacts.

AC interference: Alternating current (AC) interference causes *rapid and regular* vibrations of the baseline at a rate of 60 times per second (360 per minute).

Unstable baseline. Changes in resistance between the electrode and the patient's skin cause *slow shifts* of the baseline.

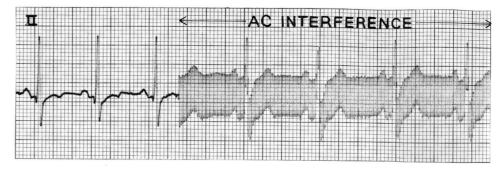

Fig. 18-2. Sinus arrhythmia. After the first three beats, marked AC interference causes rapid and regular vibrations of the baseline at a rate of 60 times per second.

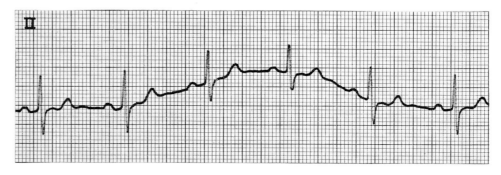

Fig. 18-3. Normal sinus rhythm. There is unstable baseline.

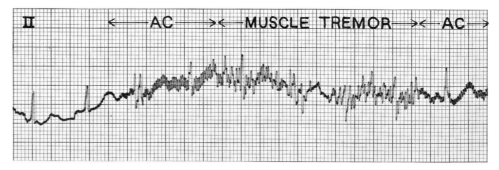

Fig. 18-4. Sinus tachycardia at a rate of 105 per minute. There are muscle tremor artifacts preceded and followed by regular vibrations due to AC interference. There is also unstable baseline. All three common artifacts are therefore present in this tracing.

Artifacts mimicking cardiac arrhythmias

Sudden shifts of the baseline cause artifacts that may closely resemble atrial or ventricular arrhythmias. The following electrocardiographic manifestations are often helpful in the recognition of the artifacts:

Rhythm. The rhythm of artifacts is usually irregular.

Configuration. The shape and amplitude of artifacts often varies. Their width is usually narrower than that of the P waves or QRS-T complexes. Sometimes artifacts occur in bursts of rapid oscillations resembling a toothbrush.

Relationship between artifacts and the P-QRS-T deflections. Artifacts do not change or interrupt the atrial or ventricular rhythm. They often occur on top of the QRS complexes or at an interval too short to allow double depolarization of the ventricles.

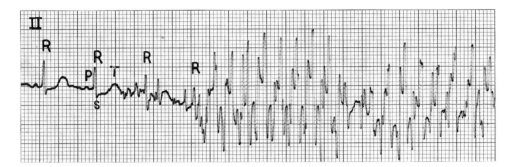

Fig. 18-7. Same patient as in Figure 18-4. Artifacts occur in bursts of rapid oscillations resembling a toothbrush.

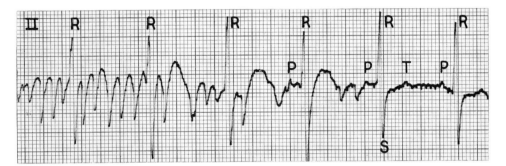

Fig. 18-5. Normal sinus rhythm at a rate of 75 per minute. Sudden shifts of the baseline cause artifacts that resemble atrial ectopic waves. The artifacts vary in shape and amplitude and their rhythm is irregular; they deform the P waves and QRS complexes but do not interrupt the atrial and ventricular rhythm.

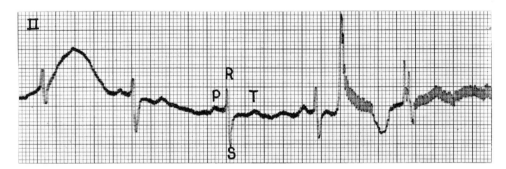

Fig. 18-8. Normal sinus rhythm at a rate of 62 per minute. In addition to an artifact resembling a ventricular extrasystole, unstable baseline and AC interference are clearly seen.

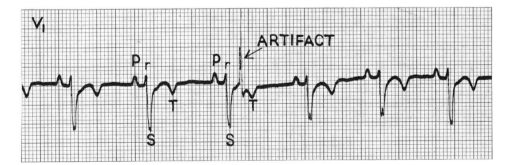

Fig. 18-6. Normal sinus rhythm. A sudden shift of the baseline causes an artifact resembling a ventricular extrasystole. Note that the artifact: (a) is separated from the preceding QRS complex by an interval too short to allow double depolarization of the ventricles, (b) does not interrupt the ventricular rhythm, and (c) has a width narrower than that of a QRS complex.

Association with other artifacts. Artifacts resembling atrial or ventricular arrhythmias are often associated with muscle tremor, AC interference and unstable baseline.

Causes of artifacts

Patient. A frequent source of artifacts is the patient himself. Voluntary or involuntary movements such as respiration, muscle tremor, hiccups, chills, cough, tics, generate voltages that become superimposed on the normal ECG waves.

ECG machine. Artifacts caused by the ECG machine include AC interference, standardization deflection falling on the P, QRS or T deflection, distortions of the ECG tracing due to momentary power failure, to varying speed of the recording paper or tape, to concussion of the machine while in use, etc.

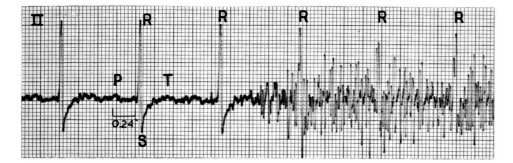

Fig. 18-9. Sinus rhythm with first-degree A-V block (P-R interval 0.24 sec.). Muscle tremor artifacts cause irregular vibrations of the baseline that become much more pronounced in the second half of the strip.

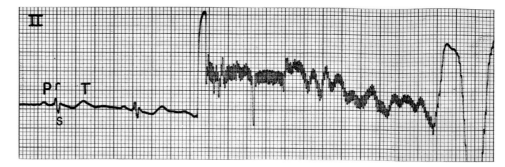

Fig. 18-12. Normal sinus rhythm. A loose connection in a monitoring electrode is responsible for sudden loss of the ECG signal, AC interference and chaotic oscillations of the baseline which might be confused with ventricular fibrillation.

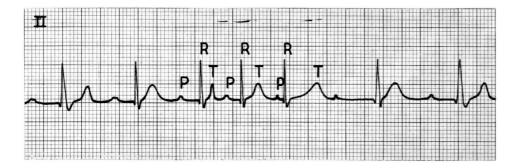

Fig. 18-10. Varying speed of the recording paper causes apparently irregular rhythm and marked changes in duration of the P waves, P-R interval and QRS-T deflections.

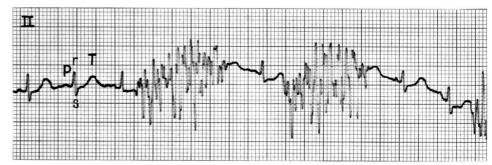

Fig. 18-13. Sinus tachycardia at a rate of 120 per minute. A vacuum cleaner used by the patient while wearing a monitoring apparatus (Holter monitor manufactured by Avionics) caused intermittent artifacts. Bursts of rapid vibrations occurred whenever the vacuum cleaner was drawn closer to the monitoring device.

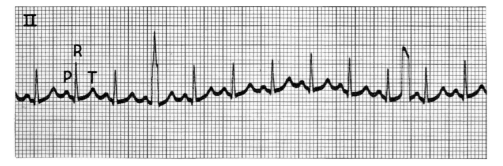

Fig. 18-11. Sinus tachycardia. The first of two standardization deflections falls on a QRS complex, making it appear taller and wider.

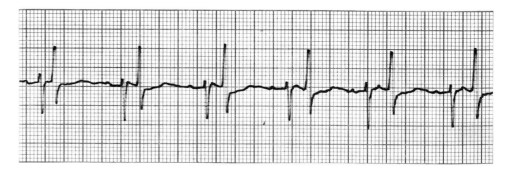

Fig. 18-14. Electrocardiographic potentials from a nurse touching the patient are superimposed on the patient's own ECG waves, mimicking a bigeminal rhythm. Note that one rhythm does not change or interrupt the other and that the first few deflections occur too close to each other, separated by an interval too short to allow double depolarization of the ventricles.

Electrodes. Monitoring electrodes and cables are other frequent sources of artifacts. A broken patient cable with intermittent contact, a loose connection in the electrodes, an improper contact between the electrodes and the patient, drags on the electrode or a swinging cable, may cause shifts of the baseline that frequently mimic cardiac arrhythmias.

Environmental factors. Signals extraneous to the patient and the ECG recording equipment may cause artifacts. Devices such as dial telephones, suction machines, hypothermia or diathermy machines, electric saws or buzzers, vacuum cleaners, ventilators, may cause more or less marked artifacts when close enough to the ECG monitor or recorder. Electrocardiographic potentials from a nurse or technician touching the patient may become superimposed on the patient's own ECG waves.

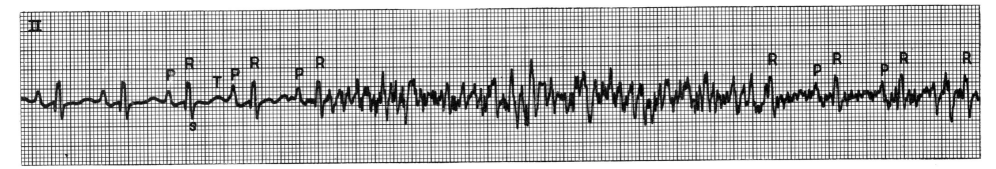

Fig. 18-15. Normal sinus rhythm at a rate of 88 per minute. Gross artifacts due to muscle tremor mimic atrial fibrillation. When the irregular vibrations are less marked, the P-QRS-T deflections of the basic rhythm can be seen to occur undisturbed.

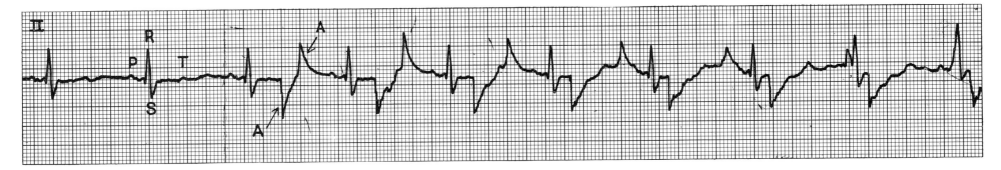

Fig. 18-16. Sinus bradycardia and artifacts (A) mimicking ventricular extrasystoles in bigeminy. Sudden negative shifts of the baseline resemble ectopic QRS complexes, positive shifts resemble their T waves. The artifacts do not disturb the cardiac rhythm. Note that the negative shifts become progressively closer to the preceding QRS complex, while the positive shifts become gradually closer to the following QRS complex.

Artifacts Mimicking Atrial Arrhythmias

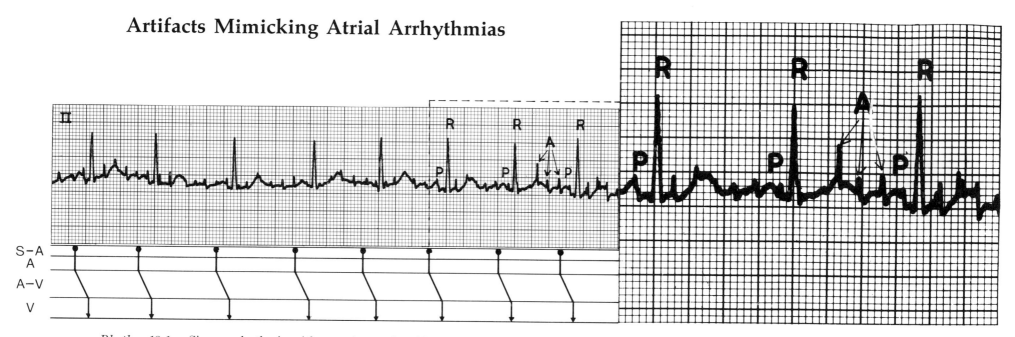

Rhythm 18-1,a. Sinus arrhythmia with superimposed artifacts (A) mimicking a rapid atrial mechanism. The rhythm of the artifacts is irregular and their rate varies between 280 and 750 per minute. The artifacts vary in size and shape and do not interrupt the P wave rhythm.

A. Rate of artifacts: variable

B. Rhythm of artifacts: usually irregular.

C. Configuration of artifacts:

    1. Varying shape.

    2. Varying amplitude.

    3. Occurring in bursts of rapid oscillations resembling a toothbrush.

D. Relationship between artifacts and P waves:

artifacts do not change or interrupt the P wave rhythm.

E. Artifacts mimicking atrial arrhythmias are often associated with muscle tremor, AC interference or unstable baseline.

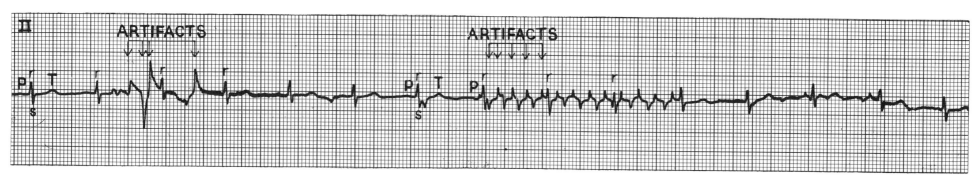

Rhythm 18-1,b. Sinus rhythm with artifacts at times mimicking atrial flutter.

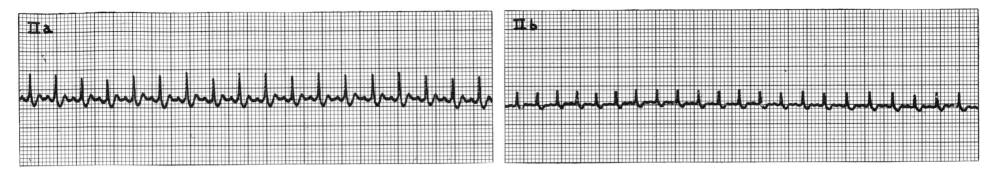

Rhythm 18-1,c. Both strips were obtained from a patient in normal sinus rhythm through a defective monitoring device recording at progressively slower speed and lower voltage. The ECG waves are artificially compressed and the rhythm resembles supraventricular tachycardia (apparent rate in IIa, 210 per minute; in IIb, 250 per minute).

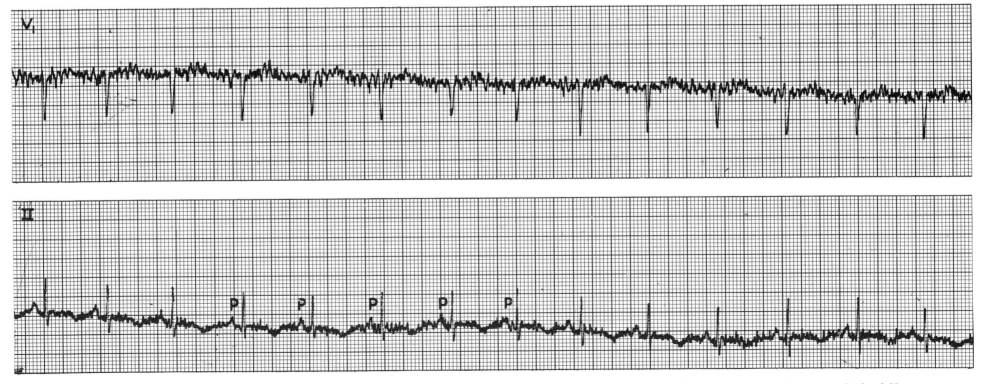

Rhythm 18-1,d. Simultaneous recording of leads V_1 and II in a patient with normal sinus rhythm and artifacts due to muscle tremor. In lead V_1 the artifacts are more marked and mimic atrial fibrillation; the P waves cannot be discerned and the ventricular rhythm is regular. In lead II the sinus P waves can be clearly seen.

Artifacts Mimicking Ventricular Arrhythmias

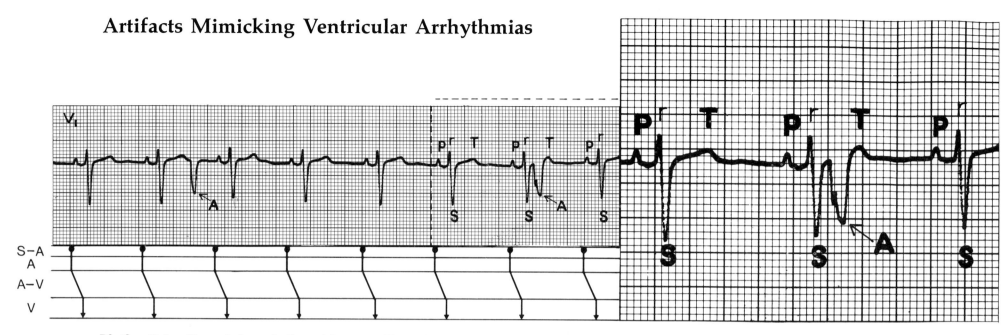

Rhythm 18-2,a. Normal sinus rhythm with two artifacts (A) mimicking ventricular extrasystoles. Neither artifact interrupts the cardiac rhythm and the second one is separated from the preceding QRS complex by an interval too short to allow double depolarization of the ventricles.

A. Rate of artifacts: variable.

B. Rhythm of artifacts: usually irregular.

C. Configuration of artifacts:
1. Varying shape.
2. Varying amplitude.
3. Width of artifacts often narrower than that of the QRS-T complexes.

4. Occurring in bursts of rapid oscillations resembling a toothbrush.

D. Relationship between artifacts and QRS complexes:
1. Artifacts do not change or interrupt the ventricular rhythm.
2. Artifacts often occur on top of the QRS complex or at an interval too short to allow double depolarization of the ventricles.

E. Artifacts mimicking ventricular arrhythmias are often associated with other artifacts due to muscle tremor, AC interference or unstable baseline.

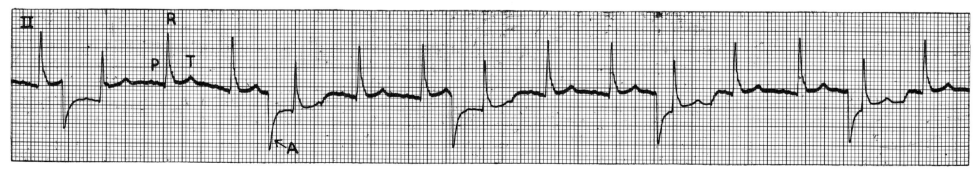

Rhythm 18-2,b. Normal sinus rhythm with artifacts (A) mimicking ventricular extrasystoles. The artifacts do not change or interrupt the ventricular rhythm. AC interference is intermittently present.

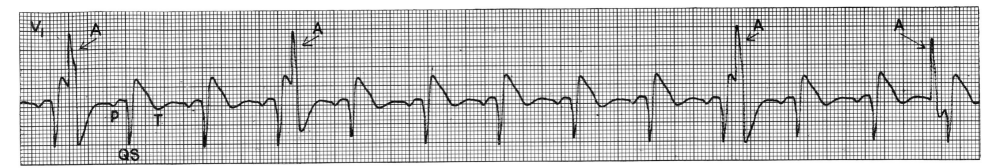

Rhythm 18-2,c. Normal sinus rhythm with four artifacts (A) mimicking ventricular extrasystoles. The artifacts occur either immediately after or immediately before a QRS complex, at an interval too short to allow double depolarization of the ventricles. In addition, they do not change or interrupt the ventricular rhythm.

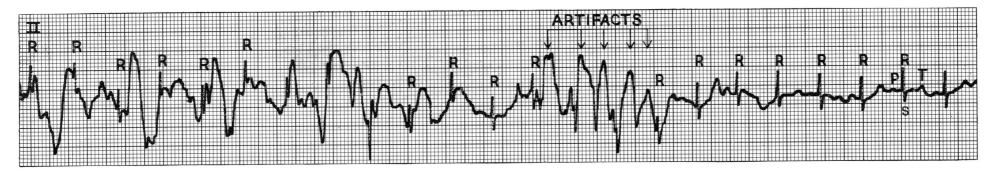

Rhythm 18-2,d. Sinus tachycardia at a rate of 135 per minute. Sudden shifts of the baseline cause artifacts mimicking ventricular tachycardia. The artifacts do not interrupt the cardiac rhythm, and most QRS complexes can still be identified.

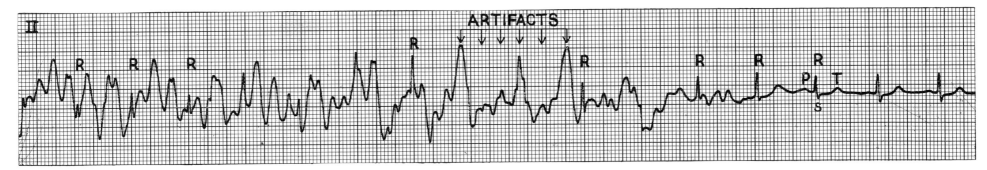

Rhythm 18-2,e. Normal sinus rhythm with gross artifacts mimicking ventricular fibrillation. Some QRS complexes can be identified among the chaotic waves caused by the artifacts.

Self-Assessment Tracings

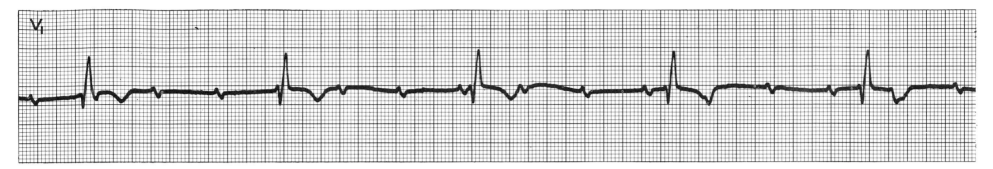

Case 1. *Question:* This strip was recorded from a 74-year-old male with ischemic heart disease. *What is your interpretation of the rhythm?*

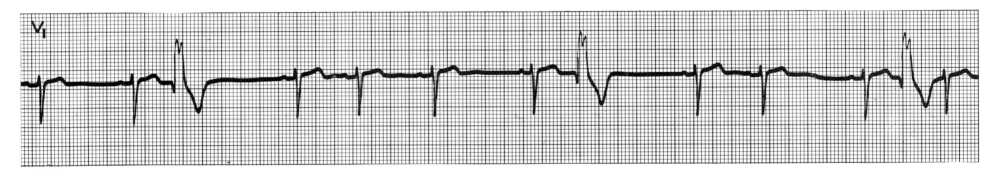

Case 2. *Question:* This ECG strip was obtained from a 20-year-old man with no evidence of heart disease. *What is your interpretation of the rhythm?*

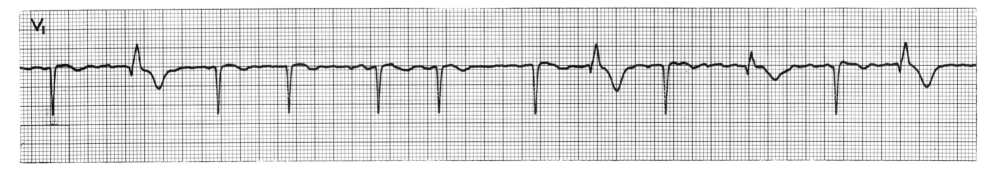

Case 3. *Question:* This ECG strip was recorded from a 62-year-old woman with rheumatic heart disease. *What is your interpretation of the rhythm?*

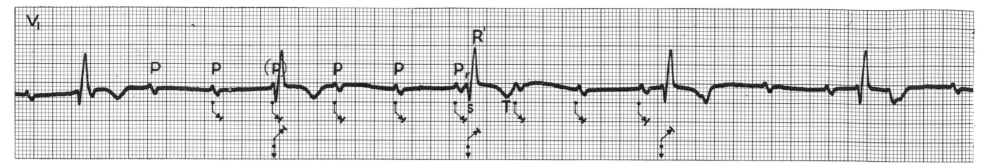

Case 1. *Interpretation:* The strip shows sinus rhythm with complete A-V block and idioventricular escape rhythm at a rate of 29 per minute. The P waves bear no constant relationship to the QRS complexes and the apparent "P-R interval" continuously changes in duration. The ventricular rhythm is regular and the QRS complexes are wide and bizarre with a configuration resembling *right* bundle branch block: the escape focus therefore is situated in the *left* ventricle.

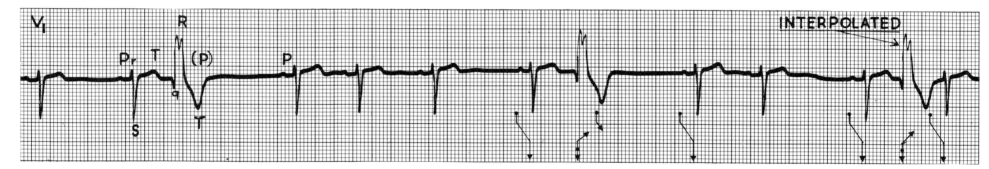

Case 2. *Interpretation:* There is respiratory sinus arrhythmia and unifocal *left* ventricular extrasystoles (their QRS complex resembles *right* bundle branch block). The first 2 ventricular extrasystoles are followed by a pause whereas the third is sandwiched between 2 consecutive sinus beats (interpolated VPC). The average ventricular rate is 60 per minute.

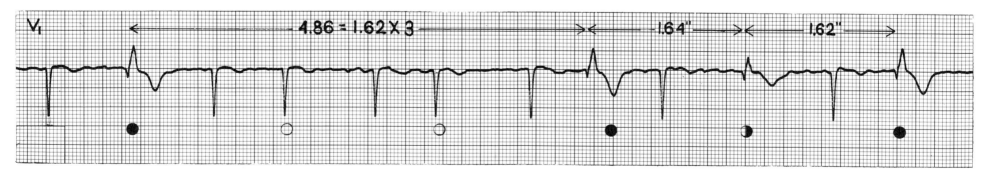

Case 3. *Interpretation:* There is atrial fibrillation with average ventricular rate of 60 per minute and ventricular parasystole. The ectopic beats could be interpreted as ventricular extrasystoles or as atrial fibrillation impulses with aberrant ventricular conduction. Close observation, however, reveals that while they have a similar configuration the coupling interval is variable. Furthermore, the long interectopic interval is a multiple of the shorter ones. The third ectopic QRS complex is a fusion beat. The position of the parasystolic impulses is indicated by black dots (pure parasystolic beats), open circles (nonmanifest parasystolic discharges) and half-shaded circles (fusion beats).

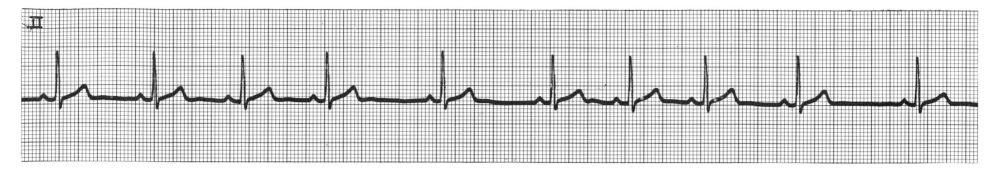

Case 4. *Question:* This strip was obtained from a 16-year-old girl with no demonstrable heart disease. *What is your interpretation of the rhythm?*

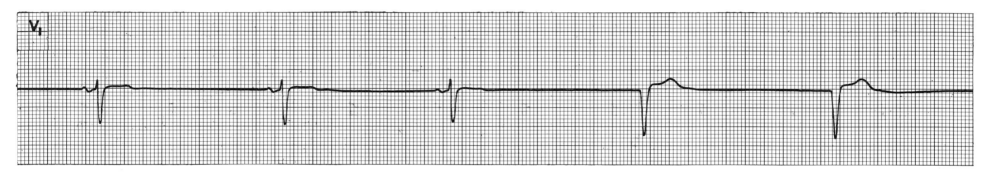

Case 5. *Question:* This ECG tracing was obtained from an 85-year-old male with arteriosclerotic heart disease. *What is your interpretation of the rhythm?*

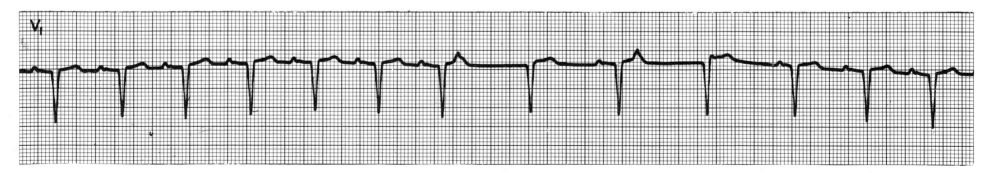

Case 6. *Question:* This rhythm strip was recorded from a 79-year-old man with congestive heart failure. *What is your interpretation of the rhythm?*

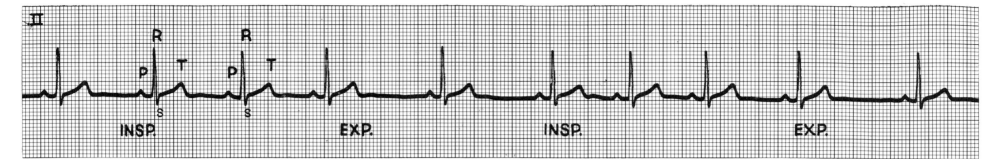

Case 4. *Interpretation:* The strip shows respiratory sinus arrhythmia. The sinus beats occur irregularly with P-P and R-R intervals varying more than 0.16 second. The rate increases for a few beats during inspiration, then decreases for the next few beats during expiration.

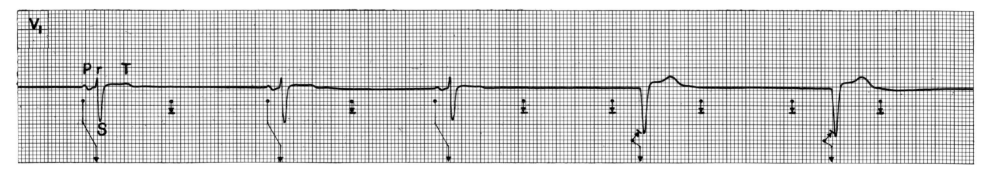

Case 5. *Interpretation:* The first 3 beats show apparent sinus bradycardia of marked degree with a rate of about 30 per minute; then sinus activity ceases completely and 2 idionodal escape beats occur. The rhythm is probably type II sinoatrial block, 2:1 at first, then complete. Retrograde block is likely to be present, because there is no evidence of atrial captures following the idionodal escape beats.

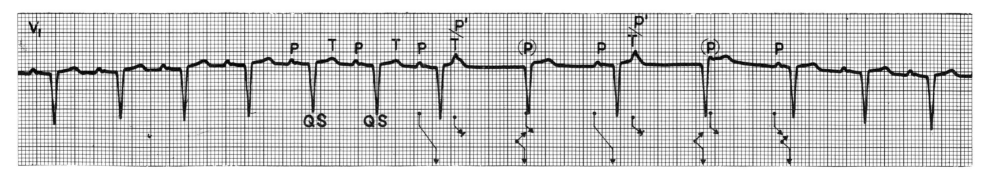

Case 6. *Interpretation:* There is sinus rhythm at a rate of 88 per minute with first degree A-V block (P-R interval 0.22 second) and nonconducted atrial extrasystoles. The extrasystolic P' wave deforms the T wave of the preceding beat. The ventricular pause caused by each nonconducted atrial ectopic impulse is terminated by an A-V nodal escape beat. The P-R interval of the beat preceding the final two is shorter than that of the other sinus beats, suggesting that this beat is also an A-V nodal escape (the A-V node has fired a second escape impulse before the sinus impulse has had a chance to reach the ventricles).

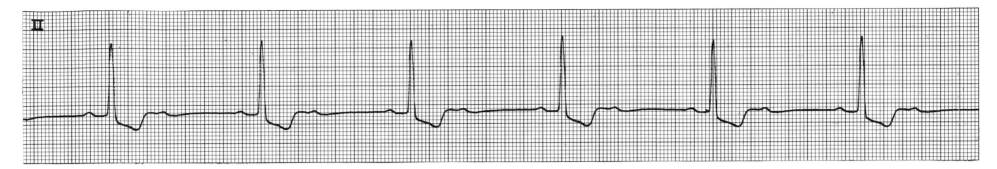

Case 7. *Question:* This rhythm strip was obtained from a 64-year-old woman with hypertension. *What is your interpretation of the rhythm?*

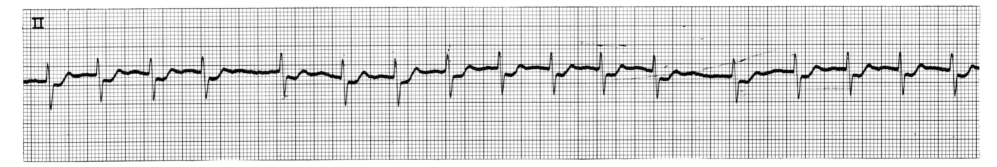

Case 8. *Question:* This ECG strip was obtained from a 72-year-old female with hypertensive cardiovascular disease, receiving digitalis and diuretics. *What is your interpretation of the rhythm?*

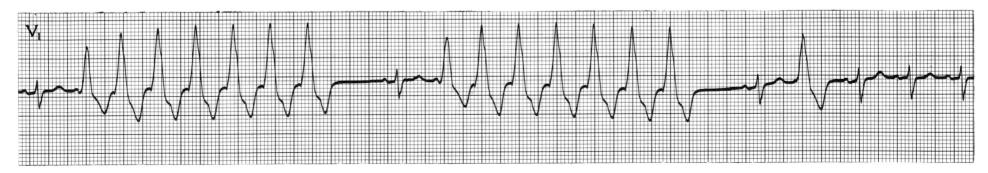

Case 9. *Question:* This rhythm strip was recorded from a 79-year-old man with acute myocardial infarction. *What is your interpretation of the rhythm?*

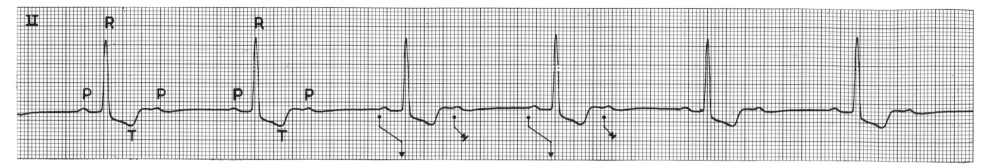

Case 7. *Interpretation:* This ECG strip shows sinus rhythm with 2:1 second degree A-V block. Second degree A-V block with 2:1 conduction ratio may be either type (Wenckebach) or type II (Mobitz). In this case, long and repeated strips failed to show Wenckebach sequences so that the 2:1 block was considered to be type II (Mobitz).

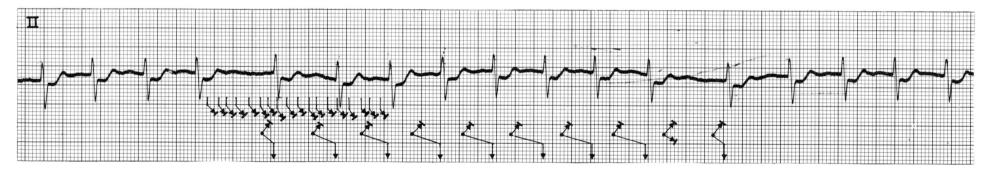

Case 8. *Interpretation:* The basic rhythm is atrial fibrillation, but the ventricular rhythm is regularly irregular with groups of QRS complexes separated by pauses (group beating). In some areas the R-R interval becomes progressively shorter while approaching the pause. The tracing represents atrial fibrillation with high grade or complete A-V block and nonparoxysmal A-V nodal tachycardia. There is intermittent exit block and the conducted A-V nodal impulses reach the ventricles with second degree A-V block type I (Wenckebach). The most likely cause of this arrhythmia is digitalis toxicity.

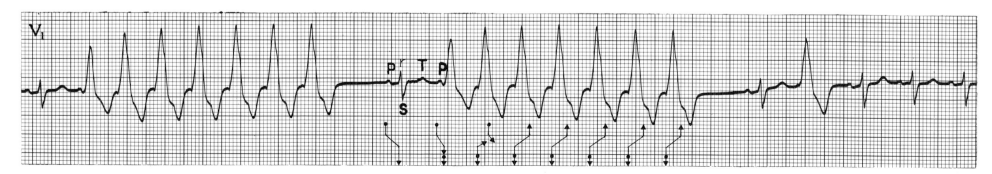

Case 9. *Interpretation:* The strip shows sinus tachycardia at a rate of 110 per minute and repetitive ventricular tachycardia at a rate of 150 per minute. The first QRS complex of each run of ventricular tachycardia is a fusion beat (between the sinus and the ectopic ventricular impulse); the last 5 QRS complexes of each run are followed by retrograde conduction to the atria (atrial captures).

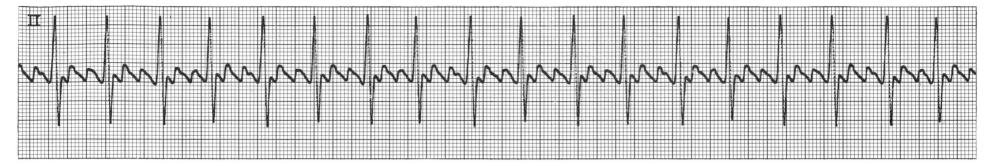

Case 10. *Question:* This tracing was obtained from a 60-year-old woman with hypertensive cardiovascular disease. *What is your interpretation of the rhythm?*

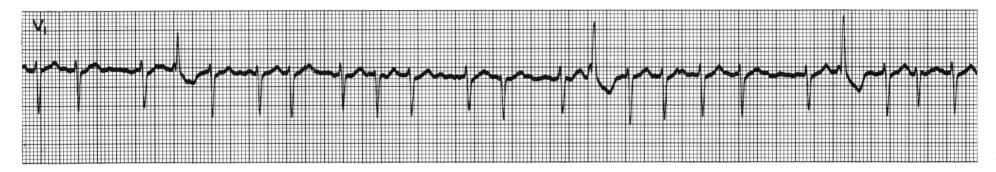

Case 11. *Question:* This strip was recorded from a 63-year-old woman with essential hypertension. *What is your interpretation of the rhythm?*

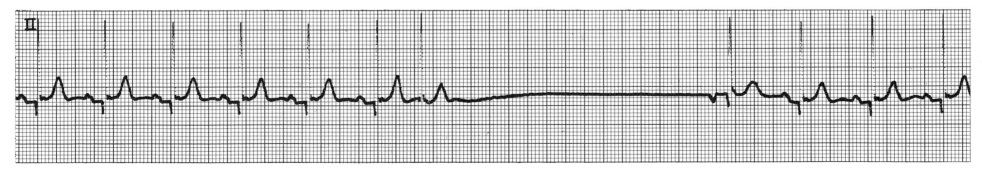

Case 12. *Question:* This ECG strip was obtained from a 68-year-old woman with recurrent syncopal episodes. *What is your interpretation of the rhythm?*

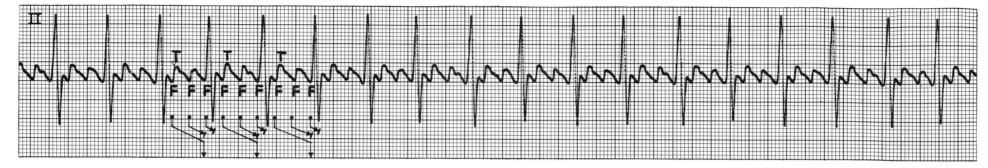

Case 10. *Interpretation:* The tracing shows atrial flutter with 3:1 A-V block and   ventricular rate of 110 per minute.

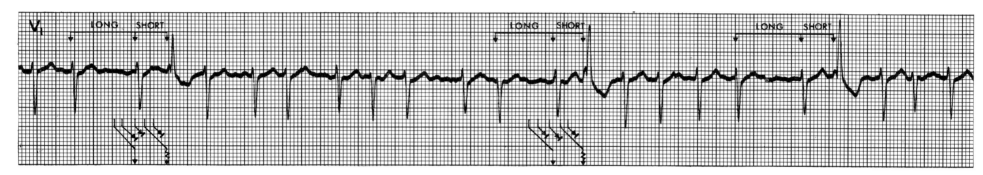

Case 11. *Interpretation:* The strip shows atrial fibrillation with average ventricular rate of 130 per minute. The 3 anomalous beats represent aberrant ventricular conduction of atrial fibrillation impulses and not ventricular extrasystoles. The following electrocardiographic manifestations are helpful in recognizing aberrant ventricular conduction in this tracing: right bundle branch block configuration; direction of the initial portion of the QRS complex (initial vector) same as in the normal beats; long-short sequence terminated by the aberrant beat (Ashman phenomenon), and absence of a significant pause following the aberrant beat.

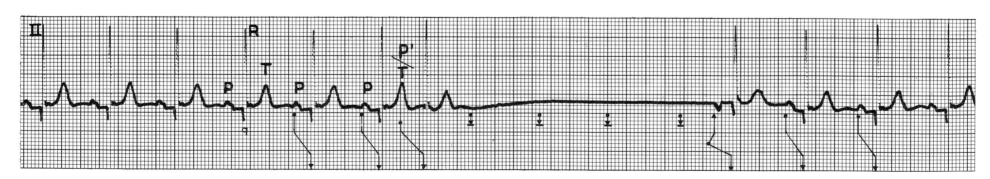

Case 12. *Interpretation:* Sinus rhythm at a rate of 85 per minute is present in the first half of the strip. Following an atrial extrasystole there is a 3.26-second pause with no evidence of atrial or ventricular activity. The pause is caused by the block of 4 consecutive sinus impulses at the S-A junction (2nd degree sino-atrial block, type II) and is terminated by an A-V nodal escape beat. The patient had the so-called "sick sinus syndrome" and was treated with artificial pacing.

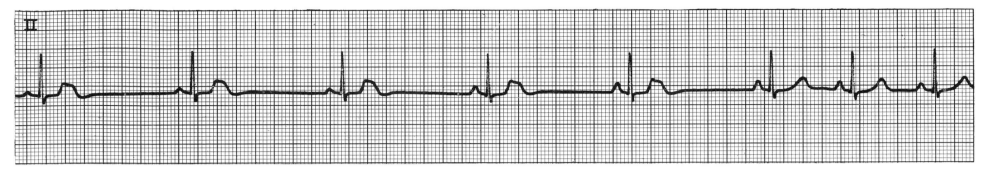

Case 13. *Question:* This strip was obtained from a 40-year-old male with idiopathic cardiomyopathy. *What is your interpretation of the rhythm?*

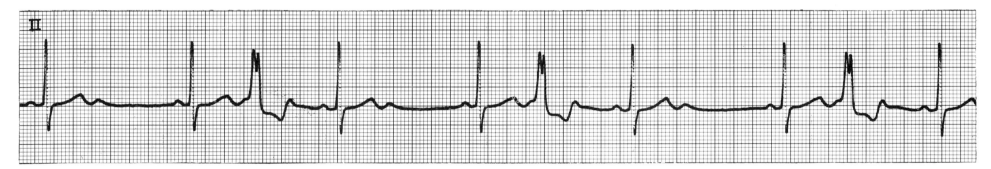

Case 14. *Question:* This strip is from a 59-year-old male with hypertension, on treatment with rauwolfia and thiazide diuretics. *What is your interpretation of the rhythm?*

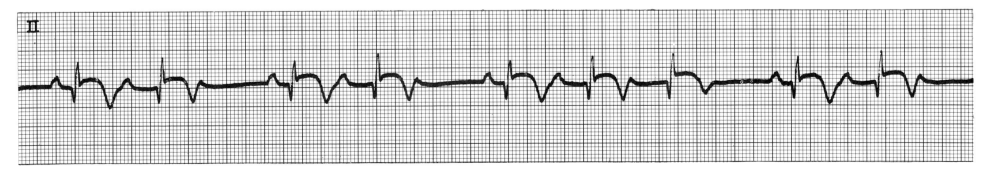

Case 15. *Question:* This tracing was obtained from a 44-year-old male with acute inferior wall infarction. *What is your interpretation of the rhythm?*

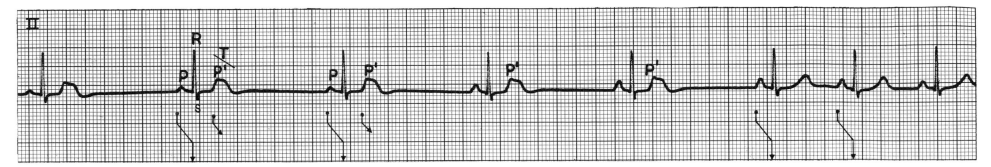

Case 13. *Interpretation:* Each of the first 5 sinus beats is followed by an atrial extrasystole which is not conducted to the ventricles because it is very premature. The run of nonconducted atrial bigeminy causes a ventricular rate of only 38 per minute. The last 3 beats show normal sinus rhythm at a rate of 70 per minute.

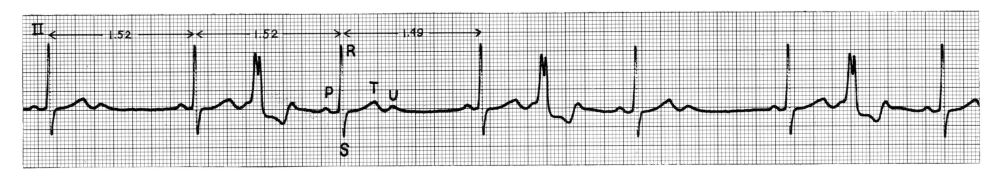

Case 14. *Interpretation:* Marked sinus bradycardia at a rate of 39 per minute with interpolated unifocal ventricular extrasystoles. The ectopic impulses have no effect on the dominant rhythm and each extrasystole is sandwiched between 2 consecutive sinus beats. Note the prominent U waves.

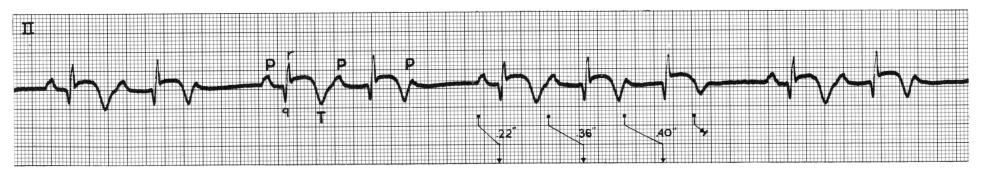

Case 15. *Interpretation:* Sinus rhythm at the rate of 83 per minute with second degree A-V block type I (Wenckebach). The P-R interval grows progressively longer until a P wave is blocked and a ventricular pause occurs. The conduction ratio is 3:2 or 4:3.

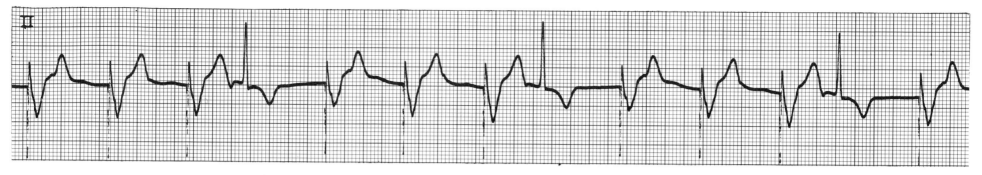

Case 16. *Question:* 63-year-old male with sick sinus syndrome. This ECG strip was recorded a few days after implantation of a permanent transvenous pacemaker. *What type of pacemaker was used? What is your interpretation of the rhythm?*

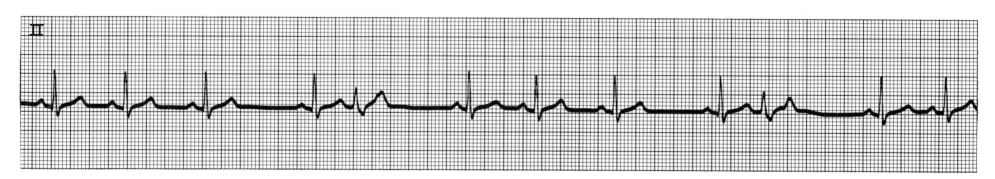

Case 17. *Question:* Strip obtained from a 22-year-old man with no evidence of heart disease. *What is your interpretation of the rhythm?*

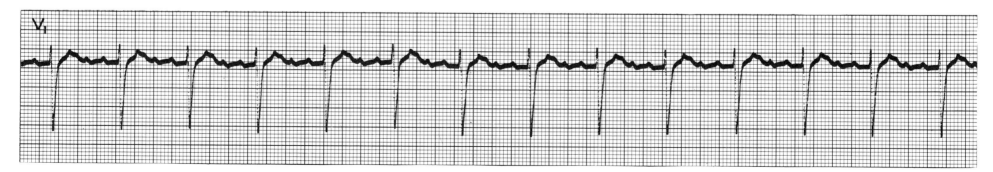

Case 18. *Question:* This tracing was obtained from a 43-year-old female with rheumatic heart disease on treatment with digoxin. *What is your interpretation of the rhythm?*

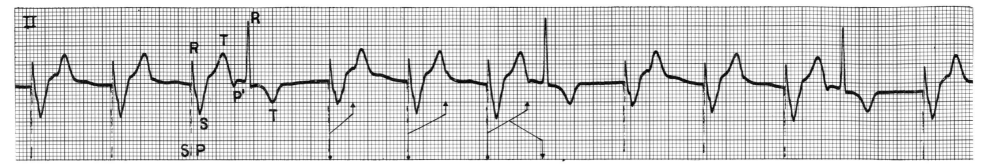

Case 16. *Interpretation:* An artificial pacemaker is pacing the heart at the rate of 70 per minute (SP, spike). Three spontaneous QRS-T complexes are sensed and temporarily inhibit pacemaker activity. The pacemaker, therefore, is a ventricular-inhibited unit. An inverted P' wave follows each paced beat and there is no evidence of sinus activity. The 3 spontaneous QRS-T complexes are reciprocal beats: the artificial pacemaker impulse activates the ventricles, spreads retrogradely to the atria with a progressively longer R-P' interval (retrograde Wenckebach phenomenon) and, when the R-P' interval becomes sufficiently prolonged, the impulse returns in a forward direction to re-excite the ventricles.

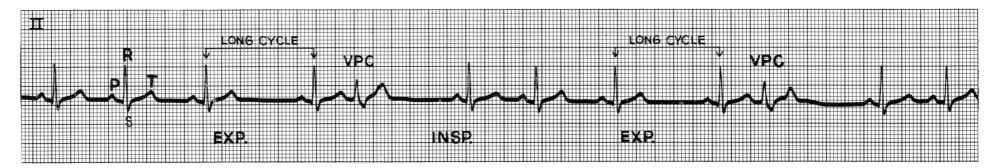

Case 17. *Interpretation:* Respiratory sinus arrhythmia. The rate increases for a few beats during inspiration (INSP.) and decreases for the next few beats during expiration (EXP.). Isolated unifocal VPC's occur after a long ventricular cycle; this phenomenon could be attributed to the so-called "rule of bigeminy" (Chap. 3).

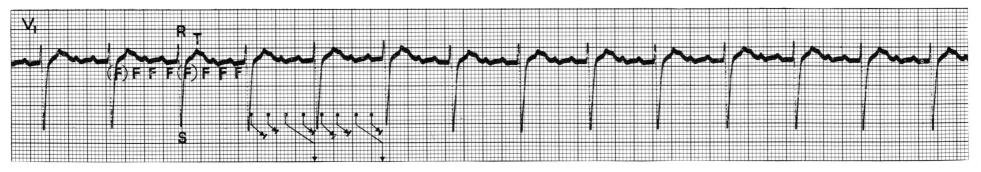

Case 18. *Interpretation:* Atrial flutter with 4:1 A-V block. A flutter wave is hidden within each QRS complex. The flutter wave responsible for the ventricular excitation is not the one immediately preceding the QRS complex ("skipped" F wave) but the one before that. The QRS complex has a normal width of 0.10 second.

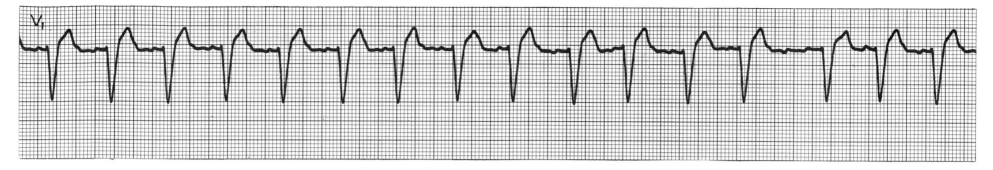

Case 19. *Question:* Electrocardiogram recorded from an 81-year-old male with arteriosclerotic heart disease on treatment with digitalis. *What is your interpretation of
the rhythm?*

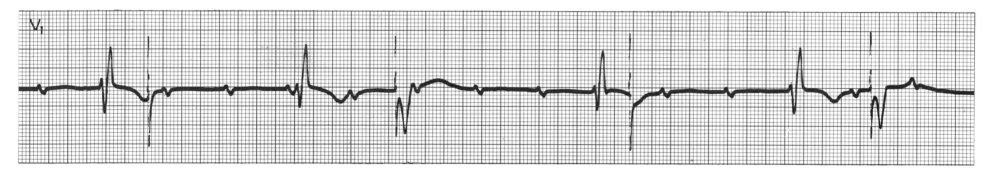

Case 20. *Question:* Tracing obtained from a 77-year-old woman with arteriosclerotic
heart disease. A permanent transvenous ventricular-inhibited pacemaker had been
implanted 12 months earlier. *What is your interpretation of the rhythm?*

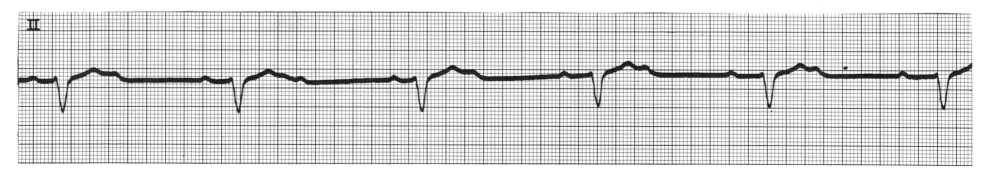

Case 21. *Question:* This ECG tracing was obtained from a 79-year-old male with
arteriosclerotic heart disease. *What is your interpretation of the rhythm?*

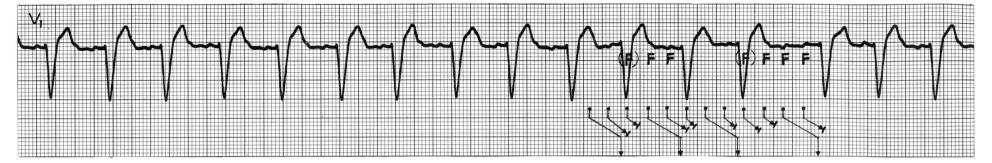

Case 19. *Interpretation:* Atrial flutter with variable A-V block (3:1, occasionally 4:1) and left bundle branch block. While 3:1 block is present the rhythm resembles normal sinus; when the A-V block becomes 4:1, two consecutive flutter waves are clearly seen (atrial rate 280 per minute). The F wave immediately preceding the QRS complex is not the wave that is conducted to the ventricles ("skipped" F wave).

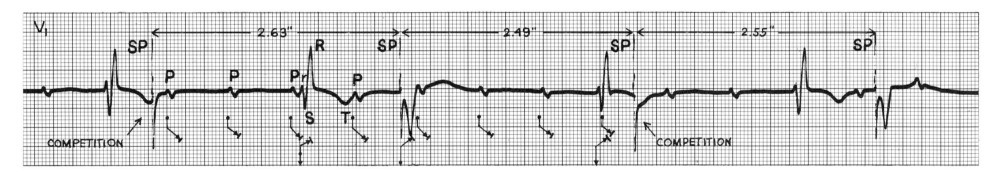

Case 20. *Interpretation:* The spontaneous cardiac activity is sinus rhythm with complete A-V block and idioventricular escape rhythm at a rate of 28 per minute. The artificial pacemaker is malfunctioning and displays a very slow and irregular pacing rhythm. In addition, the pacemaker has lost its sensing function and a spike falls twice on the T wave of a spontaneous ventricular beat (competition). SP, pacemaker spike.

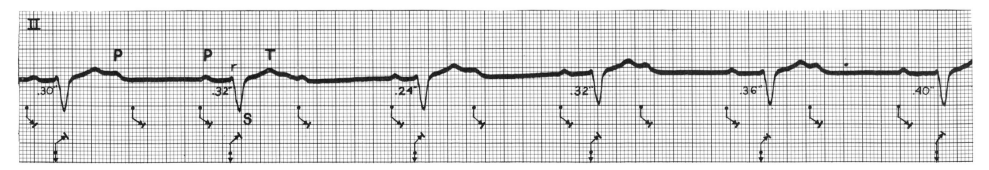

Case 21. *Interpretation:* The rhythm superficially resembles 2:1 second degree A-V block; close observation, however, reveals that the "P-R interval" continuously changes in duration. The correct interpretation therefore is sinus rhythm with complete A-V block and idioventricular escape rhythm at a rate of 33 per minute.

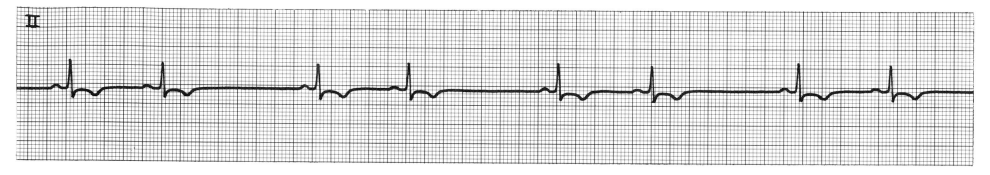

Case 22. *Question:* Rhythm strip recorded from a 65-year-old woman with congestive heart failure. *What is your interpretation of the rhythm?*

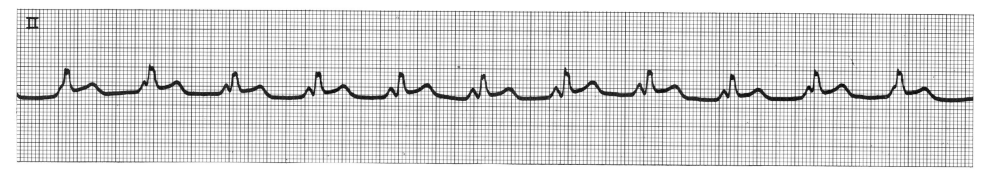

Case 23. *Question:* Electrocardiogram recorded in the Cardiac Care Unit from a 52-year-old man with severe chest pain. *What is your interpretation of the rhythm?*

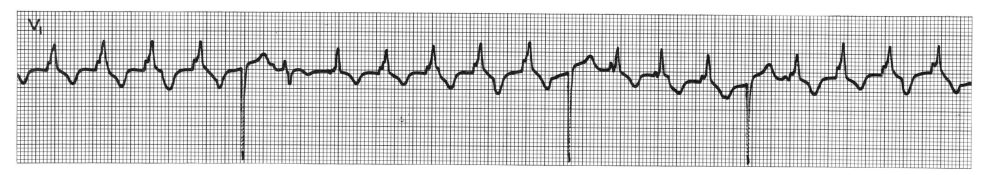

Case 24. *Question:* This ECG strip was obtained from a 44-year-old woman with idiopathic cardiomyopathy. *What is your interpretation of the rhythm?*

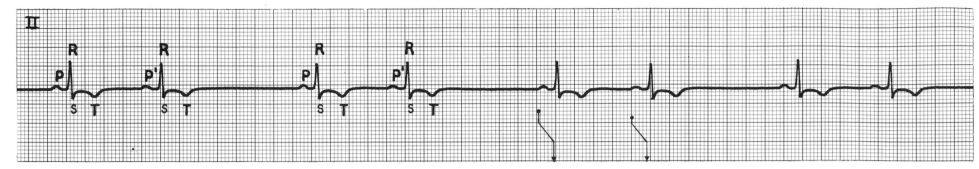

Case 22. *Interpretation:* Sinus rhythm with atrial extrasystoles in bigeminy and average ventricular rate of 45 per minute. The configuration of the P′ waves, different from that of the sinus P waves, is evidence of their ectopic atrial origin.

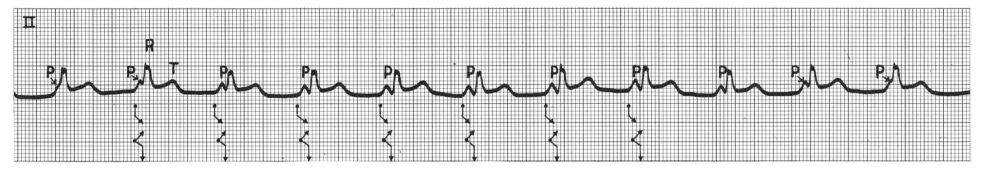

Case 23. *Interpretation:* The tracing shows A-V dissociation between the sinus and the A-V node. The P waves "travel" away from, then toward the QRS complex. The sinus and the A-V node have nearly identical rates of about 68 per minute ("isorhythmic dissociation") and there are no ventricular captures by the sinus impulses.

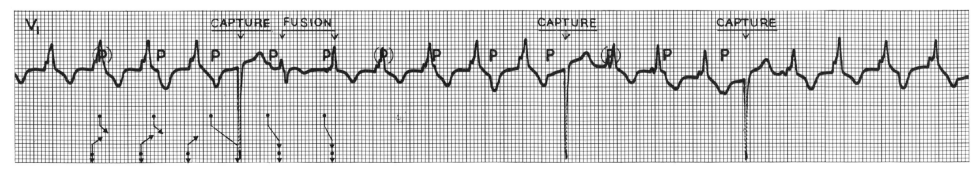

Case 24. *Interpretation:* The tracing shows paroxysmal ventricular tachycardia at a rate of 120 per minute. The atria are under the control of sinus rhythm and there is obvious A-V dissociation. Ventricular captures by sinus impulses and fusion beats between sinus and ectopic ventricular impulses are clearly seen.

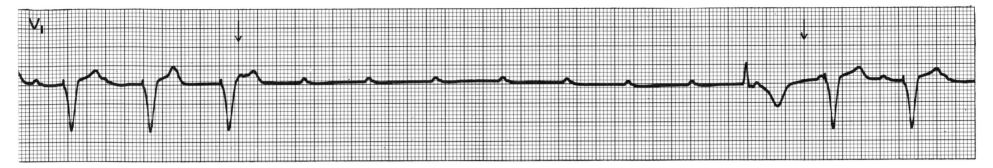

Case 25. *Question:* Electrocardiogram recorded from a 77-year-old female with a temporary transvenous pacemaker. The pacemaker was turned off (first arrow) then turned on again (second arrow). *What is your interpretation of the rhythm?*

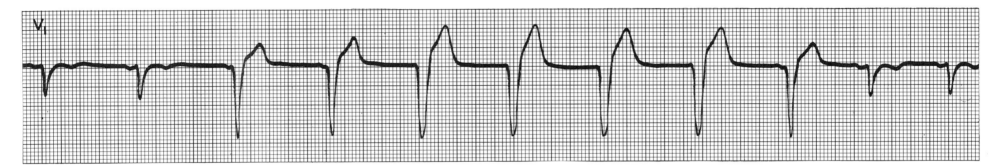

Case 26. *Question:* This rhythm strip was recorded in the Cardiac Care Unit from a 56-year-old male with acute myocardial infarction. *What is your interpretation of the rhythm?*

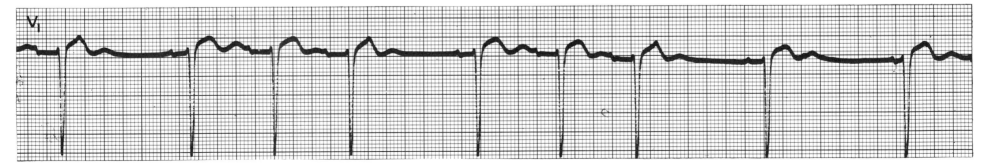

Case 27. *Question:* This ECG strip was obtained from a 55-year-old male with hypertension and congestive heart failure. *What is your interpretation of the rhythm?*

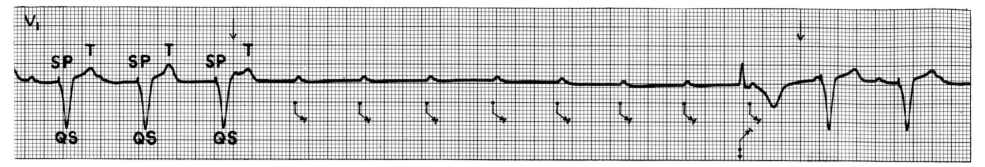

Case 25. *Interpretation:* Normally functioning transvenous pacemaker at a rate of 70 per minute. The atria are under the control of the sinus rhythm. When the unit is turned off, a 5.56-second pause results (ventricular standstill). The pause reveals the presence of complete A-V block and of a very sluggish ventricular escape mechanism.

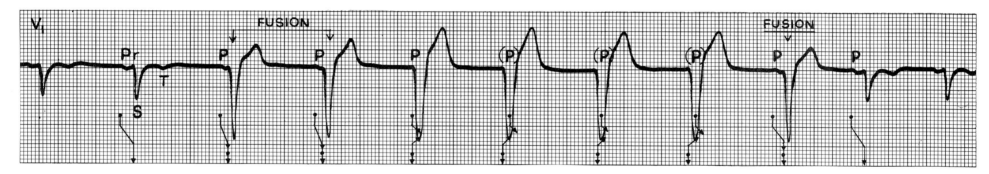

Case 26. *Interpretation:* The strip shows sinus bradycardia at a rate of 58 per minute and a run of nonparoxysmal ventricular tachycardia at a rate of 62 per minute. The sinus P waves "travel" toward, inside and away from the QRS complexes of ventricular origin (A-V dissociation). Three ventricular fusion beats are seen.

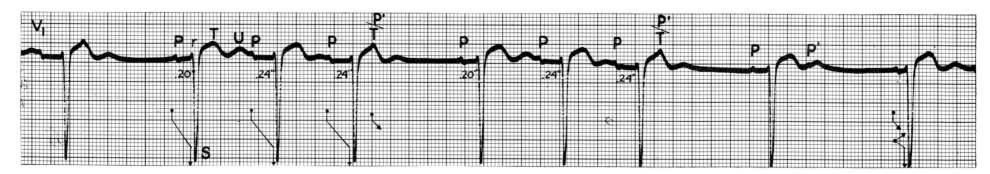

Case 27. *Interpretation:* The strip shows sinus rhythm, P-R interval of varying duration and ventricular pauses. The arrhythmia superficially resembles second degree A-V block type I (Wenckebach). Close observation, however, reveals that the P-R interval does not become progressively longer and that each pause is caused by a premature P′ wave deforming the T wave of the preceding beat (nonconducted APC's or reversed reciprocal beats). The ensuing pause enables the A-V node to conduct the following sinus impulse with a shorter P-R interval (0.20 sec. instead of 0.24 sec.). The last QRS complex is an A-V nodal escape beat. The correct interpretation, therefore, is sinus rhythm with first degree A-V block, nonconducted atrial extrasystole (or reversed reciprocal beats) and one A-V nodal escape beat.

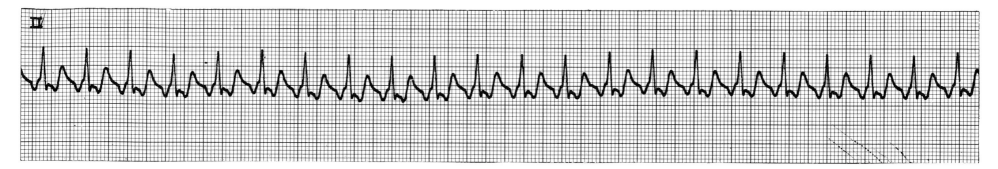

Case 28. *Question:* This electrocardiogram was recorded from a 26-year-old woman with rheumatic heart disease. *What is your interpretation of the rhythm?*

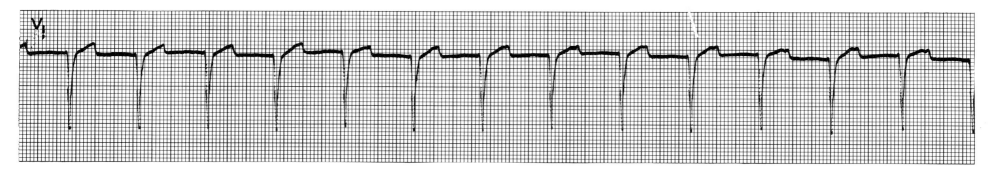

Case 29. *Question:* This rhythm strip was recorded in the Cardiac Care Unit from a 57-year-old male with acute inferior wall myocardial infarction. *What is your interpretation of the rhythm?*

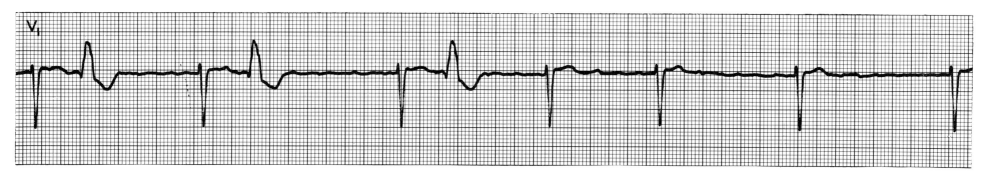

Case 30. *Question:* Rhythm strip obtained from a 75-year-old woman with arteriosclerotic heart disease on treatment with digoxin and furosemide. *What is your interpretation of the rhythm?*

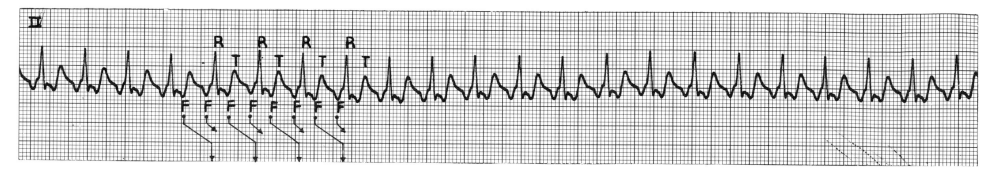

Case 28. *Interpretation:* The rhythm is atrial flutter with 2:1 conduction and ventricular rate of 130 per minute.

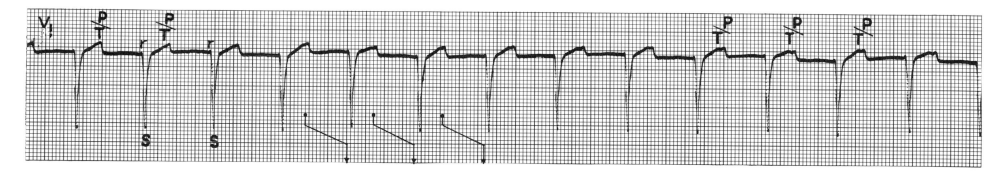

Case 29. *Interpretation:* Sinus rhythm at the rate of 80 per minute with first degree A-V block. The PR interval measures 0.44 second and the P wave is superimposed on the preceding T wave ("P on T").

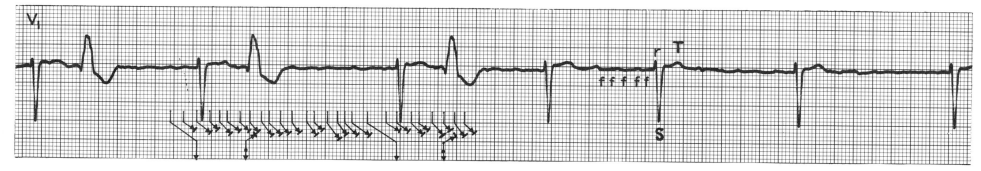

Case 30. *Interpretation:* The strip shows atrial fibrillation with 3 unifocal left ventricular extrasystoles in bigeminy and average ventricular rate of 55 per minute. Both the extrasystoles and the slow ventricular response suggest digitalis toxicity.

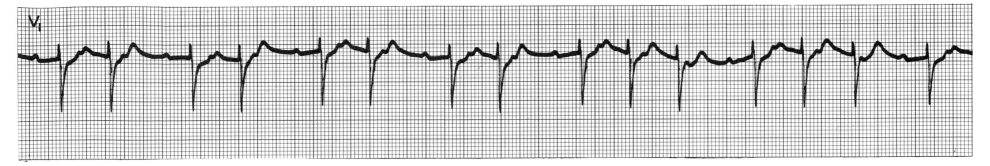

Case 31. *Question:* This strip was obtained in the Cardiac Care Unit from a 59-year-old male with acute inferior wall infarction. *What is your interpretation of the rhythm?*

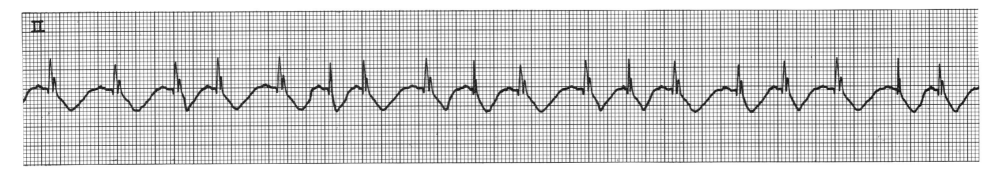

Case 32. *Question:* This rhythm strip was recorded from a 50-year-old male with rheumatic heart disease on treatment with quinidine and digoxin. *What is your interpretation of the rhythm?*

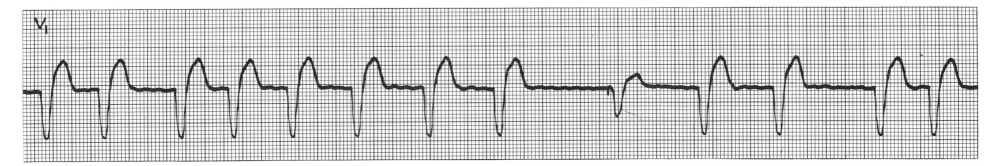

Case 33. *Question:* ECG strip recorded in the Coronary Care Unit from a 69-year-old male with acute anterior wall infarction. A temporary transvenous pacemaker had been inserted. *What is your interpretation of the rhythm? What type of pacemaker was employed?*

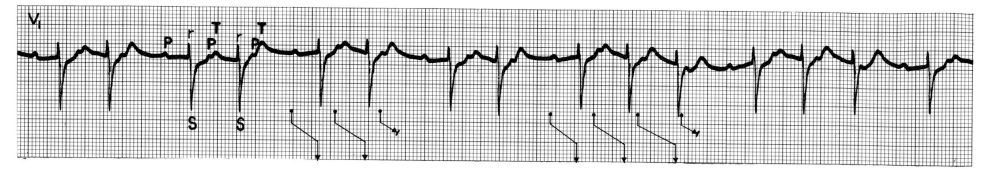

Case 31. *Interpretation:* The rhythm is sinus tachycardia at 130 per minute with second degree A-V block type I (Wenckebach). There are 3:2 and 4:3 Wenckebach sequences. The average ventricular rate is 90 per minute.

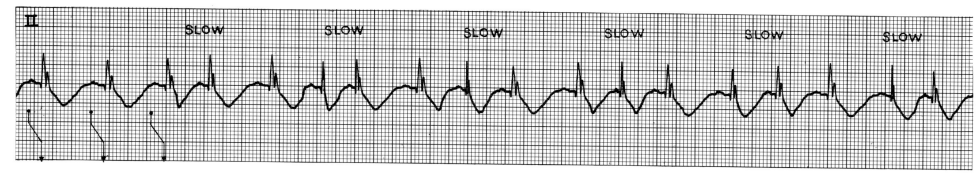

Case 32. *Interpretation:* The rhythm is normal sinus at the rate of 85 per minute. Varying speed of the recording paper is responsible for the apparently irregular rhythm and the marked changes in the duration of the P-R interval, QRS complex and T wave. The artifacts were caused by a defective paper roller in the ECG machine.

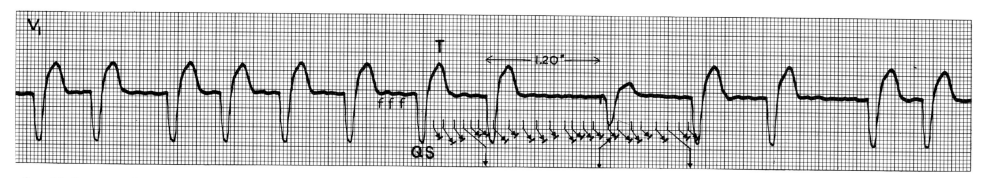

Case 33. *Interpretation:* The strip shows atrial fibrillation with average ventricular rate of 80 per minute and left bundle branch block. A long ventricular pause is terminated by a paced beat. The pacemaker is of the ventricular-inhibited (demand) type and fires only when the spontaneous ventricular beats fail to occur for 1.20 second (pacemaker escape interval).

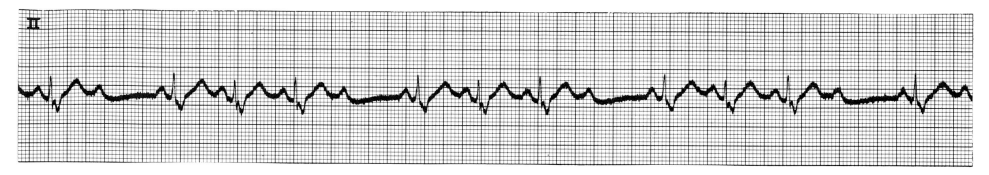

Case 34. *Question:* This rhythm strip was recorded from a 48-year-old male with coronary heart disease. *What is your interpretation of the rhythm?*

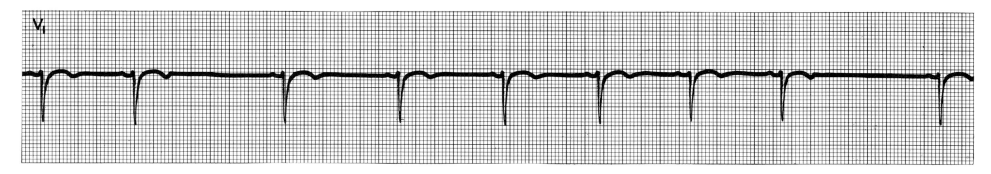

Case 35. *Question:* This rhythm strip was recorded from a 66-year-old woman with arteriosclerotic heart disease and congestive heart failure. *What is your interpretation of the rhythm?*

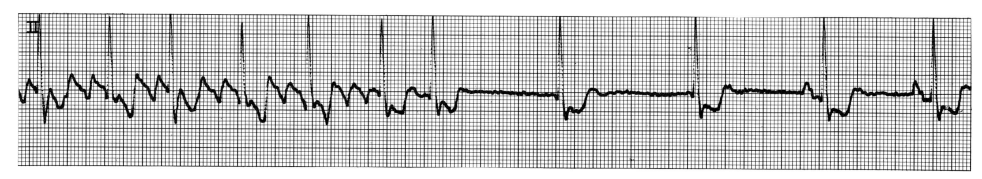

Case 36. *Question:* This ECG strip was recorded from a 79-year-old male with hypertensive cardiovascular disease and congestive heart failure. *What is your interpretation of the rhythm?*

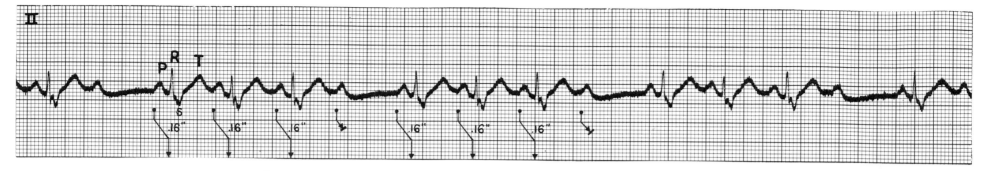

Case 34. *Interpretation:* The strip shows sinus rhythm at the rate of 90 per minute, 4:1 second degree A-V block type II (Mobitz) and bundle branch block. The P-R interval of the conducted beats is of constant duration and measures 0.16 second.

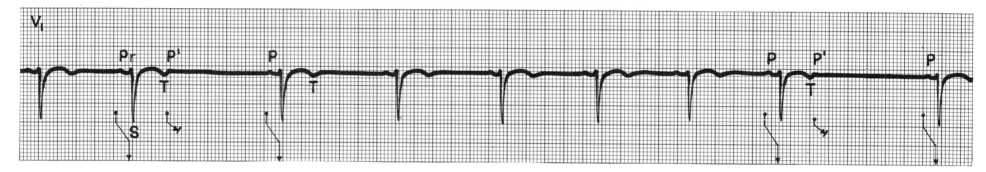

Case 35. *Interpretation:* Sinus bradycardia and sinus arrhythmia with nonconducted atrial extrasystoles causing long ventricular pauses. The premature P′ wave of each nonconducted APC deforms the T wave of the preceding beat. The average ventricular rate is 50 per minute.

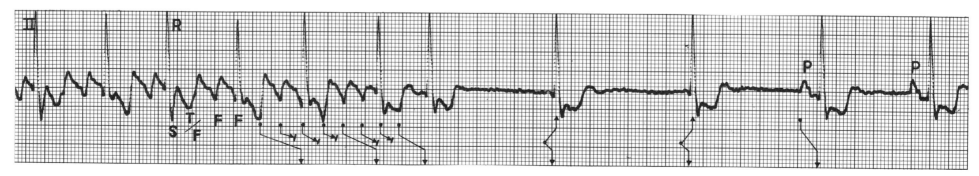

Case 36. *Interpretation:* The first half of the strip shows atrial flutter with variable A-V block. Suddenly the ectopic atrial rhythm ceases and, following 2 A-V nodal escape beats, sinus bradycardia takes control of the heart.

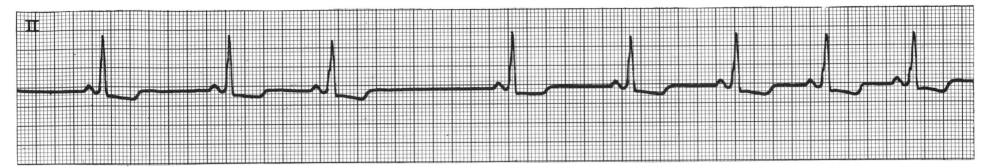

Case 37. *Question:* This ECG strip was recorded from a 70-year-old woman with hypertensive cardiovascular disease and episodes of paroxysmal atrial fibrillation, on treatment with digitalis. *What is your interpretation of the rhythm?*

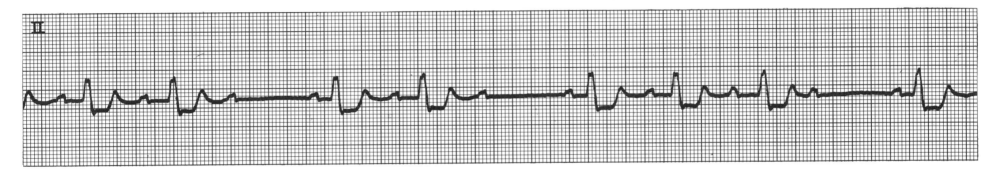

Case 38. *Question:* This rhythm strip was recorded in the Cardiac Care Unit from a 58-year-old male with acute anterior wall infarction. *What is your interpretation of the rhythm?*

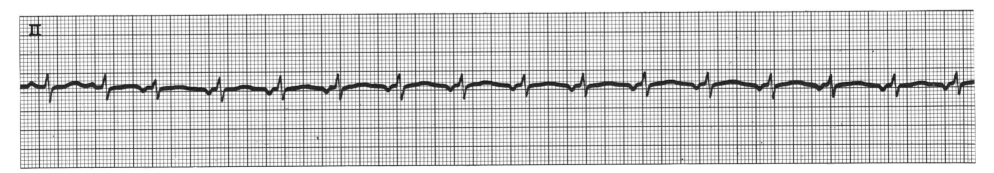

Case 39. *Question:* This tracing was recorded from a 60-year-old woman with coronary heart disease and congestive heart failure, on treatment with digitalis and diuretics. *What is your interpretation of the rhythm?*

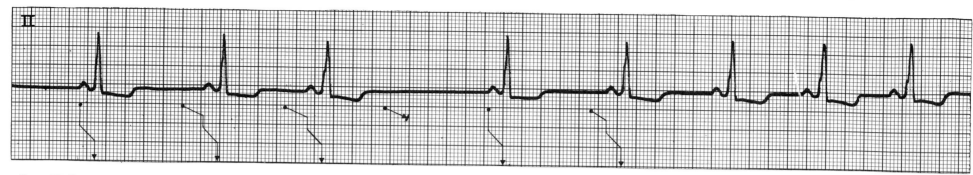

Case 37. *Interpretation:* The strip shows sinus bradycardia with second degree S-A block type I (Wenckebach). A long pause is seen in the middle of the strip. The P-P intervals before the pause become progressively shorter and the pause measures less than twice the preceding P-P interval. After the pause the P-P intervals again become progressively shorter. The arrhythmia in this patient was caused by digitalis toxicity.

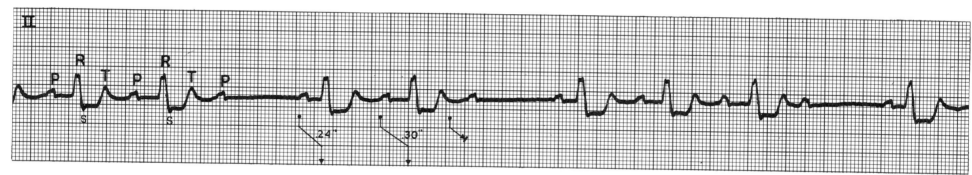

Case 38. *Interpretation:* Sinus rhythm with second degree A-V block type I (Wenckebach) and bundle branch block. The P-R interval becomes progressively longer until a P wave is blocked and a ventricular pause occurs. Second degree A-V block associated with bundle branch block may be caused by incomplete bilateral bundle branch block: the conduction disturbance responsible for the A-V block may be occurring in the other bundle branch rather that in the A-V node.

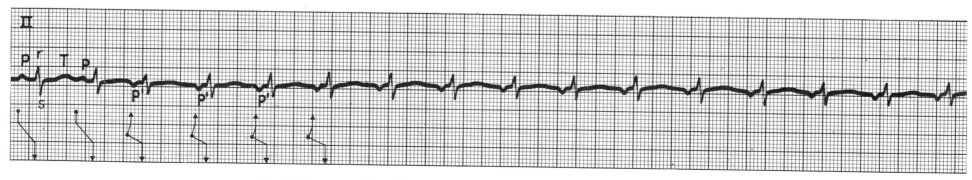

Case 39. *Interpretation:* Sinus rhythm (the first 2 beats) interrupted by nonparoxysmal "high" nodal tachycardia at a rate of 95 per minute. The arrhythmia in this patient was caused by digitalis toxicity.

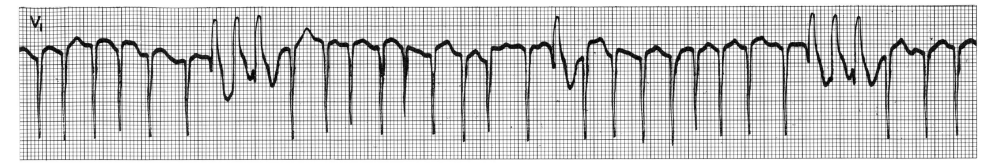

Case 40. *Question:* This strip was recorded in the Cardiac Care Unit from a 68-year-old male with acute pulmonary edema. *What is your interpretation of the rhythm?*

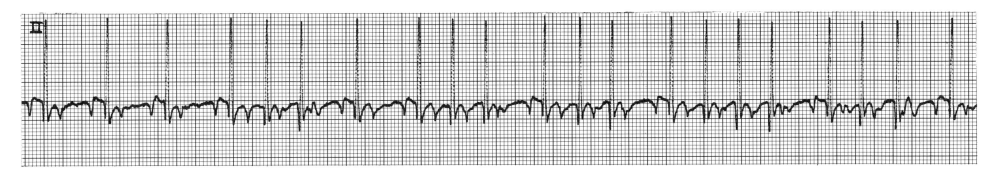

Case 41. *Question:* This strip was recorded from a 72-year-old woman with hypertensive cardiovascular disease. *What is your interpretation of the rhythm?*

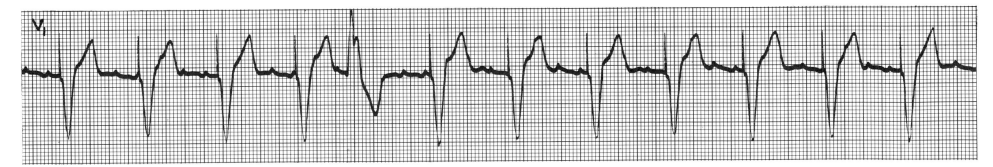

Case 42. *Question:* This rhythm strip was recorded from a 66-year-old male with arteriosclerotic heart disease. A permanent transvenous pacemaker had been implanted 6 months earlier. *What is your interpretation of the rhythm? What type of pacemaker was used?*

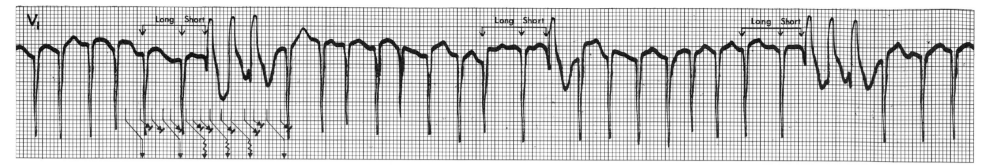

Case 40. *Interpretation:* Atrial fibrillation is present with rapid ventricular response averaging 200 per minute. The anomalous beats, occurring isolated or in triplets, are not ventricular extrasystoles but represent aberrant ventricular conduction of atrial fibrillation impulses. The following electrocardiographic manifestations are helpful in the recognition of aberrant ventricular conduction in this tracing: the anomalous beats have right bundle branch block configuration and an initial vector with the same direction as in the normally conducted beats; a long-short sequence precedes the appearance of aberrant conduction (Ashman phenomenon), and there is no significant pause following the aberrant beats.

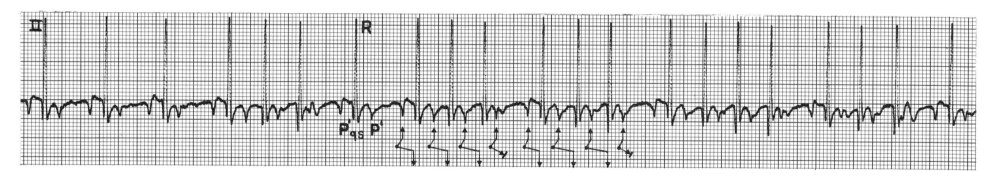

Case 41. *Interpretation:* Paroxysmal A-V nodal tachycardia at the rate of 180 per minute with second degree A-V block type I (Wenckebach) occurring below the A-V nodal focus. The average ventricular rate is 130 per minute.

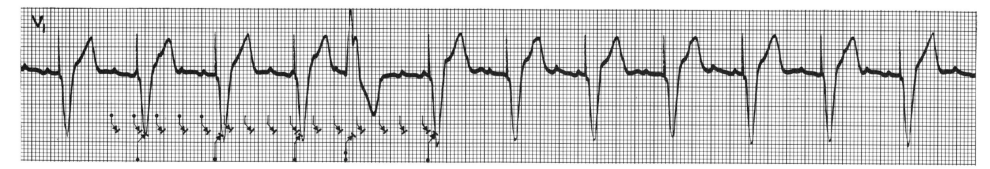

Case 42. *Interpretation:* Atrial flutter is present and the ventricles are under the control of a transvenous pacemaker (the QRS complex resembles left bundle branch block, indicating right ventricular stimulation). A ventricular extrasystole is sensed and temporarily inhibits the pacemaker activity; the pacemaker therefore is of the ventricular-inhibited type and is normally functioning at a rate of 70 per minute.

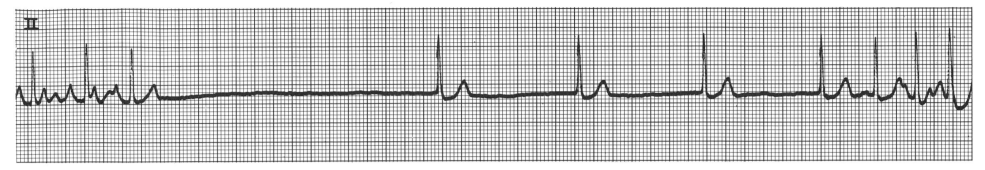

Case 43. *Question:* This strip was obtained from a 71-year-old woman with syncopal episodes. *What is your interpretation of the rhythm? What is the most likely diagnosis?*

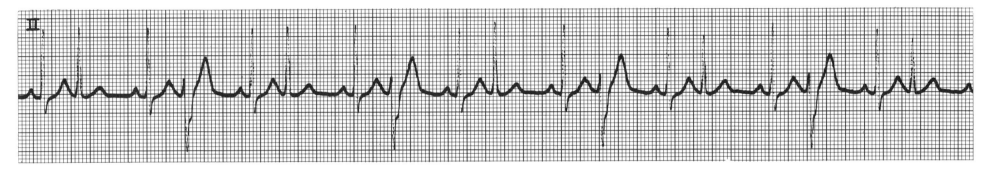

Case 44. *Question:* This tracing was recorded from a 74-year-old man with coronary heart disease and congestive heart failure. *What is your interpretation of the rhythm?*

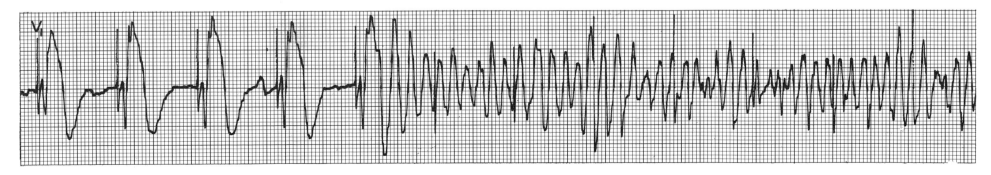

Case 45. *Question:* This strip was recorded from a 67-year-old woman with acute myocardial infarction. Temporary transvenous pacing had been instituted because of high grade A-V block. *What is your interpretation of the rhythm?*

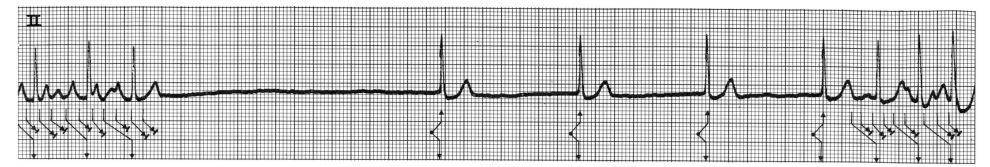

Case 43. *Interpretation:* Atrial fibrillation is present at the beginning of the strip. The ectopic atrial rhythm suddenly ceases and a long pause occurs. After 3.26 seconds of cardiac standstill, 4 idionodal escape beats occur in succession, followed by recurrence of atrial fibrillation. There is no evidence of sinus activity. The patient had Stokes-Adams attacks due to the sick sinus syndrome and was treated with artificial pacing in addition to quinidine and digitalis.

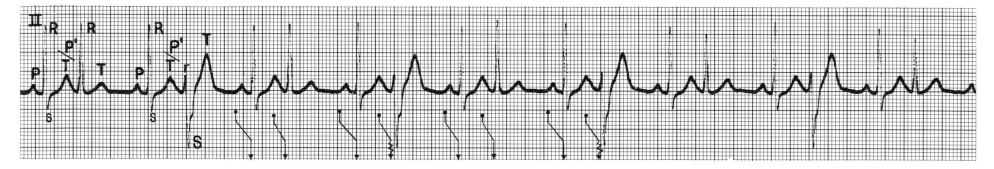

Case 44. *Interpretation:* The tracing shows sinus rhythm with atrial extrasystoles in bigeminy. Every other atrial extrasystole displays aberrant ventricular conduction mimicking a ventricular extrasystole.

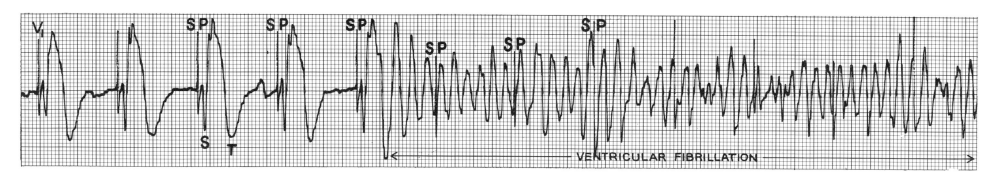

Case 45. *Interpretation:* The first 5 beats show normally functioning pacemaker at a rate of 70 per minute. Suddenly ventricular fibrillation ensues. Note the pacemaker spikes, now ineffective, which continue to occur during ventricular fibrillation. SP, pacemaker spike.

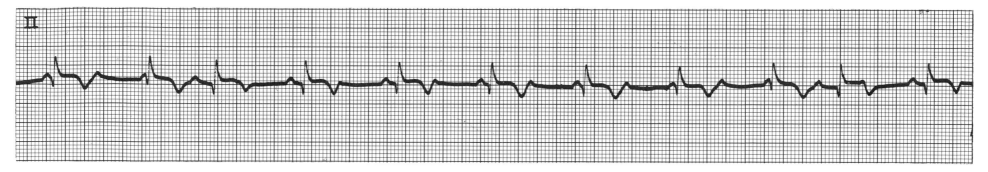

Case 46. *Question:* This strip was recorded in the Cardiac Care Unit from a 48-year-old male with acute inferior wall infarction. *What is your interpretation of the rhythm?*

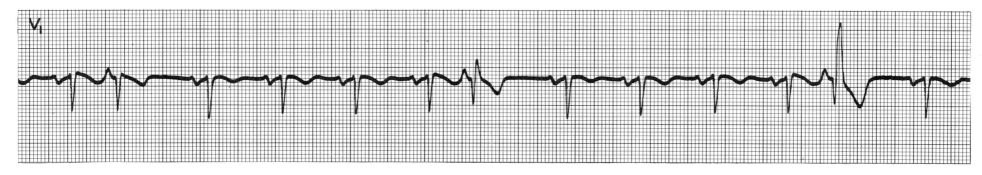

Case 47. *Question:* This ECG strip was recorded from a 79-year-old woman with congestive heart failure. *What is your interpretation of the rhythm?*

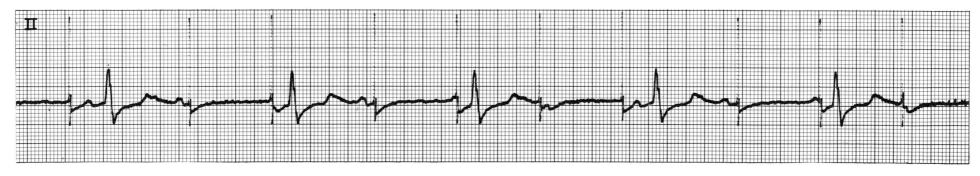

Case 48. *Question:* This tracing was obtained from a 74-year-old man with arteriosclerotic heart disease. A transvenous pacemaker had been implanted 2 years before. *What is your interpretation of the rhythm? What type of pacemaker had been used?*

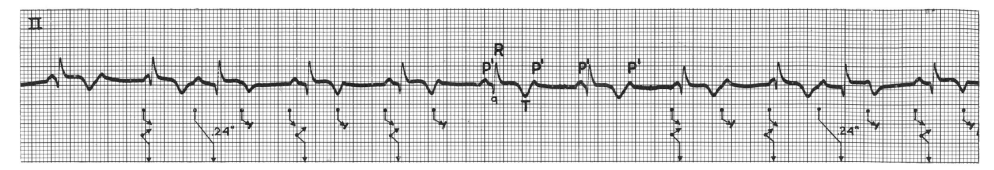

Case 46. *Interpretation:* The strips shows A-V dissociation between sinus tachycardia and A-V nodal escape rhythm, superimposed on 2:1 A-V block. The two premature QRS complexes preceded by a P wave are both ventricular captures by sinus impulses.

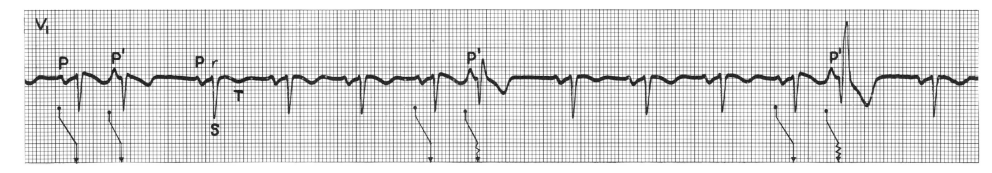

Case 47. *Interpretation:* The tracing shows sinus rhythm at a rate of 78 per minute and 3 atrial extrasystoles; the second and third atrial extrasystole show varying degrees of aberrant ventricular conduction.

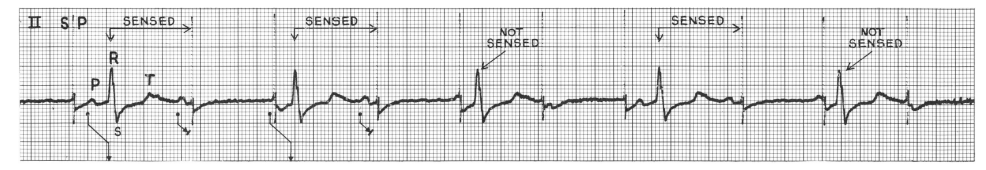

Case 48. *Interpretation:* The spontaneous rhythm is sinus with 2:1 A-V block and bundle branch block (probable incomplete bilateral bundle branch block). The pacemaker spikes are ineffective owing to complete loss of pacing function. The pacemaker sensing function, however, is preserved, and spontaneous QRS complexes occurring at an interval greater than 0.20 second from the preceding spike (refractory period of this unit) are sensed and temporarily inhibit the pacemaker activity. Those beats which fall closer than 0.20 second from the preceding spike are not sensed and the pacemaker fires at the expected time. SP, pacemaker spike.

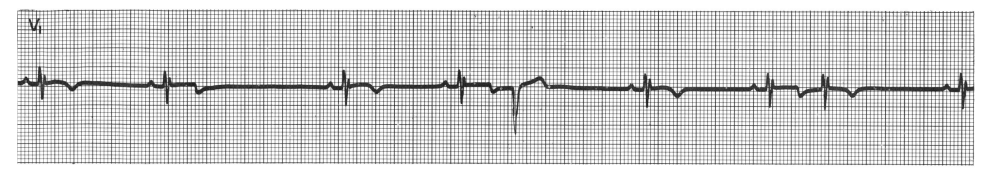

Case 49. *Question:* This ECG strip was recorded from a 40-year-old man with idiopathic cardiomyopathy. *What is your interpretation of the rhythm?*

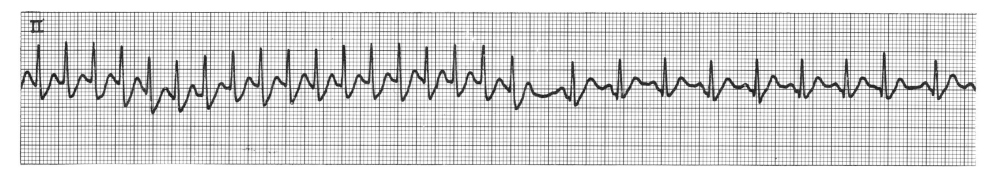

Case 50. *Question:* This strip was obtained from a 39-year-old woman with the so-called midsystolic click-mitral valve dysfunction syndrome. *What is your interpretation of the rhythm?*

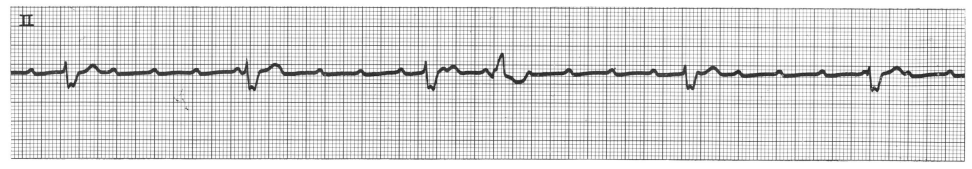

Case 51. *Question:* This tracing was recorded from a 76-year-old male with syncopal episodes. *What is your interpretation of the rhythm?*

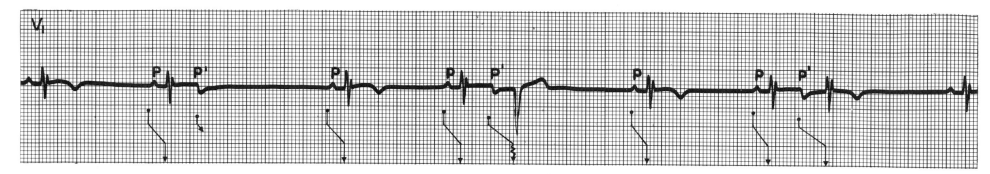

Case 49. *Interpretation:* The strip shows sinus bradycardia at a rate of 45 per minute, and 3 atrial extrasystoles: the first one is nonconducted, the second displays aberrant ventricular conduction, and the third is normally conducted to the ventricles.

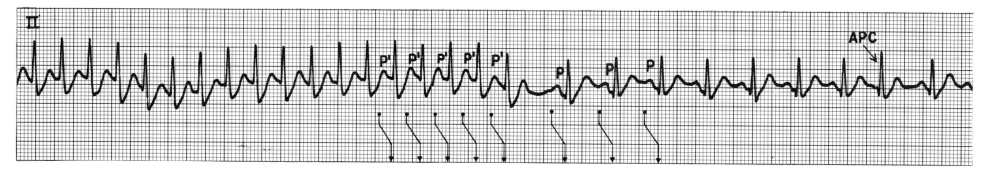

Case 50. *Interpretation:* The rhythm is atrial tachycardia at a rate of 200 per minute with 1:1 conduction and spontaneous conversion to sinus tachycardia at a rate of 125 per minute. One atrial extrasystole is seen near the end of the strip.

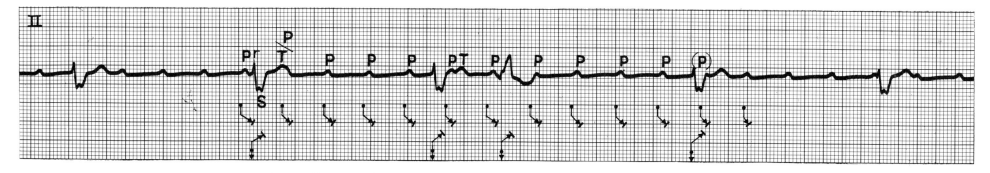

Case 51. *Interpretation:* The tracing shows sinus tachycardia with complete A-V block and idioventricular escape rhythm at a rate of 31 per minute. One ventricular extrasystole is seen in the middle of the strip.

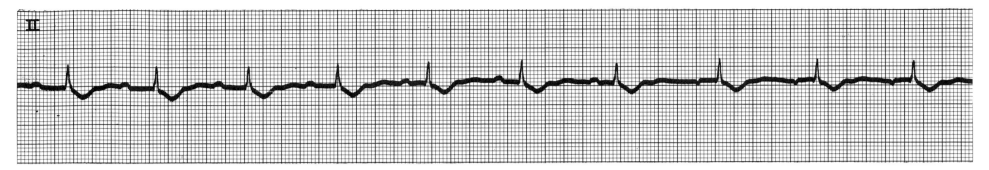

Case 52. *Question:* This ECG strip was obtained from a 70-year-old woman with arteriosclerotic heart disease on treatment with digoxin. *What is your interpretation of the rhythm?*

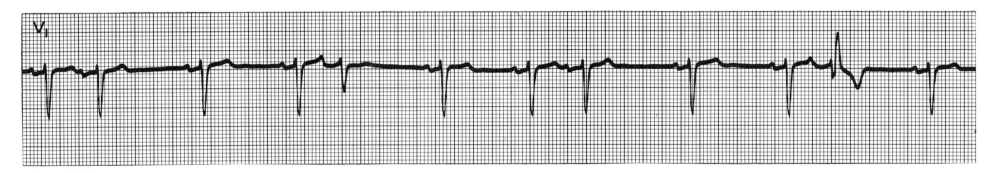

Case 53. *Question:* This strip was recorded from a 51-year-old man with arteriosclerotic heart disease. *What is your interpretation of the rhythm?*

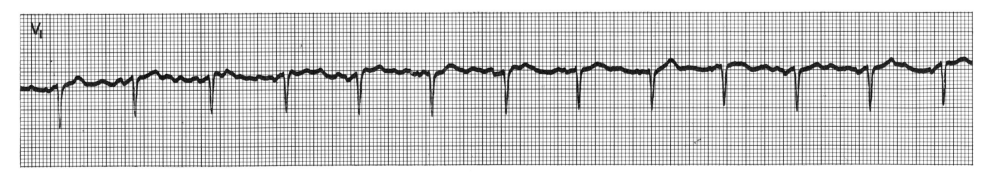

Case 54. *Question:* This strip was recorded from a 33-year-old woman with no evidence of heart disease. *What is your interpretation of the rhythm?*

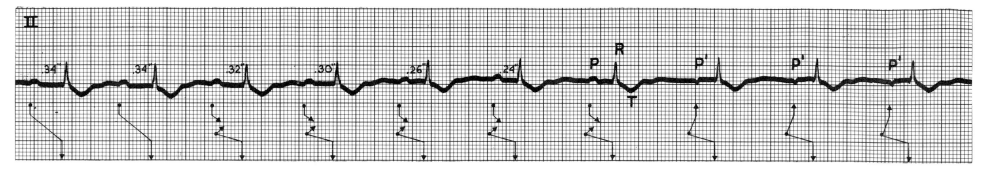

Case 52. *Interpretation:* The first 2 beats show sinus rhythm with first degree A-V block and P-R interval of 0.34 second. The P-R interval of the following beats becomes progressively shorter and the sinus P wave gradually closer to the QRS complex, owing to A-V dissociation between the sinus and the A-V node. The last 3 beats are "high" nodal escape beats preceded by inverted P' waves. The arrhythmia was caused by digitalis toxicity.

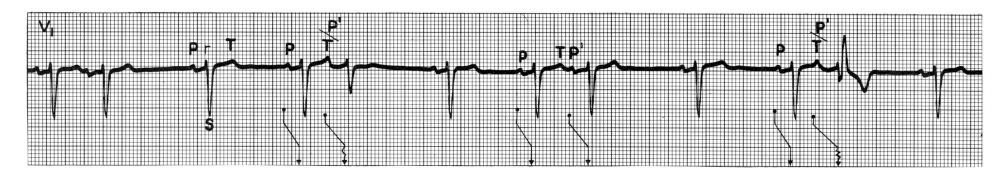

Case 53. *Interpretation:* The strip shows sinus rhythm and 4 atrial extrasystoles. The second and fourth atrial extrasystoles show varying degrees of aberrant ventricular conduction.

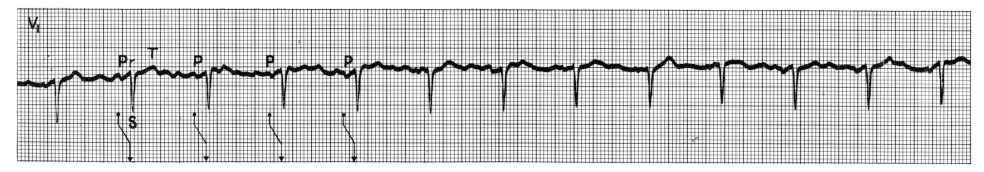

Case 54. *Interpretation:* Sinus rhythm at the rate of 78 per minute is present throughout. Gross artifacts mimic atrial fibrillation; the normal sinus P waves, however, can be discerned among the artifacts, and the ventricular rhythm is regular.

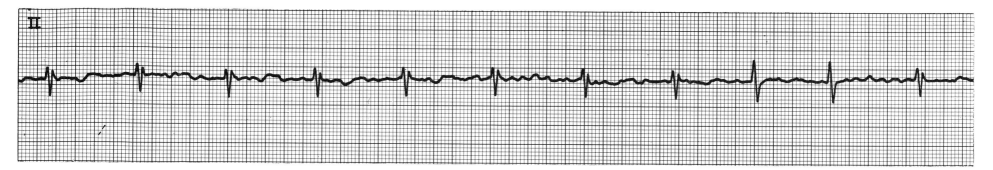

Case 55. *Question:* This electrocardiogram was recorded from a 78-year-old man with arteriosclerotic heart disease on treatment with digoxin and furosemide. *What is your interpretation of the rhythm?*

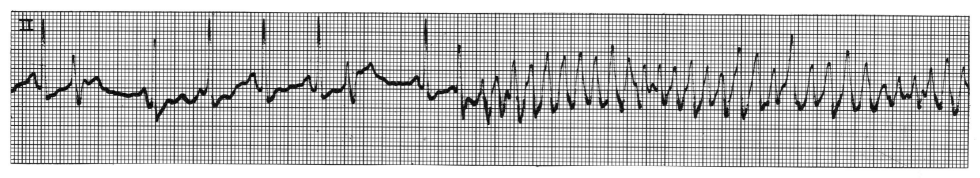

Case 56. *Question:* This strip was recorded in the Cardiac Care Unit from a 64-year-old man with subendocardial infarction. *What is your interpretation of the rhythm?*

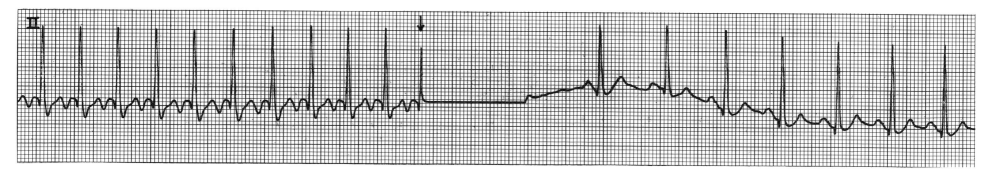

Case 57. *Question:* This strip was recorded from a 64-year-old man with arteriosclerotic and hypertensive cardiovascular disease. At the arrow an electrical shock of 25 watts per second was delivered to the precordium with appropriate synchronization. *What is your interpretation of the rhythm?*

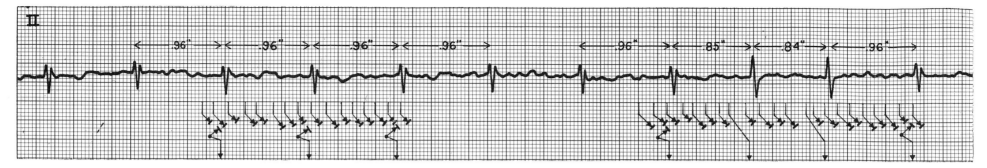

Case 55. *Interpretation:* The tracing shows atrial fibrillation with high grade A-V block, idionodal escape rhythm at a rate of about 60 per minute, and 2 ventricular captures by atrial fibrillation impulses. The arrhythmia was the result of digitalis toxicity.

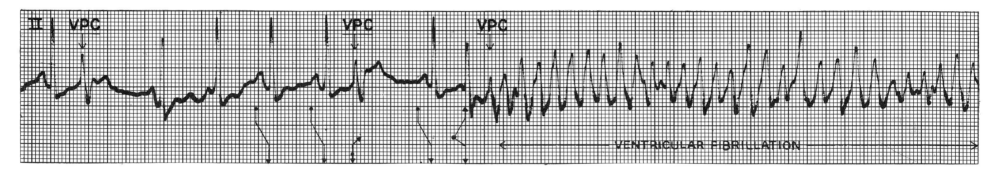

Case 56. *Interpretation:* The strip shows sinus rhythm with "malignant" ventricular extrasystoles and one A-V nodal extrasystole. One ventricular extrasystole falls on the T wave of the preceding A-V nodal extrasystole and induces ventricular fibrillation. There are minor artifacts caused by muscle tremor and unstable baseline.

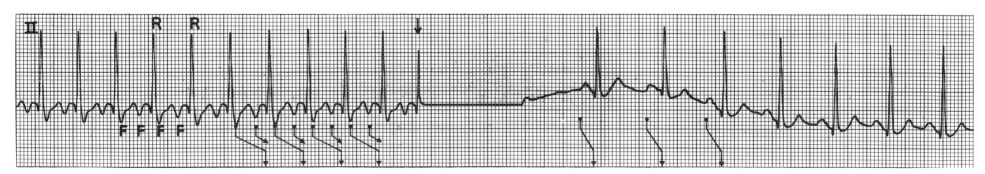

Case 57. *Interpretation:* The strip shows atrial flutter with 2:1 conduction (atrial rate 300 per minute and ventricular rate 150 per minute). The precordial shock induced conversion to normal sinus rhythm.

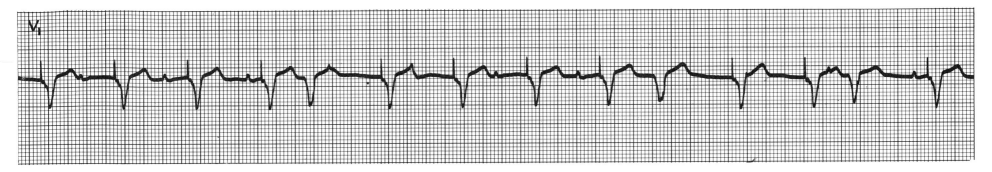

Case 58. *Question:* This tracing was obtained from an 81-year-old man with arterio-sclerotic heart disease. A transvenous pacemaker had been implanted 8 months earlier. *What is your interpretation of the rhythm? What type of pacemaker had been used?*

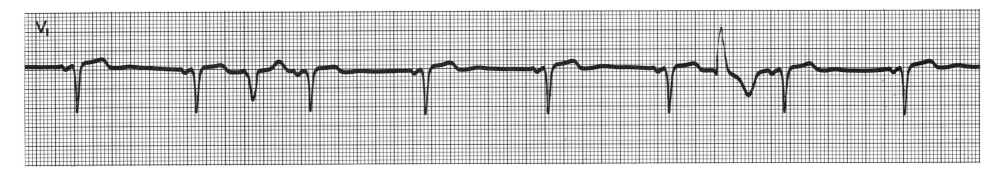

Case 59. *Question:* This tracing was recorded from a 58-year-old man with arterio-sclerotic heart disease, angina and old myocardial infarction, on treatment with propranolol and nitrates. *What is your interpretation of the rhythm?*

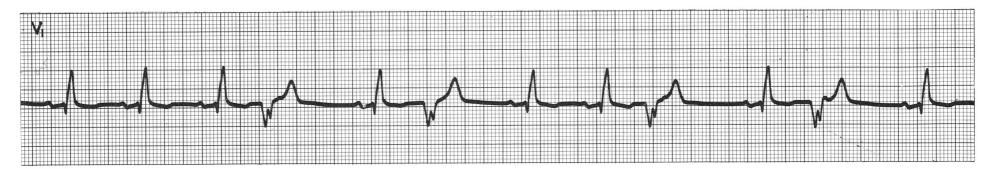

Case 60. *Question:* This ECG strip obtained from a 69-year-old man with essential hypertension. *What is your interpretation of the rhythm?*

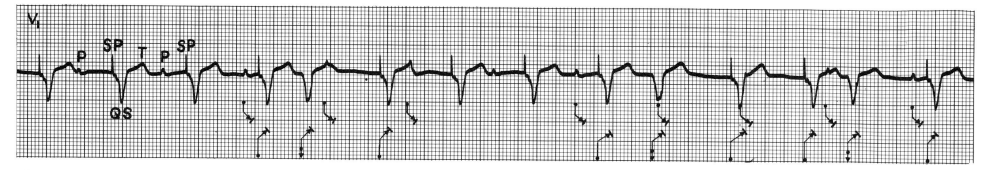

Case 58. *Interpretation:* An artificial pacemaker is pacing the heart at the rate of 80 per minute (SP, spike). Two spontaneous QRS complexes, representing unifocal right ventricular extrasystoles, inhibit the pacemaker activity. The pacemaker, therefore, is of the ventricular-inhibited type. The spontaneous atrial activity is sinus rhythm.

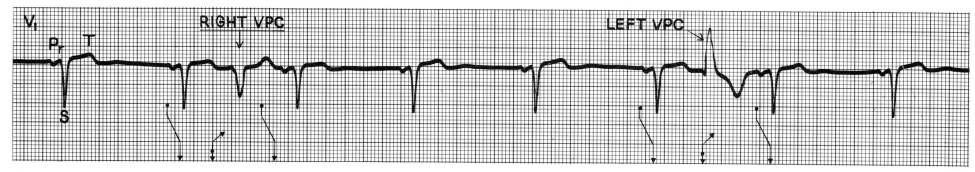

Case 59. *Interpretation:* The tracing shows sinus bradycardia and 2 multifocal ventricular extrasystoles, one right and one left. Both extrasystoles are interpolated.

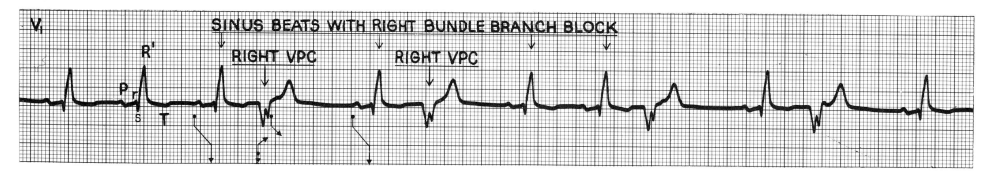

Case 60. *Interpretation:* The strip shows sinus rhythm at a rate of 75 per minute, right bundle branch block and unifocal right ventricular extrasystoles occurring mostly in bigeminy.

Practice Strips

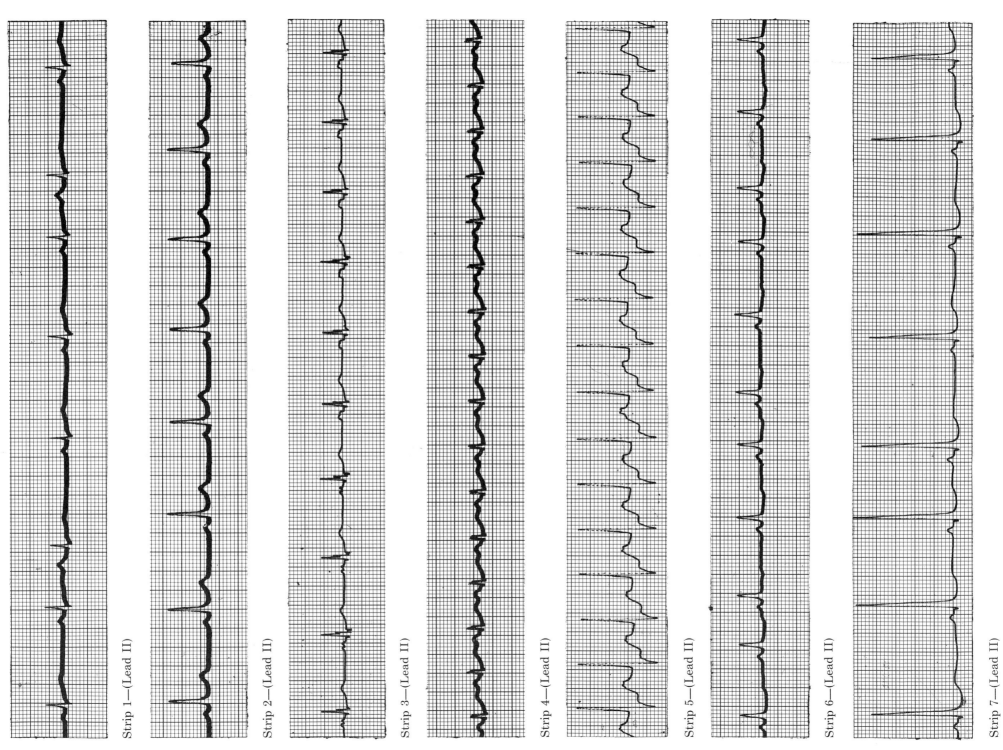

Strip 1—(Lead II)

Strip 2—(Lead II)

Strip 3—(Lead II)

Strip 4—(Lead II)

Strip 5—(Lead II)

Strip 6—(Lead II)

Strip 7—(Lead II)

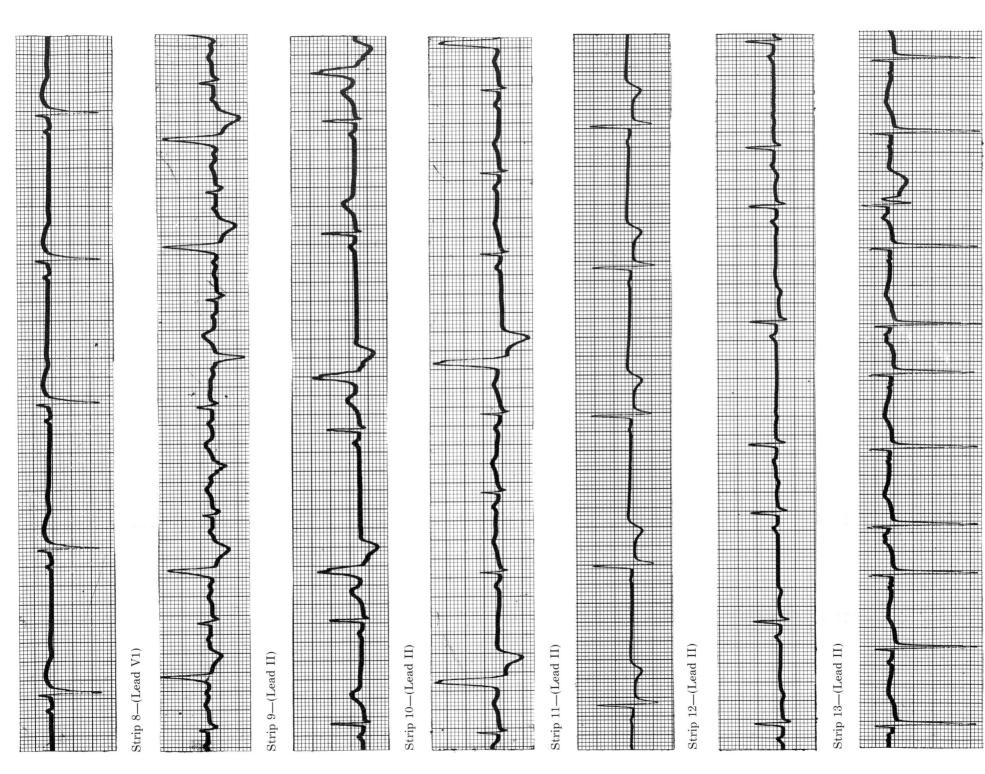

Strip 8—(Lead V1)

Strip 9—(Lead II)

Strip 10—(Lead II)

Strip 11—(Lead II)

Strip 12—(Lead II)

Strip 13—(Lead II)

Strip 14—(Lead V1)

195

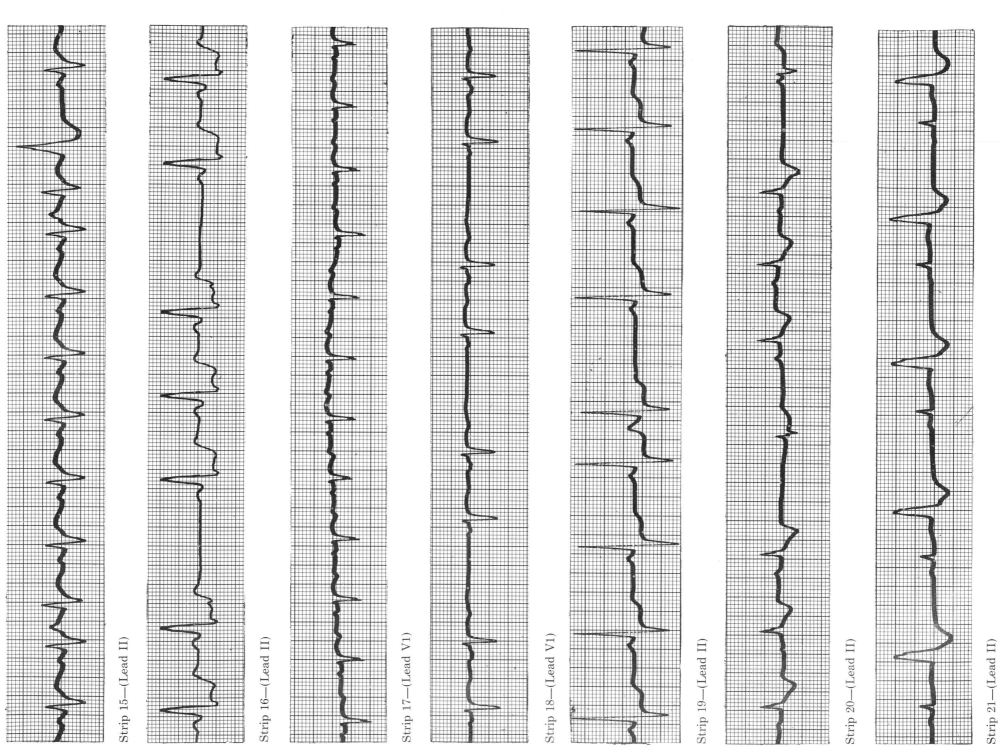

Strip 15—(Lead II)

Strip 16—(Lead II)

Strip 17—(Lead V1)

Strip 18—(Lead V1)

Strip 19—(Lead II)

Strip 20—(Lead II)

Strip 21—(Lead II)

196

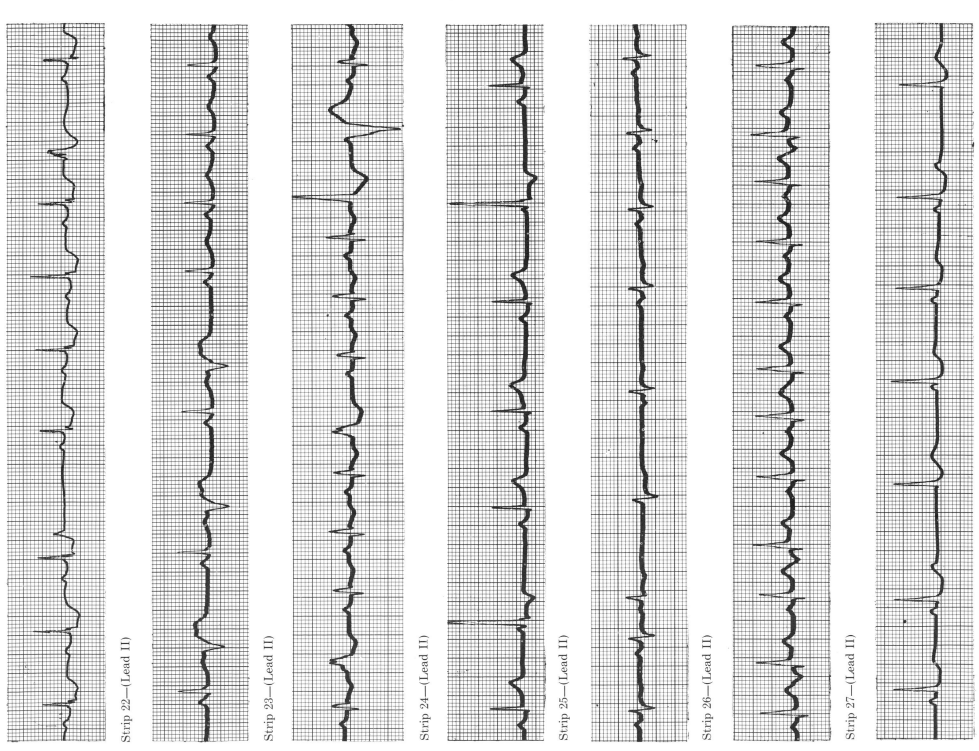

Strip 22—(Lead II)

Strip 23—(Lead II)

Strip 24—(Lead II)

Strip 25—(Lead II)

Strip 26—(Lead II)

Strip 27—(Lead II)

Strip 28—(Lead II)

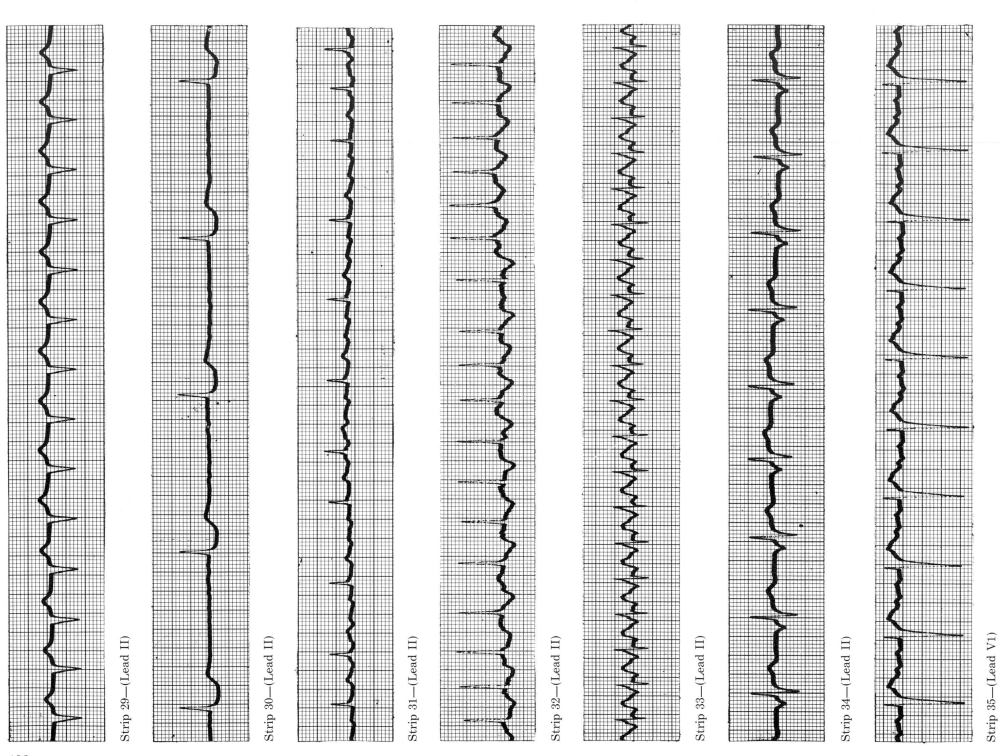

Strip 29—(Lead II)

Strip 30—(Lead II)

Strip 31—(Lead II)

Strip 32—(Lead II)

Strip 33—(Lead II)

Strip 34—(Lead II)

Strip 35—(Lead V1)

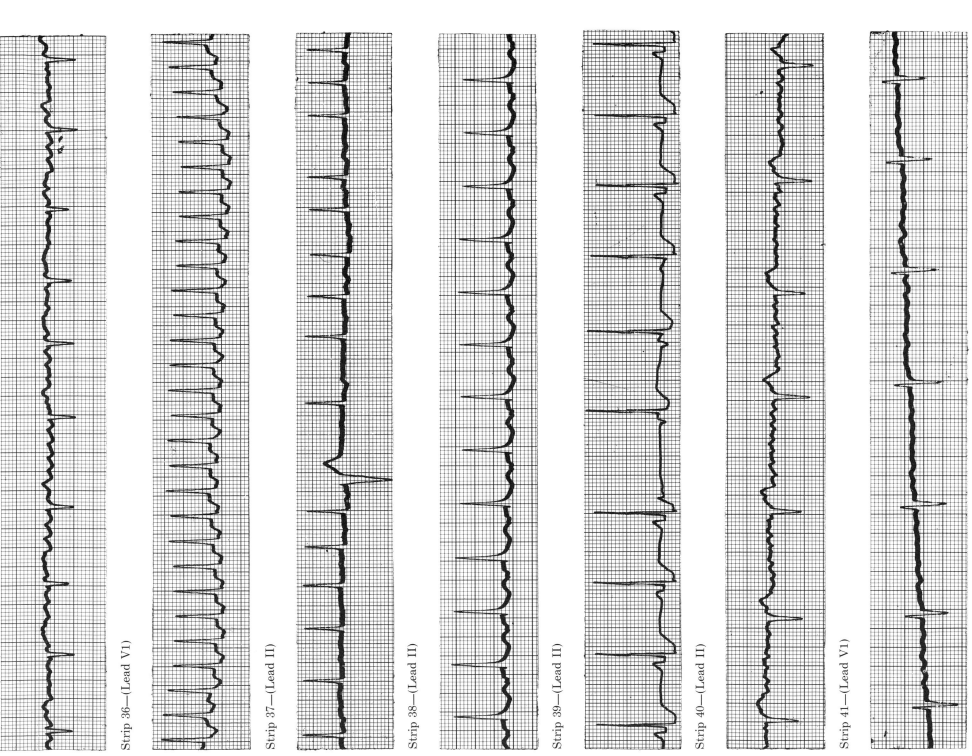

Strip 36—(Lead V1)

Strip 37—(Lead II)

Strip 38—(Lead II)

Strip 39—(Lead II)

Strip 40—(Lead II)

Strip 41—(Lead V1)

Strip 42—(Lead V1)

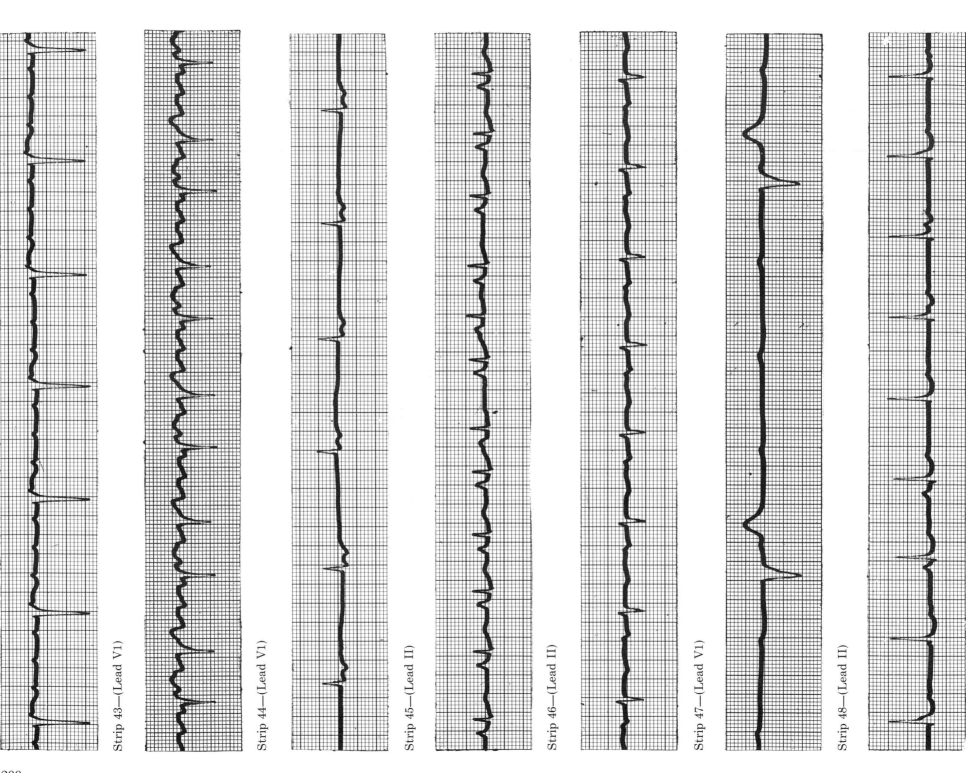

Strip 43—(Lead V1)

Strip 44—(Lead V1)

Strip 45—(Lead II)

Strip 46—(Lead II)

Strip 47—(Lead V1)

Strip 48—(Lead II)

Strip 49—(Lead II)

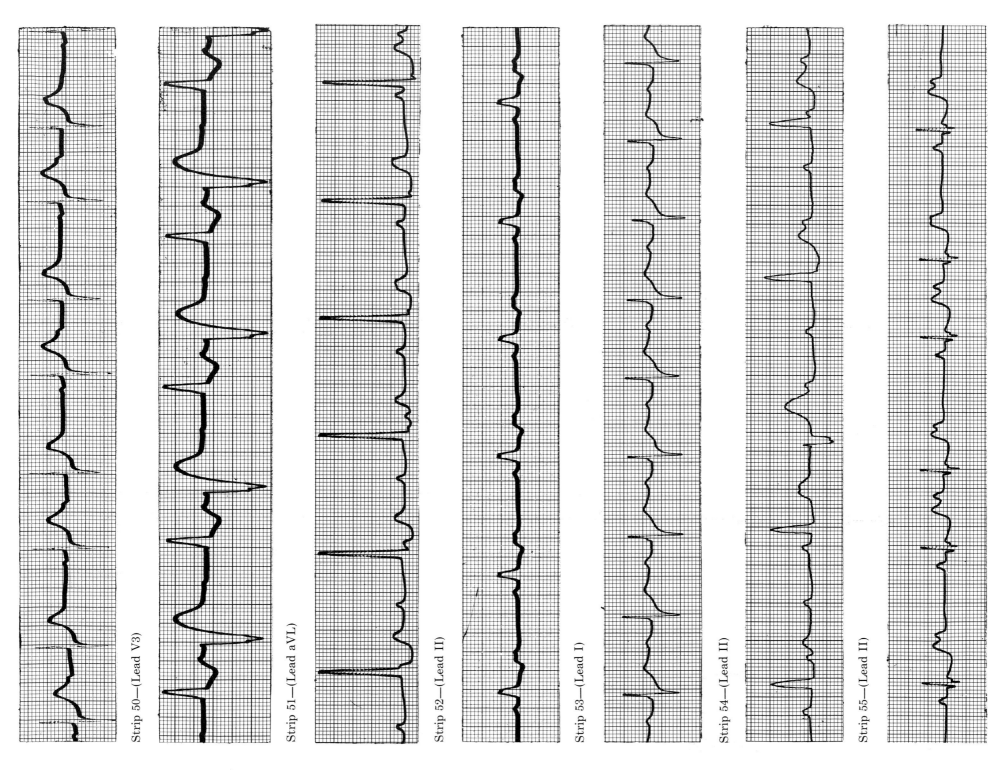

Strip 50—(Lead V3)

Strip 51—(Lead aVL)

Strip 52—(Lead II)

Strip 53—(Lead I)

Strip 54—(Lead II)

Strip 55—(Lead II)

Strip 56—(Lead II)

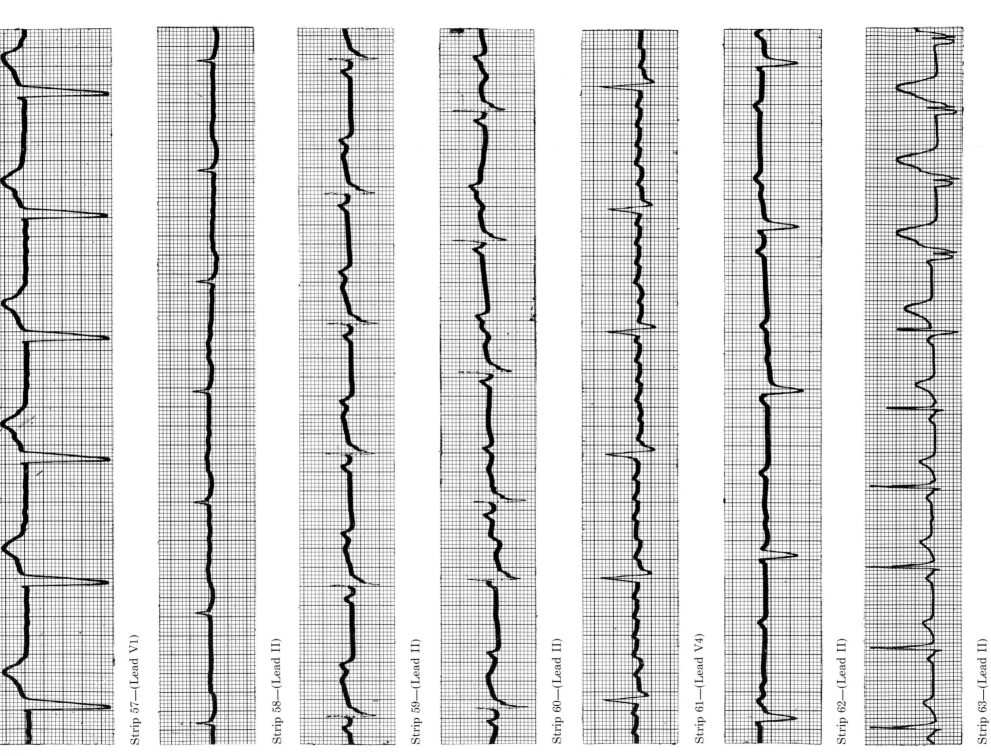

Strip 57—(Lead V1)

Strip 58—(Lead II)

Strip 59—(Lead II)

Strip 60—(Lead II)

Strip 61—(Lead V4)

Strip 62—(Lead II)

Strip 63—(Lead II)

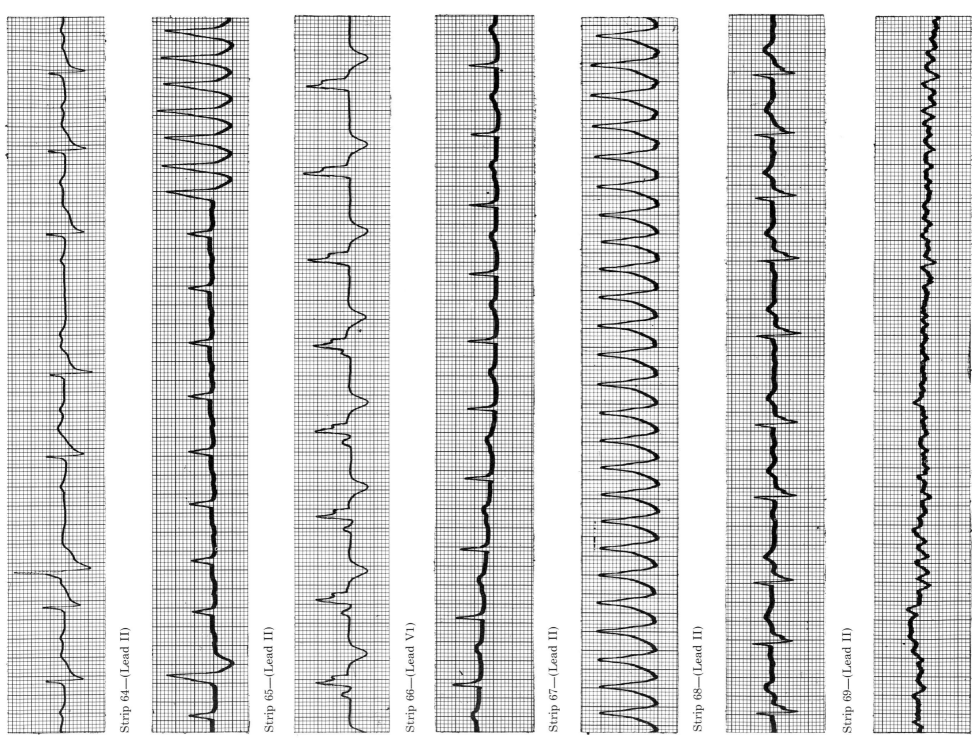

Strip 64—(Lead II)

Strip 65—(Lead II)

Strip 66—(Lead V1)

Strip 67—(Lead II)

Strip 68—(Lead II)

Strip 69—(Lead II)

Strip 70—(Lead II)

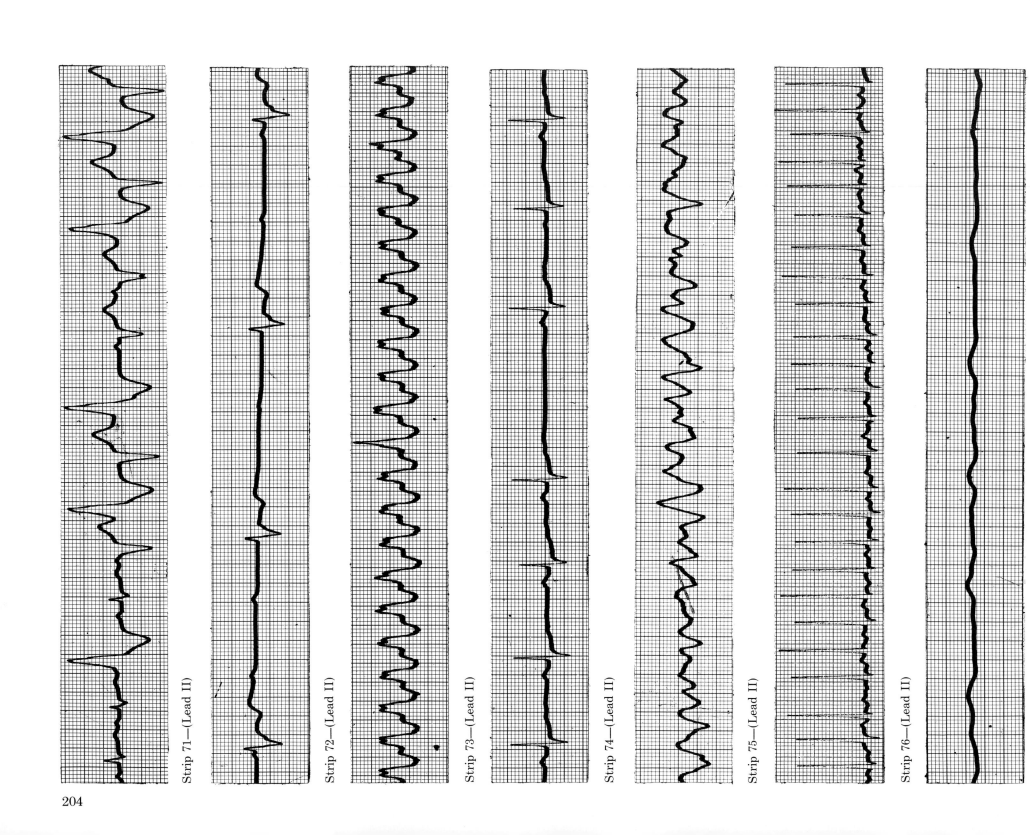

Strip 71—(Lead II)

Strip 72—(Lead II)

Strip 73—(Lead II)

Strip 74—(Lead II)

Strip 75—(Lead II)

Strip 76—(Lead II)

Strip 77—(Lead II)

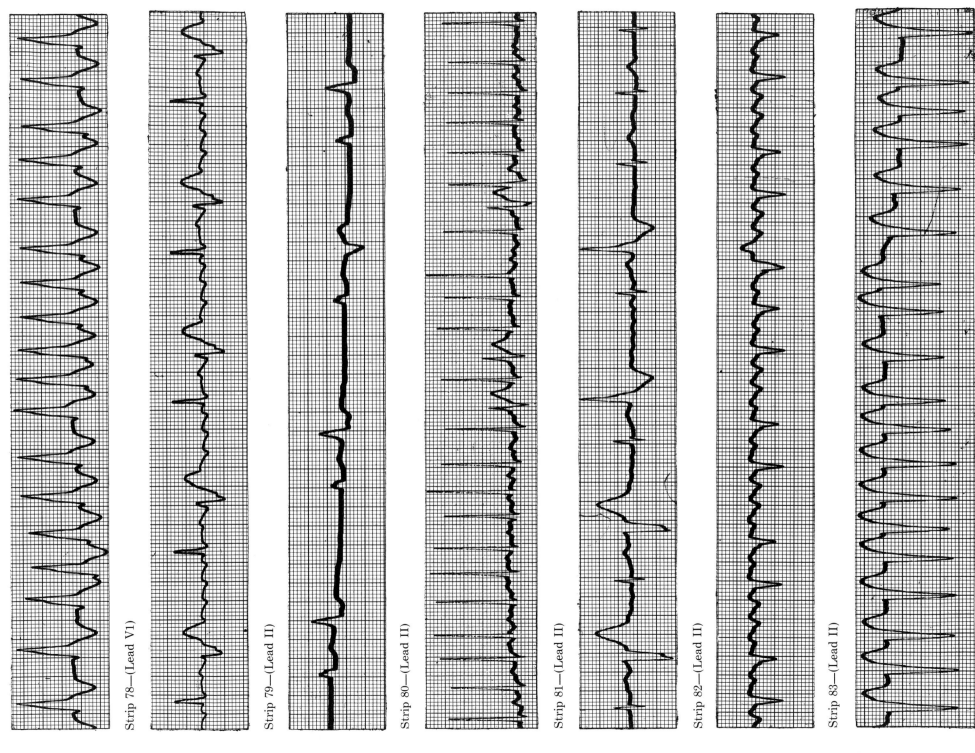

Strip 78—(Lead V1)

Strip 79—(Lead II)

Strip 80—(Lead II)

Strip 81—(Lead II)

Strip 82—(Lead II)

Strip 83—(Lead II)

Strip 84—(Lead V1)

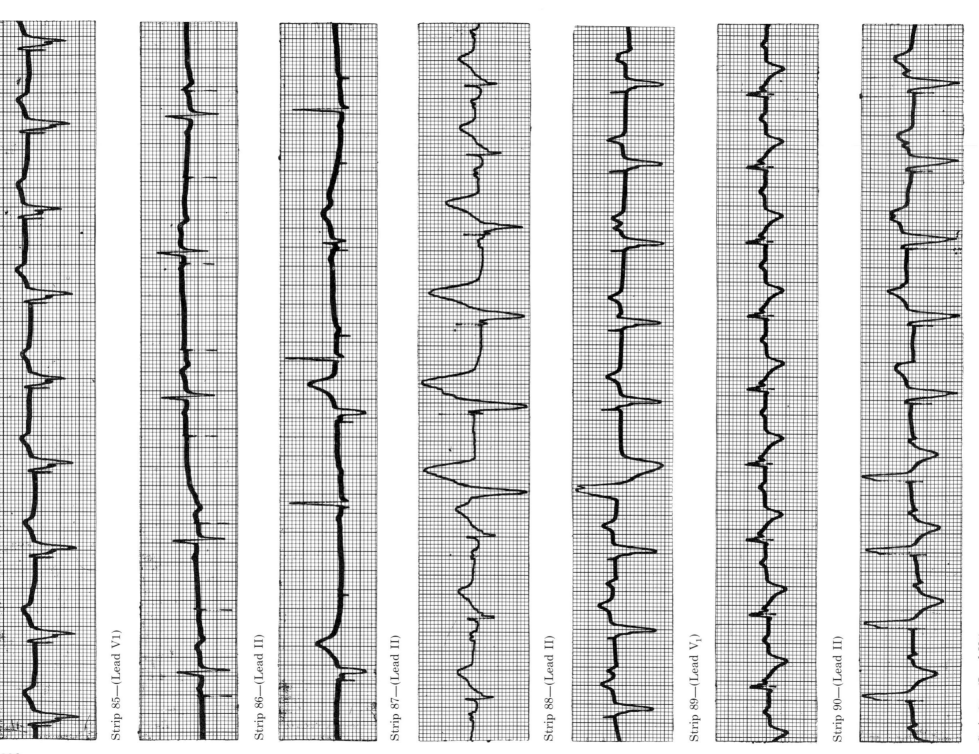

Strip 85—(Lead V1)

Strip 86—(Lead II)

Strip 87—(Lead II)

Strip 88—(Lead II)

Strip 89—(Lead V₁)

Strip 90—(Lead II)

Strip 91—(Lead V1)

Practice Strips: Interpretations

Strip 1: Sinus bradycardia with two atrial extrasystoles.

Strip 2: Normal sinus rhythm.

Strip 3: Shifting pacemaker within the sinus node.

Strip 4: Sinus tachycardia.

Strip 5: Sinus tachycardia.

Strip 6: Sinus rhythm with atrial extrasystoles in trigeminy.

Strip 7: Sinus arrhythmia and shifting pacemaker within the sinus node. There are respiratory changes in QRS voltage.

Strip 8: Sinus bradycardia.

Strip 9: Sinus tachycardia and multifocal end-diastolic ventricular extrasystoles.

Strip 10: Sinus bradycardia and unifocal ventricular extrasystoles with retrograde conduction to the atria.

Strip 11: Sinus rhythm with unifocal ventricular extrasystoles in quadrigeminy.

Strip 12: Sinus bradycardia.

Strip 13: Sinus rhythm with 2 atrial extrasystoles.

Strip 14: Sinus rhythm with 3 atrial extrasystoles, the last one with aberrant ventricular conduction.

Strip 15: Sinus rhythm with 2 atrial extrasystoles and 1 ventricular extrasystole.

Strip 16: Sinus rhythm with 2 nonconducted atrial extrasystoles.

Strip 17: Sinus tachycardia.

Strip 18: Sinus rhythm with atrial extrasystoles in bigeminy.

Strip 19: Sinus rhythm with 1 atrial extrasystole.

Strip 20: Sinus rhythm with 2 nonconducted supraventricular extrasystoles deforming the T wave and causing a sudden pause. Each pause is terminated by an A-V nodal escape beat.

Strip 21: Sinus rhythm with unifocal ventricular extrasystoles in bigeminy.

Strip 22: Sinus rhythm with first degree A-V block, one nonconducted atrial extrasystole and one ventricular extrasystole.

Strip 23: Sinus rhythm with 3 unifocal ventricular extrasystoles in bigeminy.

Strip 24: Sinus rhythm with multifocal ventricular extrasystoles, isolated or in pairs.

Strip 25: Sinus bradycardia with 2 unifocal end-diastolic ventricular extrasystoles.

Strip 26: Sinus rhythm with 1 A-V nodal extrasystole followed by 2 A-V nodal escape beats.

Strip 27: Sinus tachycardia with 3 A-V nodal extrasystoles and 1 atrial extrasystole.

Strip 28: Sinus rhythm with 2 nonconducted atrial extrasystoles. The third, the fourth and the last QRS complexes are A-V nodal escape beats.

Strip 29: Nonparoxysmal "mid" nodal tachycardia.

Strip 30: Atrial fibrillation with complete A-V block and idionodal escape rhythm.

Strip 31: Atrial flutter with variable A-V block.

Strip 32: Atrial fibrillation with fast ventricular response.

Strip 33: Atrial flutter with 2:1 conduction.

Strip 34: Nonparoxysmal "high" nodal tachycardia.

Strip 35: Atrial flutter with 4:1 A-V block.

Strip 36: "Coarse" atrial fibrillation.

Strip 37: Supraventricular tachycardia, probably atrial flutter, with 1:1 conduction.

Strip 38: Atrial fibrillation with 1 ventricular extrasystole.

Strip 39: Nonparoxysmal "high" nodal tachycardia.

Strip 40: Sinus rhythm with 1 nonconducted atrial extrasystole followed by 3 A-V nodal escape beats. The P waves preceding the second and the third escape beats are atrial fusions between the sinus and the A-V nodal impulses.

Strip 41: Atrial fibrillation with slow ventricular response.

Strip 42: Atrial fibrillation with slow ventricular response.

Strip 43: Atrial tachycardia with 4:1 A-V block.

Strip 44: Atrial flutter with variable (2:1, 4:1) A-V block.

Strip 45: "Low" idionodal escape rhythm.

Strip 46: Sinus rhythm with atrial extrasystoles, isolated or in pairs.

Strip 47: Sinus rhythm with first degree A-V block.

Strip 48: Sinus bradycardia with complete A-V block and idioventricular escape rhythm at a very slow rate.

Strip 49: A-V dissociation between the sinus and the A-V node.

Strip 50: Sinus tachycardia with 3:2 second degree A-V block type I

Strip 51: Sinus rhythm with first degree A-V block, bundle branch block and unifocal ventricular extrasystoles in bigeminy.

Strip 52: Sinus rhythm with second degree (or complete) A-V block and idionodal escape rhythm.

Strip 53: Sinus rhythm with 2:1 second degree A-V block and bundle branch block.

Strip 54: Sinus rhythm with first degree A-V block.

Strip 55: Sinus rhythm with complete A-V block, idioventricular escape rhythm and one ventricular extrasystole.

Strip 56: Sinus rhythm with second degree A-V block type I (Wenckebach). There are 2:1 and 3:2 Wenckebach sequences.

Strip 57: Atrial fibrillation with high grade or complete A-V block. There is probably idionodal escape rhythm with bundle branch block.

Strip 58: Atrial fibrillation with high grade or complete A-V block and idionodal escape rhythm.

Strip 59: Sinus rhythm with 2:1 second degree A-V block and bundle branch block.

Strip 60: A-V dissociation between sinus and A-V node, superimposed on 2:1 second degree A-V block and bundle branch block. The third QRS complex is a ventricular capture by a sinus impulse.

Strip 61: Atrial flutter with high grade or complete A-V block. The ventricles are probably under the control of an idionodal escape rhythm with bundle branch block.

Strip 62: Sinus rhythm with complete A-V block and idioventricular escape rhythm.

Strip 63: Sinus rhythm with a run of nonparoxysmal ventricular tachycardia. The fifth and sixth QRS complexes are fusion beats between the sinus and the ventricular impulses.

Strip 64: Sinus rhythm with second degree A-V block type I (Wenckebach) and 1 "malignant" VPC.

Strip 65: Atrial fibrillation with 1 ventricular extrasystole and a run of ventricular flutter.

Strip 66: A-V dissociation between sinus rhythm and nonparoxysmal ventricular tachycardia (or A-V nodal tachycardia with bundle branch block).

Strip 67: Sinus rhythm with first degree A-V block.

Strip 68: Ventricular flutter.

Strip 69: Atrial fibrillation with bundle branch block.

Strip 70: Ventricular fibrillation.

Strip 71: Sinus tachycardia, 1 ventricular extrasystole, and a run of bidirectional ventricular tachycardia. There are fusion beats between the sinus and the ectopic ventricular impulses.

Strip 72: Shifting pacemaker within the sinus node, complete A-V block and idioventricular escape rhythm.

Strip 73: Ventricular tachycardia.

Strip 74: Sinus rhythm with sino-atrial block, type II.

Strip 75: "Coarse" ventricular fibrillation.

Strip 76: Atrial fibrillation with very fast ventricular response.

Strip 77: "Fine" ventricular fibrillation.

Strip 78: Atrial fibrillation with right bundle branch block.

Strip 79: Atrial flutter with ventricular extrasystoles in bigeminy.

Strip 80: Atrial fibrillation with slow ventricular response and multifocal ventricular extrasystoles in bigeminy.

Strip 81: Atrial fibrillation with fast ventricular response and intermittent aberrant ventricular conduction.

Strip 82: Atrial fibrillation and multifocal ventricular extrasystoles in bigeminy.

Strip 83: Atrial flutter with variable (2:1, 4:1) A-V block and 1 ventricular extrasystole.

Strip 84: Atrial fibrillation with left bundle branch block.

Strip 85: Normally functioning transvenous pacemaker, type unknown. There is no spontaneous atrial or ventricular activity.

Strip 86: Malfunctioning pacemaker, type unknown, firing ineffective spikes in a continuous-asynchronous manner. The spontaneous cardiac rhythm is marked sinus bradycardia (or 2:1 sino-atrial block).

Strip 87: Malfunctioning continuous-asynchronous pacemaker. There is competition and intermittent exit block. The spontaneous cardiac rhythm is sinus bradycardia. The next to the last QRS complex is a fusion beat between the sinus and the pacemaker impulse.

Strip 88: Sinus rhythm. A ventricular-inhibited pacemaker manifests its activity (one pure paced beat and two fu-

sion beats) when a ventricular extrasystole causes a pause longer than the pacemaker escape interval.

Strip 89: Normally functioning ventricular-inhibited pacemaker. The spontaneous atrial activity is sinus rhythm. One ventricular extrasystole is sensed by the pacemaker.

Strip 90: Normally functioning ventricular-triggered pacemaker. The spontaneous rhythm is normal sinus with first degree A-V block and the pacemaker delivers a "sensing" spike on top of each QRS complex.

Strip 91: Normally functioning ventricular-inhibited pacemaker. The spontaneous rhythm is sinus with second degree A-V block type I (Wenckebach) and right bundle branch block. The first 4 QRS complexes are of sinus origin and display a "sensing" spike; the others are pacemaker-induced.

References

Books

1. Bilitch M: A Manual of Cardiac Arrhythmias. Boston, Little, Brown and Company, 1971
2. Bradlow BA: How to Produce a Readable Electrocardiogram. Springfield, Illinois, Charles C Thomas, 1964
3. Burch GE, Winsor T: A Primer of Electrocardiography. Philadelphia, Lea & Febiger, 1955
4. Castellanos A, Lemberg L: Electrophysiology of Pacing and Cardioversion. New York, Appleton-Century-Crofts, 1969
5. Chung EK: Principles of Cardiac Arrhythmias. Baltimore, Williams & Wilkins, 1971
6. Dreifus LS, Likoff W, Moyer JH: Mechanism and Therapy of Cardiac Arrhythmias. New York, Grune & Stratton, 1966
7. Hoffman BF, Cranefield PF: The Electrophysiology of the Heart. New York, McGraw-Hill, 1960
8. Katz LN: Electrocardiography. Philadelphia, Lea & Febiger, 1946
9. Katz LN, Pick A: Clinical Electrocardiography: The Arrhythmias. Philadelphia, Lea & Febiger, 1956
10. Lepeschkin E: Modern Electrocardiography. Baltimore, Williams & Wilkins, 1951
11. Marriott HJL: Armchair Arrhythmias. Oldsmar, Florida, Tampa Tracings, 1963
12. Marriott HJL: Practical Electrocardiography. Baltimore, Williams & Wilkins, 1972
13. Marriott HJL: Workshop in Electrocardiography. Oldsmar, Florida, Tampa Tracings, 1972
14. Massie E, Walsh TJ: Clinical Vectorcardiography and Electrocardiography. Chicago, Year Book Medical Publishers, 1960
15. Meltzer LE, Kitchell JR: Current Concepts of Cardiac Pacing and Cardioversion. A Symposium. Philadelphia, The Charles Press, 1971
16. Ritota MC: Diagnostic Electrocardiography. Philadelphia, Lippincott, 1969
17. Rosenbaum MB, Elizari MV, Lazzari JO: The Hemiblocks. Oldsmar, Florida, Tampa Tracings, 1970
18. Schamroth L: The Disorders of Cardiac Rhythm. Oxford, Blackwell Scientific Publications, 1971
19. Scherf D, Cohen J: The Atrio-ventricular Node and Selected Cardiac Arrhythmias. New York, Grune & Stratton, 1964
20. Schlant RC, Hurst JW: Advances in Electrocardiography. New York, Grune & Stratton, 1972
21. Sodi-Pallares D, Calder RM: New Bases of Electrocardiography. St. Louis, Mosby, 1956
22. Stock JPP: Diagnosis and Treatment of Cardiac Arrhythmias. London, Butterworth, 1970

Articles

23. Averill KH, Fosmoe RJ, Lamb LE: Electrocardiographic findings in 67,375 asymptomatic subjects. IV. Wolff-Parkinson-White syndrome. Amer J Cardiol 6:108–129, 1960
24. Burchell HB: Surgical approach to the treatment of ventricular pre-excitation. Adv Intern Med 16:43–58, 1970
25. Castellanos A, Castillo CA, Martinez A, et al: Pre-excitation and the Wolff-Parkinson-White syndrome. In: Advances in Electrocardiography (Schlant RC, Hurst JW, ed). New York, Grune & Stratton, 1972, p 249
26. Castellanos A, Lemberg L, Arcebal AG: Mechanism of slow ventricular tachycardias in acute myocardial infarction. Dis Chest 56:470–476, 1969
27. Castellanos A, Lemberg L: Diagnosis of isolated and combined blocks in the bundle branches and the divisions of the left branch. Circulation 43:971–979, 1971
28. Castellanos A, Spence MI, Chapell DE: Hemiblock and bundle branch block: A nursing approach. Heart and Lung 1:36–44, 1972
29. Chung EK: Parasystole. Progr Cardiovasc Dis 11:64–81, 1968
30. Chung EK, Walsh TJ, Massie E: Wolff-Parkinson-White syndrome. Amer Heart J 69:116–133, 1965
31. Chung EK, Walsh TJ, Massie E: Double ventricular parasystole. Amer Heart J 67:162–165, 1964
32. Cobb FR, Blumenschein SD, Sealy WC, et al: Successful surgical interruption of the bundle of Kent in a patient with Wolff-Parkinson-White syndrome. Circulation 38:1018–1029, 1968
33. Cohen HC, Gozo EG, Pick A: Ventricular tachycardia with narrow QRS complexes (left posterior fascicular tachycardia). Circulation 45:1035–1043, 1972
34. Damato AN, Lau SH: His bundle rhythm. Circulation 40:527–534, 1969
35. Davies M, Harris A: Pathological basis of primary heart block. Brit Heart J 31:219–226, 1969
36. Dreifus LS, Haiat R, Watanabe Y, et al: Ventricular fibrillation. A possible mechanism of sudden death in patients with Wolff-Parkinson-White syndrome. Circulation 43:520–527, 1971
37. Dreifus LS, Nichols H, Morse D, et al: Control of recurrent tachycardia of Wolff-Parkinson-White syndrome by surgical ligature of the A-V bundle. Circulation 38:1030–1036, 1968
38. Dreifus LS, Watanabe Y, Haiat R, et al: Atrioventricular block. Amer J Cardiol 28:371–379, 1971
39. Dressler W, Roesler H: The occurrence in paroxysmal ventricular tachycardia of ventricular complexes transitional in shape to sino-auricular beats. Amer Heart J 44:485–493, 1952
40. Durrer D, Schoo L, Schuilenburg RM, et al: The role of premature beats in the initiation and termination of supraventricular tachycardia in Wolff-Parkinson-White syndrome. Circulation 36:644–662, 1967
41. Edmonds JH, Ellison RG, Crews TL: Surgically induced A-V block as treatment for recurrent atrial tachycardia in Wolff-Parkinson-White syndrome. Circulation 39 (Suppl 1):1–105–1–111, 1969
42. Ferrer MI: The sick sinus syndrome in atrial disease. JAMA 206:645–646, 1968
43. Fisch C, Greenspan K, Anderson GJ: Exit block. Amer J Cardiol 28:402–405, 1971
44. Glushien AS, Goldblum HL: Aberrant atrio-ventricular conduction with normal P-R interval and prolonged QRS complex simulating bundle branch block. Amer Heart J 40:476–483, 1950
45. Gouaux JL, Ashman R: Auricular fibrillation with aberration simulating ventricular paroxysmal tachycardia. Amer Heart J 34:366–373, 1947
46. Greenspan K, Anderson GJ, Fisch C: Electrophysiological correlate of exit block. Amer J Cardiol 28:197–200, 1971
47. Gulotta SJ: Transvenous cardiac pacing. Technics for optimal electrode positioning and prevention of coronary sinus placement. Circulation 42:701–718, 1970
48. Haft JI, Lasser RP: ECG patterns useful in the diag-

nosis of intermittent heart block. JAMA 222:184–188, 1972

49. Hau J: The concepts of reentrant activity responsible for ectopic rhythms. Amer J Cardiol 28:402–405, 1971

50. Hejtmancik MT, Hermann GR: The electrocardiographic syndrome of short P-R interval and broad QRS complexes: A clinical study of 80 cases. Amer Heart J 54:708–721, 1957

51. James TN: Anatomy of the human sinus node. Anat Rec 141:109–139, 1961

52. James TN: The conducting pathways between the sinus node and the A-V node, and between the right and left atrium in the human heart. Amer Heart J 66:498–508, 1963

53. James TN: The specialized conducting tissue of the atria. In: Mechanism and Therapy of Cardiac Arrhythmias (Dreifus LS, Likoff W, ed). New York, Grune & Stratton, 1966

54. Javier RP, Narula OS, Samet, P: Atrial tachysystole (flutter?) with apparent exit block. Circulation 40: 179–183, 1969

55. Johnson RL, Averill KH, Lamb LE: Electrocardiographic findings in 67,375 asymptomatic individuals. Part VII: A-V block. Amer J Cardiol 6:53–61, 1960

56. Langendorf R, Pick A: Mechanism of intermittent ventricular bigeminy. II. Parasystole, and parasystole or re-entry with conduction disturbance. Circulation 11:431–439, 1955

57. Langendorf R, Pick A, Winternitz M: Mechanism of intermittent ventricular bigeminy. I. Appearance of ectopic beats dependent upon the length of the ventricular cycle, the "rule of bigeminy". Circulation 11: 422–430, 1955

58. Lopez JF: Electrocardiographic findings in patients with complete atrioventricular block. Brit Heart J 30:20–28, 1968

59. Lown B, Ganong WF, Levine SA: The syndrome of short P-R interval, normal QRS complex and paroxysmal rapid heart action. Circulation 5:693–706, 1952

60. Mangiola S: Intermittent left anterior hemiblock with Wenckebach phenomenon. Amer J Cardiol 30:892–895, 1972

61. Marriott HJL: Artifacts and pitfalls in ECG interpretations. In: Advanced Cardiac Nursing. Philadelphia, The Charles Press, 1970, p 36–50

62. Massumi RA, Amsterdam EA, Salel A, et al: Ectopic rhythms arising from anterior and posterior fascicles of the left bundle branch in anterior and posterior myocardial infarctions. Amer J Cardiol 29:278–279, 1972

63. Mower NM, Aranaga C, Tabatznik B: Unusual patterns of conduction produced by pacemaker stimuli. Amer Heart J 74:24–28, 1967

64. Norris RM, Croxson MS: Bundle branch block in acute myocardial infarction. Amer Heart J 79:728–733, 1970

65. Phillips J, Spano J, Burch G: Chaotic atrial mechanism. Amer Heart J 78:171–179, 1969

66. Pick A: Aberrant ventricular conduction of escape beats: preferential and accessory pathways in the A-V junction. Circulation 13:702–711, 1956

67. Pick A, Katz LN: Disturbances of impulse formation and conduction in the pre-excitation (W.P.W.) syndrome—their bearing on its mechanism. Amer J Med 19:759–771, 1955

68. Pryor R: Fascicular block and the bilateral bundle branch block syndrome. Editorial. Amer Heart J 83: 441–446, 1972

69. Rabbino MD, Dreifus LS, Likoff W: Cardiac arrhythmias following intracardiac surgery. Amer J Cardiol 7:681–689, 1961

70. Riseman JEF, Sagall EL: Diagnostic problems resulting from improper electrocardiographic technique. JAMA 178:806–811, 1961

71. Rosenbaum MB: Classification of ventricular extrasystoles according to form. J Electrocardiol 2:289–297, 1969

72. Rosenbaum MB, Nau GJ, Lev RJ, et al: Wenckebach periods in the bundle branches. Circulation 40:79–86, 1969

73. Rosenbaum MB, Halpern MS, Nau GJ et al: The mechanism of narrow ventricular ectopic beats. In: Symposium on Cardiac Arrhythmias. Elsinore, Denmark, April 23–25, 1970

74. Rothfeld EL, Zucker R, Parsonnet V, et al: Idioventricular rhythm in acute myocardial infarction. Circulation 37:203–209, 1968

75. Sandler AI, Marriott HJL: The differential morphology of anomalous ventricular complexes of RBBB type in lead V_1. Ventricular ectopy versus aberration. Circulation 31:551–556, 1965

76. Scanlon PJ, Pryor R, Blount SG: Right bundle branch block associated with left superior or inferior intraventricular block: Associated with acute myocardial infarction. Circulation 42:1135–1142, 1970

77. Schamroth L, Dove E: The Wenckebach phenomenon in sino-atrial block. Brit Heart J 28:350–358, 1966

78. Schamroth L, Marriott HJL: Intermittent ventricular parasystole with observations on its relationship to extrasystolic bigeminy. Amer J Cardiol 7:799–809, 1961

79. Scheidt S, Killip T: Bundle branch block complicating acute myocardial infarction. JAMA 222:919–924, 1972

80. Scherf D, Gurbuzer B: Further studies on coronary sinus rhythm. Amer J Cardiol 1:579–583, 1958

81. Scherf D, Reid EC, Chamsai DG: Intermittent parasystole. Cardiologia 30:217–228, 1957

82. Singer DH, Lazzara R, Hoffman BF: Interrelationship between automaticity and conduction in Purkinje fibers. Circ Res 21:537–558, 1967

83. Singer DH, Ten Eick RE: Aberrancy: electrophysiologic aspects. Amer J Cardiol 28:381–401, 1971

84. Truex RC: Reconstruction of the human sino-atrial node. Anat Rec 158:11–19, 1967

ECG Tracing Index

The ECG tracings listed in this index can be found as follows:
Those labeled *Fig.* and *Rhythm* between pages 8 and 149
Those labeled *Case* between pages 150 and 192
Those labeled *Strip* between pages 194 and 206